Autoimmune Diseases: Clinical Theory

Autoimmune Diseases: Clinical Theory

Edited by **Marcy Ward**

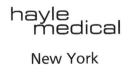

New York

Published by Hayle Medical,
30 West, 37th Street, Suite 612,
New York, NY 10018, USA
www.haylemedical.com

Autoimmune Diseases: Clinical Theory
Edited by Marcy Ward

International Standard Book Number: 978-1-63241-052-8 (Hardback)

Printed in the United States of America.

Contents

Preface

In my initial years as a student, I used to run to the library at every possible instance to grab a book and learn something new. Books were my primary source of knowledge and I would not have come such a long way without all that I learnt from them. Thus, when I was approached to edit this book; I became understandably nostalgic. It was an absolute honor to be considered worthy of guiding the current generation as well as those to come. I put all my knowledge and hard work into making this book most beneficial for its readers.

Autoimmune Disorders, a heterogeneous and multifaceted group of diseases, affect virtually any organ of the human body. This book intends to present currently accessible manifestations by providing an etiopathogenetic overview of both systemic and organ detailed autoimmune diseases, pathogenesis of systemic autoimmune disorders: genetic and environmental contributors, the intersecting communication among autoimmunity and cardiovascular morbidity.

I wish to thank my publisher for supporting me at every step. I would also like to thank all the authors who have contributed their researches in this book. I hope this book will be a valuable contribution to the progress of the field.

                                                                                      Editor

Part 1

Comorbidities of Autoimmune Disorders

Chronic Periaortitis as a Systemic Autoimmune Disease

Chang-Hee Suh

Rheumatology, Ajou University School of Medicine
Korea

1. Introduction

Chronic periaortitis is an idiopathic disease whose hallmark is the presence of a fibro-inflammatory tissue arising from the adventitia of the abdominal aorta and the common iliac arteries and extending into the surrounding retroperitoneum and frequently encasing neighboring structures such as the ureters and the inferior vena cava (Mitchinson, 1984; Parums, 1990). It should be regarded as a generalized disease with three different pathophysiological entities, specifically idiopathic retroperitoneal fibrosis, inflammatory abdominal aortic aneurysms, and perianeurysmal retroperitoneal fibrosis (Vaglio et al., 2003; Jois et al., 2004).

Idiopathic retroperitoneal fibrosis is characterized by periaortic fibroinflammatory tissue, which often causes obstruction of the ureters and other adjacent abdominal structures by extending into the retroperitoneum (Mitchinson, 1970; Gilkeson & Allen, 1996). A dilated aorta is usually not present in idiopathic retroperitoneal fibrosis. Its initial signs and symptoms are often nonspecific, such as malaise, anorexia, weight loss, fever, and flank, back, or abdominal pain. Inflammatory abdominal aortic aneurysms characteristically develop the mass around a dilated aorta, but usually do not cause obstructions (Crawford et al., 1985; Pennell et al., 1985). It usually presents with typical symptoms and signs characterized by the triad of abdominal or back pain, a pulsatile and sometimes tender abdominal mass, and an elevated erythrocyte sedimentation rate. Perianeurysmal retroperitoneal fibrosis, which represents a link between these two diagnoses, involves an abdominal aortic aneurysms surrounded by fibroinflammatory tissue that encases other abdominal organs (Serra et al, 1980).

These definitions may be a little confusing, and it would probably be more appropriate to distinguish aneurysmal from nonaneurysmal forms of chronic periaortitis; idiopathic retroperitoneal fibrosis may be referred as non-aneurysmal chronic periaortitis, where as inflammatory abdominal aortic aneurysms and perianeurysmal retroperitoneal fibrosis as aneurysmal chronic periaortitis (Vaglio et al., 2006).

It is important to diagnose chronic periaortitis early in its course in order to attempt to prevent the severe secondary complication of renal failure due to ureteric obstruction and the potentially fatal consequence of aortic rupture (Jois et al., 2004). Although most studies have considered these entities separately, these conditions have common clinical and histopathologic findings, and thus probably represent different manifestations of the same disease.

2. Epidemiology

The prevalence of chronic periaortitis is not well known; the only available epidemiological data concern idiopathic retroperitoneal fibrosis and inflammatory abdominal aortic aneurysms. Reports from Duke University and the Mayo Clinic estimate that the incidence of idiopathic retroperitoneal fibrosis is less than 1 per 10,000 patients (Gilkeson & Allen 1996). A recent study conducted in Finland on idiopathic retroperitoneal fibrosis has demonstrated that its incidence and prevalence are 1/1,000,000 person-year and 1.38 cases/100,000 inhabitants (Uibu et al., 2004). On the other hand, data regarding the incidence of the aneurysmal forms of chronic periaortitis in the whole population are lacking, however they represent about 4% to 10% of all abdominal aortic aneurysms (Rasmussen et al, 1997; von Fritschen et al., 1999; Yusuf et al., 2007).

Chronic periaortitis frequently develops in middle-aged adults with a mean age of approximately 60 years, but it may also occur in children (Miller et al. 2003; Uibu et al., 2004; Vaglio et al., 2006). Men are affected two to three times as often as women and that is even more pronounced in the inflammatory abdominal aortic aneurysms (Gilkeson & Allen 1996; Uibu et al., 2004; Vaglio et al., 2006).

There is no evidence of a clear ethnic predisposition or familial clustering, and the disease has been reported in twins and siblings only in anecdotal cases (Duffy et al., 1984; Doolin et al. 1987). A few studies have addressed the question whether genetic factors may contribute to the development of chronic periaortitis. Recent studies have suggested that immunogenetic factors may be involved in the pathogenesis of the disease (Rasmussen et al., 1997; Martorana et al., 2006).

A case-control study evaluated the prevalence of HLA alleles in patients with inflammatory abdominal aortic aneurysms compared with healthy subjects found that in the inflammatory abdominal aortic aneurysms a genetic risk determinant mapping at the HLA-DRB1 locus (Rasmussen et al., 1997). Additionally, they identified HLA-DRB1*15 and B1*0404 as predisposing alleles.

Another recent case-control study on patients with chronic periaortitis and healthy controls in order to investigate the role of HLA in the susceptibility to chronic periaortitis revealed that the frequency of the HLA-DRB1*03 allele was markedly higher in patients with chronic periaortitis than in the controls (Martorana et al., 2006). The HLA-DRB1*03 allele is a well-known marker of autoimmunity, since it is associated with a number of autoimmune diseases, which include systemic lupus erythematosus and autoimmune thyroid disease (Davidson and Diamond, 2001). Also, the HLA-B*08 allele was significantly associated with chronic periaortitis and it is itself linked to a wide range of immune-mediated diseases. Furthermore, the comparison of the clinical and laboratory characteristics of HLA-DRB1*03-positive and HLA-DRB1*03-negative patients showed that the HLA-DRB1*03-positive patients with chronic periaortitis have higher acute-phase reactant levels at the time of diagnosis (Martorana et al., 2006). These results could imply that the HLA system not only confers susceptibility to the development of the disease but also plays a role in the modulation of the inflammatory response.

More recently, CC chemokine receptor 5 (CCR5) gene delta 32 polymorphism has been mapped in 100 patients with chronic periaortitis (Boiardi L et al., 2011). The distribution of the CCR5 gene delta 32 genotype differed between patients with chronic periaortitis and controls (P = 0.01). The CCR5 gene delta 32 allele was more frequent in patients with chronic periaortitis [P = 0.02, odds ratio (OR) 2.8 (95% CI 1.2, 6.4)]. Furthermore, CCR5 gene delta 32 allele occurred more frequently in patients with inflammatory abdominal aortic aneurysms than in patients with idiopathic retroperitoneal fibrosis [P = 0.001, OR 6.4 (95% CI 2.1, 19.1)]. The CCR5 gene delta 32 allele frequency was higher in inflammatory abdominal aortic aneurysms patients without established atherosclerotic disease compared with controls [66.7 vs 5.6%, P = 0.00001, OR 34.0 (95% CI 7.4, 156.3)]. The CC chemokine receptor 5 is expressed on many immune cells, particularly Th1 cells, and acts by binding to different chemokines, including RANTES, MIP-1α and MIP-1β. The CCR5 gene delta 32 polymorphism creates a truncated, nonfunctional receptor and probably shifts the immune response toward a Th2 pattern. Interestingly, the association between the CCR5 gene delta 32 polymorphism and aneurysmal chronic periaortitis is even stronger in patients without overt atherosclerotic disease, which suggests that immune mechanisms independent of atherosclerosis play a role in the pathogenesis of chronic periaortitis (Vaglio et al., 2011).

Additionally, environmental and occupational agents have been shown to contribute to susceptibility to chronic periaortitis. In a recent study, it has been demonstrated that asbestos exposure is associated with a markedly increased risk of developing the chronic periaortitis, and smoking is also a significant risk factor (Uibu et al., 2004; Hellmann et al., 2007). Although smoking is an established risk factor for classical atherosclerotic abdominal aortic aneurysms, its frequency is even higher in patients with inflammatory abdominal aortic aneurysms (Nitecki et al., 1996; Hellmann et al., 2007).

3. Pathology

Chronic periaortitis affects the aortic wall and the surrounding retroperitoneum. The classical macroscopic appearance of chronic periaortitis is grossly a whitish and hard periaortic mass which extends between the origin of the renal arteries and the bifurcation of the common iliac vessels and often distorting medially the ureters but histologically there is a continuum of lesions ranging from acute changes to chronic damage (Mitchinson, 1970).

In the early stages of chronic periaortitis, or in patients with a prominent acute-phase reaction, the tissue is highly inflammatory, with numerous lymphocytes, plasma cells, macrophages and scattered eosinophils and loose deposits of collagen matrix in thick, irregular bands (Mitchinson, 1970; Corradi et al., 2007). In late disease, these aspects evolve, either spontaneously or after glucocorticoid therapy, into a relatively acellular fibrous tissue. Perivascular involvement of the thoracic aorta is not uncommon, while rarely atypical localizations such as peri-duodenal, peri-pancreatic and pelvic sites have also been found (Hughes & Buckley, 1993; Corradi et al., 2007).

Microscopic examination shows signs of active mononuclear cell inflammation in a framework of fibrous tissue and fibroblasts (Serra et al, 1980; Gilkeson & Allen, 1996). The background of chronic periaortitis consists of varying degrees of fibrosis, characterized by a mild-to-moderate and mitotically inactive fibroblasts and myofibroblasts, which are immuno-histochemically positive for vimentin and, in the more cellular areas, for α-smooth muscle actin (Vaglio et al., 2006). The fibrous component is particularly abundant in the late stages when the tissue becomes relatively avascular and acellular; its distribution is usually diffuse, but sometimes perivascular and perineural.

The inflammatory infiltrate includes mononuclear cells such as T and B lymphocytes, macrophages and plasma cells, although scattered eosinophils can also be found

(Mitchinson, 1970). The majority of lymphocytes, macrophages and most vascular endothelial cells are HLA-DR-positive. The Ki67 and BerH2 staining is found in B cells and T-helper cells, indicating that these cells were proliferating and activated (Meier et al., 2007). Two main inflammatory patterns are usually seen, perivascular and diffuse. The perivascular aggregates consist mainly of B lymphocytes and a smaller component of plasma cells, macrophages, and T lymphocytes, most of which are CD4+ (Corradi et al., 2007). Sometimes, these follicular aggregates show a germinal center architecture. The sclerotic component consists of thick fascicles of type-I collagen, irregularly distributed along the lesion; a pathological hallmark is the presence of a regular circumferential fibrous bundle surrounding blood vessels and nerves. On the other hand, the diffuse infiltrate has an equal percentage of T cells and B cells. Scattered eosinophils are common, whereas neutrophils are rare (Mitchinson, 1970; Vaglio et al., 2003). In cases of severe inflammation, there may be focal infiltration of the small and medium-sized retroperitoneal vessels, with frank vasculitis and fibrinoid necrosis.

The aortic wall also shows particular changes, such as atherosclerotic degeneration of the intima, medial thinning, and marked adventitial inflammation and fibrosis. The composition of the inflammatory infiltrate in the aortic wall is similar to the retroperitoneal one, with diffuse and perivascular patterns. The adventitial inflammatory infiltrate is often organized in lymphoid follicles (Sakata et al., 2008), which are examples of ectopic lymphoneogenesis and expression of a highly structured inflammatory or immune-mediated response. Adventitial vasa vasorum in aortas of chronic periaortitis show inflammatory infiltration up to frank necrotizing vasculitis, endarteritis obliterans, or obliterative phlebitis (Vaglio et al., 2003; Sakata et al., 2008). These aortic wall changes are found in all chronic periaortitis disease entities, regardless of the presence of aneurysmal dilatation.

It is interesting to note that autopsy studies have documented the presence of adventitial inflammation in aortic sections lacking periaortic fibrosis, which may suggest that aortitis could precede the development of adventitial and periadventitial fibrosis (Mitchinson, 1970). Another autopsy studies have shown that moderate adventitial inflammation and fibrosis may not be limited to the abdominal aorta, but may also involve its thoracic aorta (Mitchinson, 1972).

Molecular analysis of aortic biopsies in patients with chronic periaortitis shows gene transcripts consistent with lymphocyte activation, such as IFN-γ, IL-1α, IL-2 and IL-4, in keeping with the concept that chronic periaortitis is an active inflammatory aortic disease (Ramshaw et al., 1994).

4. Pathogenesis

Chronic periaortitis is idiopathic in nature, and its pathogenesis remains a matter of debate. Initially, it was postulated to represent a local inflammatory reaction to antigens such as ceroid and oxidised low-density lipoproteins (LDL), which can be found in the atherosclerotic plaques of the abdominal aorta (Parums et al., 1986; Parums et al., 1990; Ramshaw & Parums, 1994). Since an intact media constitutes an immunoprivileged site, the capacity of lipids deposited in the intima and media to elicit an inflammatory reaction in the adventitia may depend on the thinning or breach of the media itself, with consequent transit of the lipids. These can be processed by adventitial macrophages and presented to B and T cells, thus eliciting a local inflammatory reaction which eventually leads to adventitial and peri-aortic inflammation and fibrosis.

Morphologic and experimental findings showed that adventitial inflammation also seems to be more marked where the media is thinner (Mitchinson, 1972; Mitchinson 1984; Parums et al., 1990). IgG has been detected in close apposition to extracellular ceroid, and serum antibodies to oxidized LDL and ceroid were more common in patients with chronic periaortitis than in healthy individuals (Parums et al., 1986; Parums et al., 1990). Furthermore, a wide spectrum of adhesion molecules and gene products for cytokines, such as interleukin-1α, interleukin-2, interleukin-4, and interferon-γ, have been detected in the aortic adventitia, thus strengthening the hypothesis that chronic periaortitis is associated with active adventitial chronic inflammation (Ramshaw & Parums, 1994; Ramshaw et al., 1994).

According to this hypothesis, advanced atherosclerosis is a *sine qua non* for the development of chronic periaortitis, which may be an exaggerated local immune response to plaque antigens. The notion that chronic periaortitis is secondary to atherosclerosis is challenged by several findings. There was no substantial difference in the incidence of advanced atherosclerosis between patients with chronic periaortitis and healthy controls (Uibu et al., 2004; Breems et al., 2000). Also, chronic periaortitis may affect patients without atherosclerosis, and it has been reported in pediatric patients (Miller et al., 2003). A recent study showed no significant differences in anti-ox-LDL antibody levels between patients with chronic periaortitis and controls (van Bommel et al., 2011).

Furthermore, a number of findings support the hypothesis that chronic periaortitis may be a manifestation of systemic disease rather than the result of a local reaction. These include its constitutional symptoms, the high acute-phase reactant levels, autoantibody positivity, and the frequent association with other autoimmune diseases (Gilkeson & Allen, 1996; Demko et al., 1997; Vaglio et al., 2003; Marcolongo et al., 2004). Additionally, the association with HLA-DRB1, a marker of autoimmune diseases, is an additional clue to its autoimmune origin (Martorana et al., 2006).

Chronic periaortitis also has histologic similarities to large vessel vasculitis such as giant cell arteritis and Takayasu's arteritis; prominent adventitial inflammation and the involvement of the vasa vasorum (Ramshaw et al., 1994; Vanoli et al., 2005; Vaglio et al., 2006; Salvarani et al., 2008), and sometimes extends beyond the abdominal aorta (Mitchinson 1972; Cid et al., 1998; Jois et al., 2004). In addition, in some patients with chronic periaortitis the disease involves not only the abdominal aorta and the iliac vessels, but also other vascular territories such as the thoracic aorta. This finding was already observed long time ago by autopsy studies (Mitchinson, 1972). Recently, in a study using 18F-fluorodeoxyglucose positron emission tomography, it have also shown that in some patients with chronic periaortitis the high 18F-fluorodeoxyglucose uptake in the abdominal aorta and in the common iliac arteries coexists with a pathologic uptake in the thoracic aorta and its main branches, which confirms the idea that chronic periaortitis is a systemic disease in some cases (Salvarani et al., 2005).

These findings strengthen the idea that chronic periaortitis may originate as a primary arteritis involving the aorta. The perivascular- and sometimes transmural-involvement of vasa vasorum may represent the initial event of the disease. Its centrifugal extension could induce a fibro-inflammatory periaortic reaction, whereas its centripetal spreading could promote atherosclerosis, medial thinning and aneurysm formation (Vaglio & Buzio, 2005; Vaglio et al., 2006).

Structural alterations of the aortic wall seen in chronic periaortitis result in part from degradation of the macromolecules, such as collagen and elastin. These changes are associated with excessive production of matrix metalloproteinases (MMPs), which are assumed to orchestrate the widespread matrix destruction (Freestone et al., 1995). The inflammatory infiltrate is thought to play an etiologic role in aneurysm formation by direct local production of matrix-degrading enzymes and production of cytokines that induce resident mesenchymal cell production of MMPs (Newman et al., 1994). Recent findings suggest that both the local mesenchymal cell expression and the macrophage expression of MMPs are required for aneurysm formation (Longo et al., 2002).

Both fibrillar collagen and elastin are highly organized in the lamellar structure of the aortic media. One potential mechanism for the complementary role of MMP-2 and MMP-9 is that MMP-2 primarily acts as a collagenase-initiating cleavage of the triple helix into one- and three-quarter lengths. The single α chains could then be degraded by MMP-9, releasing the coiled elastin and causing it to become fattened and attenuated. Rupture and expansion rates of abdominal aortic aneurysms have been linked to MMP-2 and MMP-9 levels in tissue and plasma (Petersen et al., 2000). Such observations appear consistent with the increased medial atrophy observed within inflammatory abdominal aortic aneurysms, because activated MMPs may weaken the media by causing destruction of elastic and collagen fibers and smooth muscle cells.

As in many other immune-mediated diseases, environmental and infectious agents probably contribute to the pathogenesis of chronic periaortitis. As mentioned above, asbestos exposure and smoking are established risk factors (Uibu et al., 2004). It has been hypothesized that inflammation within the aortic wall may be a response to infection. Both herpes and cytomegalovirus have been described as potential agents (Tanaka et al., 1994). Recent interest has been focused on Chlamydia pneumoniae, which was found to be more prevalent in aneurysmal than in normal aortic tissue (Tang et al., 2005).

5. Clinical features

The clinical presentation of chronic periaortitis is insidious and vague. Lumbar, abdominal or flank pain is present in about 80% of the patients. It has been described as insidious, persistent and dull, poorly localized, unmodified by movement or rest. If the ureters are involved, the pain may be acute and colic-like (Baker et al., 1987; Vaglio et al., 2003; van Bommel et al., 2009). During the initial phases, patients may find relief using non-steroidal anti-inflammatory drugs, but the beneficial effect of these agents is transient (Gilkeson & Allen, 1996; Vaglio et al., 2006).

In addition to pain, the commonest clinical manifestations are systemic symptoms, most likely related to the inflammatory nature of the disease: about 40 to 80% of patients complain of fatigue, anorexia, weight loss and low-grade fever (Baker et al., 1987; Kardar et al., 2002; Vaglio et al., 2003; Scheel et al., 2009). Ureteral obstruction is the most frequent complication of idiopathic retroperitoneal fibrosis. It involves both ureters in a high percentage of cases (50–80%) and may occur simultaneously (Kardar et al., 2002; van Bommel et al., 2007). Ureteric obstruction is commonly due to edema or inflammation rather than fibrosis. This observation is supported by the fact that the obstruction can improve rapidly with corticosteroid therapy (Baker et al., 1987; Nitecki et al., 1996).

In cases of advanced bilateral ureteral obstruction, oliguria and symptoms secondary to uremic syndrome occur (Baker et al., 1987; Sterpetti et al., 1989; Jois et al., 2004). Varicocele and hydrocele, sometimes associated with testicular pain, are not uncommon, and also probably develop because of compression of the gonadal vessels (Baker et al., 1988; Vaglio et al., 2003). Constipation and claudication are less common. Lower limb edema and deep venous thrombosis may occur, probably as a result of inferior vena cava and iliac vein involvement.

Physical examination usually reveals abdominal tenderness and sometimes a palpable, pulsatile and tender abdominal mass. A periumbilical bruit may be heard in patients with inflammatory abdominal aortic aneurysms (Crawford et al., 1985; Nitecki et al., 1996). The combination of abdominal pain, a pulsatile mass with overlying bruit, constitutional symptoms, and high levels of acute-phase reactants usually distinguish inflammatory abdominal aortic aneurysms from noninflammatory abdominal aortic aneurysms.

Laboratory examinations are useful, but not diagnostic for chronic periaortitis. Acute phase reactants such as the erythrocyte sedimentation rate and C-reactive protein are elevated in more than 80% of patients with active disease, in keeping with the presence of a systemic inflammation and are often used to monitor the clinical course of the disease (Kardar et al., 2002; Marcolongo et al., 2004; Vaglio et al., 2006). The erythrocyte sedimentation rate and C-reactive protein dramatically decrease or even normalize after a few weeks of therapy (van Bommel et al., 2007), whereas their sensitivity in heralding relapses is uncertain (Vaglio et al., 2005). A recent retrospective study investigated whether the erythrocyte sedimentation rate and C-reactive protein levels might predict response to glucocorticoid therapy, but found that baseline erythrocyte sedimentation rate and C-reactive protein did not discriminate between chronic periaortitis patients who experienced disease regression and those who showed mass stabilization or progression (Magrey et al., 2009).

Renal dysfunction is related to the severity of ureteral involvement, but only 18-21% of patients actually experiences end-stage renal failure (Baker et al., 1987; Nitecki et al., 1996). Normochromic, normocytic anemia is often present as a result of systemic chronic inflammation. Leukocytosis, eosinophilia, and polyclonal hypergammaglobulinemia may be disclosed in some patients (Gilkeson & Allen, 1996). If polyclonal hypergammaglobulinemia is present, it is worthwhile assessing serum immunoglobulin levels and, if available, IgG subclasses; IgG4 is high in chronic periaortitis patients with features of IgG4-related systemic disease (Vaglio et al, 2011; J.R. Stone, 2011).

Immunologic and autoimmune tests should always be assessed in patients with chronic periaortitis. Antinuclear antibodies have been reported in up to 60% of patients, whereas anti-dsDNA and antiextractable nuclear antigen antibodies are rare (Vaglio et al., 2003). Rheumatoid factor is not uncommon. The presence of these autoantibodies, although non-organ-specific and often positive at low titers, may be a clue to an autoimmune origin of chronic periaortitis. Alternatively, they may be the earliest manifestation of a smoldering disorder that will clinically emerge late in the course of chronic periaortitis.

On the other hand, certain autoantibodies actually indicate the presence of an associated autoimmune disease. When autoimmune thyroiditis coexists, antithyroglobulin and antithyroid microsome antibodies are positive (Vaglio et al., 2003). P-antineutrophil and C-antineutrophil cytoplasmic antibodies have been detected in a few cases of chronic periaortitis associated with small vessel vasculitis, such as Wegener granulomatosis and microscopic polyangiitis (Kaipiainen-Seppanen et al., 1996; Aslangul et al., 2003).

6. Evidence of systemic autoimmunity in chronic periaortitis

Although it has been considered a localized inflammatory disease secondary to atherosclerosis, several genetic, clinical, laboratory and pathologic findings suggest that chronic periaortitis is a systemic autoimmune disease, perhaps involving a vasculitic process of small and medium vessels (Table 1).

Autoimmune Component	Example
Genetics	Association with HLA-DRB1*03, DRB1*0404, DRB1*15 and HLA-B*08 Association with CC chemokine receptor 5 (CCR5) gene delta 32 polymorphism
Autoantibodies	Antinuclear antibody Anti-thyroid microsome and anti-thyroglobulin antibody Anti-neutrophil cytoplasmic antibody Rheumatoid factor Anti-smooth muscle antibody
Association with Autoimmune diseases	Autoimmune thyroiditis Rapidly progressive glomerulonephritis Systemic vasculitis Rheumatoid arthritis Juvenile rheumatoid arthritis Ankylosing spondylitis Systemic lupus erythematosus Antiphospholipid syndrome IgG4-related systemic disease
Histologic finding	Small vessel vasculitis of retroperitoneal vessels and aortic vasa vasorum Ectopic lymphoid follicles with germinal centers in periaortic retroperitoneum and aortic adventitia
Clinical manifestations	Constitutional symptoms, such as fever, fatigue, weight loss, anorexia and sleep disturbances Systemic involvement of large arteries
Laboratory findings	High erythrocyte sedimentation rate High C-reactive protein Anemia
Treatment response	Rapid response to corticosteroids
Prognosis	Chronic-relapsing course

Table 1. Summary of systemic autoimmune components implicated in chronic periaortitis

6.1 Genetics

Genetic association study revealed that patients with chronic periaortitis were associated with certain genetic markers, which is involved in the immune response and commonly associated with autoimmune or inflammatory disease. The HLA system plays a role in conferring susceptibility to chronic periaortitis (Rasmussen et al., 1997; Martorana et al., 2006). The bias in expression of specific HLA alleles are defining features of autoimmune disease.

The HLA-DRB1*03, DRB1*0404, DRB1*15 and HLA-B*08 alleles was significantly higher in patients with chronic periaortitis. These alleles are a well-known marker of autoimmunity, since it is associated with a number of autoimmune diseases such as systemic lupus erythematosus, rheumatoid arthritis, giant cell arteritis, autoimmune thyroiditis, type 1 diabetes mellitus and myasthenia gravis.

The CC chemokine receptor 5 (CCR5) gene delta 32 polymorphism is associated with aneurysmal chronic periaortitis, which creates a truncated, nonfunctional receptor and probably shifts the immune response toward a Th2 pattern (Boiardi L et al., 2011).

6.2 Autoantibodies
Several autoantibodies are positive in varying proportions of patients, which may be a clue to an autoimmune origin of chronic periaortitis. Antinuclear antibodies are positive in up to 50–60% of the cases, although their titer is often low (Vaglio et al., 2003). Anti-thyroid microsome and anti-thyroglobulin antibodies may be positive in 25–30% (Martorana et al., 2006). Other autoantibodies, such as antineutrophil cytoplasmic antibodies, rheumatoid factor, and anti-smooth muscle may also be positive.

6.3 Association with autoimmune disease
Chronic periaortitis are frequently associated with autoimmune diseases involving other organs or structures. Two recent studies have showed a higher incidence of systemic autoimmune diseases. A case-control study comparing inflammatory abdominal aortic aneurysms and noninflammatory abdominal aortic aneurysms showed a higher incidence of systemic autoimmune diseases in the former group (Haug et al., 2003). In another study of 16 consecutive patients with chronic periaortitis, three had antineutrophil cytoplasmic antibody-positive rapid progressive renal disease, three had autoimmune thyroiditis, and one had rheumatoid arthritis (Vaglio et al., 2003).

Another frequently reported association is systemic vasculitides, which in most cases involve small and medium-sized vessel vasculitis, such as Wegener granulomatosis and polyarteritis nodosa (Akman et al., 1983; Hautekeete et al., 1990; De Roux-Serratrice et al., 2002) or unclassifiable systemic vasculitis (Hellstrom & Perez-Stable, 1966; Littlejohn & Keystone, 1981). Antineutrophil cytoplasmic antibody-associated vasculitic syndromes are more and more often reported.

Chronic periaortitis may frequently be associated with fibroinflammatory disorders affecting other organs, IgG4-related systemic disease, which have an autoimmune origin (Matsumoto et al., 2008; Ito et al., 2008; Kasashima et al., 2008; Sakata et al., 2008). Other rheumatic diseases reported in patients with chronic periaortitis include ankylosing spondylitis, juvenile rheumatoid arthritis, systemic lupus erythematosus and antiphospholipid syndrome (Leblanc et al., 2002; Tsai et al., 1996; Okada et al., 1999; Kim et al., 2010).

6.4 Histologic findings
Two peculiar histopathological findings may be interpreted as manifestations of autoimmunity. Firstly, about half of patients with chronic periaortitis had adventitial inflammation with vasa vasoritis in the small retroperitoneal vessels and the aortic vasa vasorum with mononuclear cell infiltration and sometimes fibrinoid necrosis (Mitchinson, 1970; Vaglio et al., 2003; Lindell et al., 1987). Secondly, the inflammatory infiltrate may be organized in lymphoid structures such as lymphoid follicles with germinal centers in both periaortic retroperitoneum and aortic adventitia (Ramshaw & Parums, 1994). Ectopic lymphoid microstructures with germinal centers have been found in autoimmune disorders, such as the synovium in rheumatoid arthritis (Weyand et al., 2001).

6.5 Clinical manifestations

Most patients with chronic periaortitis often complain of constitutional symptoms, such as fever, fatigue, weight loss, anorexia and sleep disturbances, which probably reflect the systemic inflammatory status (Baker et al., 1987; Vaglio et al., 2003). At least in a subgroup of patients, chronic periaortitis is a vasculitis affecting large vessels (Vaglio et al., 2011).

6.6 Laboratory findings

Chronic periaortitis usually present with high concentrations of acute-phase reactants such as erythrocyte sedimentation rate and C-reactive protein, varying degrees of anemia and, in a high percentage of cases, azotemia , which reflect the systemic inflammation (Kardar et al., 2002; Vaglio et al., 2006). The erythrocyte sedimentation rate and C-reactive protein can also be used to monitor the disease course (van Bommel et al., 2007).

6.7 Treatment response

The clinical manifestations of chronic periaortitis promptly subside after the initiation of glucocorticoids therapy, which again is well in agreement with their inflammatory nature. In most patients, they induce remission of the clinical symptoms, normalization of the acute-phase reactant levels, reduction in size of the retroperitoneal mass and also resolution of the obstructive complications (Kardar et al., 2002; Marcolongo et al., 2004; van Bommel et al., 2007; Magrey et al., 2009).

However, glucocorticoids have various significant side effects, which sometimes limit their prolonged use. The combination of glucocorticoids and immunosuppressants such as azathioprine, cyclophosphamide and methotrexate has recently been reported to yield favorable results in patients with chronic periaortitis (Marcolongo et al., 2004; Warnatz et al., 2005).

6.8 Prognosis

As is the case in many inflammatory and autoimmune diseases, chronic periaortitis also has a chronic-relapsing course. The frequency of relapses may depend on the treatment approach, as they occur in 10% to 50% of patients treated with surgery alone and in about 10% when combined immunosuppressive and surgical therapies are used (Baker et al., 1988).

7. IgG4-related systemic disease

In recent years, numerous studies have reported chronic periaortitis in association with IgG4-related systemic disease, a group of autoimmune and fibrosing conditions characterized by high serum levels of IgG4 and tissue infiltration by IgG4-bearing plasma cells (Vaglio et al, 2011; J.R. Stone, 2011). These conditions share common histopathologic characteristics, such as diffuse lymphoplasmacytic infiltration, irregular fibrosis, eosinophilic infiltration, and obliterative phlebitis (Neild et al., 2006; Deshpande et al., 2006; Masaki et al., 2009).

7.1 Idiopathic peritoneal fibrosis with IgG4-related systemic disease

It has become clear that in a subset of patients with idiopathic retroperitoneal fibrosis, the disorder is in fact occurring in the setting of IgG4-related systemic disease. For 10 years, there were several reports that autoimmune pancreatitis could be associated with inflammatory masses within the retroperitoneum, and it was later recognized that both conditions were a manifestation of IgG4-related systemic disease (J.R. Stone, 2011).

In those reports revealed that the retroperitoneal involvement is typically not entirely diffuse, but present primarily as inflammatory masses that often primarily involve the abdominal aorta, the kidneys or the ureters (Hamano et al., 2002; Miyajima et al., 2006; Tanabe et al., 2006). The inflammatory masses are composed of lymphoplasmacytic inflammation and fibrosis with a substantial number of the plasma cells expressing IgG4. The nearly all patients revealed an aortic adventitial involvement, even in the absence of aortic aneurysm formation.

In a recent study of retroperitoneal biopsies of patients with idiopathic retroperitoneal fibrosis, 10 of 17 cases were felt to be due to IgG-related systemic disease (Zen et al., 2009). In these 10 patients, the fraction of plasma cells staining for IgG4 ranged from 35 to 76% compared with 0 to 10% for the other seven patients. Furthermore, for the patients with IgG4-related disease, the mean serum IgG4 concentration was 695 mg/dl (range 154–2330 mg/dl) compared with 30 mg/dl (range 10–53 mg/dl) for the other seven patients.

7.2 Inflammatory abdominal aortic aneurysms with IgG4-related systemic disease

There are several reports which have indicated that a subset of inflammatory abdominal aortic aneurysms cases is in fact a result of IgG4-related systemic disease (Sakata et al., 2008; Kasashima et al., 2008; Qian et al., 2009). A recent study comparing 11 cases of inflammatory abdominal aortic aneurysms to 12 cases of atherosclerotic abdominal aortic aneurysms and demonstrated that the aneurysms defined as inflammatory contained more IgG4+ plasma cells than those defined as atherosclerotic. However, in that study there was no clear delineation as to which inflammatory aneurysms actually represented involvement by IgG4-related systemic disease. In addition, the fraction of plasma cells expressing IgG4 was not reported for either aneurysms group, making it unclear if the enhanced number of IgG4+ plasma cells was simply a manifestation of more plasma cells in general being present in the aneurysms labeled as inflammatory.

There have been several cases reported of inflammatory abdominal aortic aneurysms, which were attributed to IgG4-related systemic disease, and which included pathologic evaluation of the aorta (Kasashima et al., 2008; Ito et al., 2008; Qian et al., 2009). Pathologically, most cases of IgG-4 related inflammatory abdominal aortic aneurysms showed the predominant involvement in adventitia with high fraction of IgG4+ infiltrating plasma cells and high serum IgG levels (J.R. Stone, 2011).

Kasashima et al. reported that four of 10 cases (40%) of inflammatory abdominal aortic aneurysm were due to IgG4-related systemic disease with prominent IgG4+ plasma cell infiltration and high-IgG4 serum levels, whereas the remaining six had a mild (IgG4+ and total) plasma cell infiltration. Inflammation was more evident and tissue eosinophilia predominated in the IgG4-related inflammatory abdominal aortic aneurysms, whereas some degree of neutrophilic infiltration and only rare eosinophils were found in the non-IgG4-related inflammatory abdominal aortic aneurysms. Because inflammatory aneurysms may represent 2–15% of all abdominal aortic aneurysms, this would suggest 1–6% of all abdominal aortic aneurysms could be due to IgG4-related inflammatory abdominal aortic aneurysms (J.R. Stone, 2011).

7.3 Thoracic aortitis with IgG4-related systemic disease

Until now, the six cases of thoracic aortitis due to IgG4-related systemic disease reported, which derived from surgical resections (Khosroshahi et al., 2009; J.H. Stone et al., 2009; Ishida et al., 2009; J.H. Stone et al., 2010; Kasashima et al., 2010). All six patients were men in an old age (65-74 years). The arch was the most commonly involved in five cases, with two cases having involvement of the ascending aorta, and only one case having involvement of the descending aorta. Five of the six patients presented with an aneurysm.

According to histologic assessment, all displayed a prominent lymphoplasmacytic infiltrate, with a high percentage of the plasma cells staining for IgG4 (74-89%). In addition, at least five patients showed an obstructive phlebitis within the adventitia. In three cases, there was a marked predominance for the adventitia compared with the media and intima (J.R. Stone, 2011). Serum IgG4 level was found to be markedly elevated in 2 patients who tested it and both of these patients had documented extra-aortic involvement.

Assessment of all thoracic aortitis cases surgically resected in a 5-year at one institute revealed that IgG4-related systemic disease was responsible for three of four cases of lymphoplasmacytic aortitis and 9% of all cases of thoracic aortitis (J.H. Stone et al., 2010). According to that study, IgG4-related aortitis was present in 0.5% of all thoracic aorta resections. In a subsequent study from Japan, assessment of 125 thoracic aorta resections revealed two cases of IgG4-related aortitis, indicating 1.6% of all resected thoracic aortas contained IgG4-related aortitis (Khosroshahi et al., 2010).

Although much remains to be clarified with regard to the pathogenesis of chronic periaortitis, it is conceivable that IgG4 may represent a link between chronic periaortitis and systemic fibro-inflammatory conditions. The analysis of IgG4-related cases may provide additional clues supporting the possible systemic large-vessel involvement in chronic periaortitis (Vaglio et al., 2011).

8. Conclusion

Chronic periaortitis is a chronic disease characterized by a retroperitoneal fibroinflammatory reaction surrounding the abdominal aorta, which may or may not be dilated. Although it has been considered a localized inflammatory response to advanced atherosclerosis, there is increasing evidence supporting the hypothesis of an underlying systemic autoimmune disease with vasculitic process involving small and medium vessels. Further studies are warranted in order to elucidate the potential triggers of the disease, the pathways leading to the aortic-periaortic inflammation and to the disproportionate fibrogenic reaction.

9. References

Akman N., Avanoglu Y., Karabay K., Erek E., Tokgoz A., Aras E., Girisken G., Tuzuner N. & Avanoglu H. (1983). Henoch-Schoenlein purpura and retroperitoneal fibrosis. *Acta Haematologica*, Vol.70, No.6, (December 1983), pp. 400-401, ISSN 0001-5792

Aslangul E., Ranque B. & Papo T. (2003). Pseudotumoral retroperitoneal fibrosis and localized vasculitis with very high serum levels of anti-PR3 ANCA. *The American Journal of Medicine*, Vol.105, No.3, (August 2003), pp. 250-252, ISSN 0002-9343

Baker LR., Mallinson WJ., Gregory MC., Menzies EA., Cattell WR., Whitfield HN., Hendry WF., Wickham JE. & Joekes AM. (1987). Idiopathic retroperitoneal fibrosis. A retrospective analysis of 60 cases. *British Journal of Urology*, Vol.60, No.6, (December 1987), pp. 497–503, ISSN 0007-1331

Boiardi L., Vaglio A., Nicoli D., Farnetti E., Palmisano A., Pipitone N., Maritati F., Casali B., Martorana D., Moroni G., Buzio C. & Slvarani C. (2011). CC chemokine receptor 5 polymorphism in chronic periaortitis. *Rheumatology (Oxford)*, Vol.50, No.6, (June 2010), pp. 1025-1032 ISSN 1462-0324

Breems DA., Haye H. & van der Meulen J. (2000), The role of advanced atherosclerosis in idiopathic retroperitoneal fibrosis. *The Netherlands Journal of Medicine*, Vol.56, No.2, (February 2000), pp. 38–44, ISSN 0300-2977

Cid MC., Font C., Coll-Vinent B. & Grau M. (1998). Large vessel vasculitides. *Current Opinion in Rheumatology*, Vol.10, No.1, (January 1998), pp. 18–28, ISSN 1040-8711

Corradi D., Maestri R., Palmisano A., Bosio S., Greco P., Mneti L., Ferretti S., Cobelli R., Moroni G., Dei Tos AP., Buzio C. & Vaglio A. (2007). Idiopathic retroperitoneal fibrosis: clinicopathologic features and differential diagnosis. *Kidney International*, Vol.72, No.6 (September2007), pp. 742–753, ISSN 0085-2538

Crawford JL., Stowe CL., Safi HJ., Hallman CH. & Crawford ES. (1985). Inflammatory aneurysms of the aorta. *Journal of Vascular Surgery*, Vol.2, No.1, (January 1985), pp. 113-124, ISSN 0741-5214

Davidson A. & Diamond B. (2001). Autoimmune diseases. *New England Journal of Medicine*, Vol.345, No.5, (August 2001), pp. 340–350, ISSN 0028-4793'

Demko TM., Diamond JR. & Groff J. (1997). Obstructive nephropathy as a result of retroperitoneal fibrosis: a review of its pathogenesis and associations. *Journal of American Society of Nephrology*, Vol.8, No.4, (April 1997), pp. 684–688, ISSN 1046-6673

De Roux-Serratrice C., Serratrice J., Granel B., Dsdier P., Bartoli JM., Pache X., Astoul P., Garbe L., Branchereau A. & Weiller PJ. (2002). Periaortitis heralding Wegener's granulomatosis. *Journal of Rheumatology*, Vol.29, No.2, (February 2002), pp. 392–394, ISSN 0315-162X

Deshpande V., Chicano S., Finkelberg D., Selig MK., Mino-Kenudson M., Brugge WR., Colvin RB. & Lauwers GY. (2006). Autoimmune pancreatitis: a systemic immune complex mediated disease. *The American Journal of Surgical Pathology*, Vol.20, No.12, (December 2006), pp. 1537–1545, ISSN 0147-5185

Doolin EJ., Goldstein H., Kessler B., Vinocur C. & Marchildon MB. (1987). Familial retroperitoneal fibrosis. *Journal of Pediatric Surgery*, Vol.33, No.12 (December 1987), pp. 1092–1094, ISSN 0022-3468

Duffy PG., Johnston SR. & Donaldson RA. (1984). Idiopathic retroperitoneal fibrosis in twins. *Journal of Urology*, Vol.131, No.4, (April 1984), pp. 746, ISSN 0022-5374

Freestone T., Turner RJ., Coady A., Higman DJ., Greenhalgh RM. & Powell JT. (1995). Inflammation and matrix metalloproteinases in the enlarging abdominal aortic aneurysm. *Arteriosclerosis, Thrombosis, and Vascular Biology*, Vol.15, No.8, (August 1995), pp. 1145–1151, ISSN 1079-5642

Haug, ES., Skomsvoll, JF., Jacobsen, G., Halvorson, TB., Saether, OD. & Myhre, HO. (2003). Inflammatory aortic aneurysm is associated with increased incidence of autoimmune disease. *Journal of Vascular Surgery*, Vol.38, No.3, (September 2003), pp. 492-497, ISSN 0741-5214

Hautekeete ML., Babany G., Marcellin P., Gayno S., Palazzo E., Erlinger S. & Benhamou JP.
(1990). Retroperitoneal fibrosis after surgery for aortic aneurysm in a patient with
periarteritis nodosa: successful treatment with corticosteroids. *Journal of Internal
Medicine*, Vol.228, No.5, (November 1990), pp. 533–536, ISSN 0954-6820
Hellstrom HR. & Perezstable EC. (1966). Retroperitoneal fibrosis with disseminated
vasculitis and intrahepatic sclerosing cholangitis. (1966). *The American Journal of
Medicine*, Vol.40, No.2, (February 1966), pp. 184-187, ISSN 0002-9343
Hellmann DB., Grand DJ. & Freischlag JA. (2007). Inflammatory abdominal aortic aneurysm.
JAMA, Vol.297, No.4, (January 2007), pp. 395–400, ISSN 1538-3598
Hughes D. & Buckley PJ. (1993). Idiopathic retroperitoneal fibrosis is a macrophage-rich
process. Implications for its pathogenesis and treatment. *The American Journal of
Surgical Pathology*, Vol.17, No.5, (May 1993), pp. 482–90, ISSN 0147-5185
Gilkeson GS. & Allen NB. (1996). Retroperitoneal fibrosis. A true connective tissue disease.
Rheumatic disease clinics of North America, Vol.22, No.1, (February 1996), pp. 23-38,
ISSN 0889-857X
Ishida M., Hotta M., Kushima R., Asai T. & Okabe H. (2009). IgG4-related inflammatory
aneurysm of the aortic arch. *Pathology International*, Vol.59, No.4, (April 2009), pp.
269–273, ISSN 1440-1827
Ito H., Kaizaki Y., Noda Y., Fujii S. & Yamamoto S. (2008). IgG4-related inflammatory
abdominal aortic aneurysm associated with autoimmune pancreatitis. *Pathology
International*, Vol.58, No.7, (July 2008), pp. 421-6, ISSN 1440-1827
Jagadesham VP., Scott DJ. & Carding SR. (2008). Abdominal aortic aneurysms: an
autoimmune disease? *Trends in Moleular Medicine*, Vol.14, No.12, (December 2008),
pp. 522-529, ISSN 1471-4914
Jois RN., Gaffney K., Marshall T. & Scott DGI. (2004). Chronic periaortitis. *Rheumatology
(Oxford)*, Vol.43, No.11, (November 2004), pp. 1441-1446, ISSN 1462-0324
Kaipiainen-Seppanen O., Jantunen E., Kuusisto J. & Marin S. (1996). Retroperitoneal fibrosis
with antineutrophil cytoplasmic antibodies. *Journal of Rheumatology*, Vol.23, No.4,
(April 1996), pp. 779–781, ISSN 0315-162X
Kardar AH., Kattan S., Lindstedt E. & Hanash K. (2002). Steroid therapy for idiopathic
retroperitoneal fibrosis: dose and duration. *Journal Urology*, Vol.168, No.2, (August
2002), pp. 550–555, ISSN 0022-5347
Kasashima S., Zen Y., Kawashima A., Konishi K., Sasaki H., Endo M., Kawakami K., Zen Y.
& Nakanuma Y. (2008). Inflammatory abdominal aortic aneurysm: close
relationship to IgG4-related periaortitis. *American Journal of Surgical Pathology*,
Vol.32, No.2, (February 2008), pp. 197–204, ISSN 0147-5185
Kasashima S., Zen Y., Kawashima A., Endo M., Matsumoto Y., Kasashima F., Ohtake H. &
Nakanuma Y. (2010). A clinicopathologic study of immunoglobulin G4-related
sclerosing disease of the thoracic aorta. *Journal of Vascular Surgery*, Vol.52, No.6,
(December 2010), pp. 1587-1595, ISSN 1097-6809
Khosroshahi A., Stone JR., Pratt DS., Deshpande V. & Stone JH. (2009). Painless jaundice
with serial multiorgan dysfunction. *Lancet*, Vol.373, No.9673, (April 2009), pp. 1494,
ISSN 1474-547X
Kim HA., Won JH. & Suh CH. (2010). Chronic periaortitis with antiphospholipid syndrome.
International Journal of Rheumatic Diseases, Vol.13, No.1, (February 2010), pp. 91-93,
ISSN 1756-185X

Leblanc CM., Inman R., Dent P., Smith C., Babyn P. & Laxer RM. (2002). Retroperitoneal fibrosis: an extraarticular manifestation of ankylosing spondylitis. *Arthritis Rheumatism*, Vol.47, No.2, (April 2002), pp. 210–214, ISSN 1474-547X

Lindell OI., Sariola HV. & Lehtonen TA. (1987). The occurrence of vasculitis in perianeurysmal fibrosis. *Journal of Urology*, Vol.138, No.4, (October 1987), pp. 727–729, ISSN 0022-5347

Littlejohn GO. & Keystone EC. (1981). The association of retroperitoneal fibrosis with systemic vasculitis and HLA-B27: a case report and review of the literature. *Journal of Rheumatology*, Vol.8, No.4, (July 1981), pp. 623–629, ISSN 0315-162X

Longo GM., Xiong W., Greiner TC., Zhao Y., Fiotti N. & Baxter BT. (2002). Matrix metalloproteinases 2 and 9 work in concert to produce aortic aneurysms. *The Journal of Clinical Investigation*, Vol.110, No.5, (September 2002), pp. 625–632, ISSN 0021-9783

Magrey MN., Husni ME., Kushner I. & Calabrese LH. (2009). Do acute-phase reactants predict response to glucocorticoid therapy in retroperitoneal fibrosis? *Arthritis Rheumatism*, Vol.61, No.5, (May 2009), pp. 674–679, ISSN 1474-547X

Marcolongo R., Tavolini IM., Laveder F., Busa M., Voventa F., Bassi P. & Semenzato G. (2004). Immunosuppressive therapy for idiopathic retroperitoneal fibrosis: a retrospective analysis of 26 cases. *The American Journal of Medicine*, Vol.116, No.3, (February 2004), pp. 194–197, ISSN 0002-9343

Martorana D., Vaglio A., Greco P., Zanetti A., Moroni G., Salvarani C., Savi M., Buzio C. & Neri TM. (2006). Chronic periaortitis and HLA-DRB1*03: another clue to an autoimmune origin. *Arthritis Rheumatism*, Vol.55, No.1 (February 2006), pp. 126–130, ISSN 0004-3591

Masaki Y., Dong L., Kurose N., Kitagawa K., Morikawa Y., Yamamoto M., Takahashi H., Shinomura Y., Imai K., Saeki T., Azumi A., Nakada S., Sygiyama E., Matsui S., Origuchi T., Nishiyama S., Nishimori I., Nojima T., Yamada K., Kawano M., Kneko M., Miyazaki K., Twubota K. Eguchi K., Tomoda K., Sawaki T., Kawanami T., Tanaka M., Fukushima T., Sugai S. & Umehara H. (2009). Proposal for a new clinical entity, IgG4-positive multiorgan lymphoproliferative syndrome: analysis of 64 cases of IgG4-related disorders. *Annals of the Rheumatic Disease*, Vol.68, No.8, (August 2009), pp. 1310–1315, ISSN 1468-2060

Matsumoto Y., Kasashima S., Kawashima A., Kawashima A., Sasake H., Endo M., Kawakami K., Zen Y. & Nakanuma Y. (2008). A case of multiple immunoglobulin G4-related periarteritis: a timorous lesion of the coronary artery and abdominal aortic aneurysm. *Human Pathology*, Vol.39, No.6, (June 2008), pp. 975–80, ISSN 1532-8392

Meier P., Vogt B. & Blanc E. (2007). Rethinking the Triggering Inflammatory Processes of Chronic Periaortitis. *Nephron Experimental Nephrology*, Vol.105, No.1, (January 2007), pp. e17–e23, ISSN 1660-2129

Miller OF., Snith LJ., Ferrara EX., McAleer IM. & Kaplan GW. (2003). Presentation of idiopathic retroperitoneal fibrosis in the pediatric population. *Journal of Pediatric Surgery*, Vol.38, No.11, (November 2003), pp. 1685-1688, ISSN 1531-5037

Mitchinson MJ. (1970). The pathology of idiopathic retroperitoneal fibrosis. *Journal of Clinical Pathology*, Vol.23, No.8, (November 1970), pp. 681–689, ISSN 0021-9746

Mitchinson MJ. (1984). Chronic periaortitis and periarteritis. *Histopathology*, Vol.8, No.4, (July 1984), pp. 589–600, ISSN 0309-0167

Miyajima N., Koike H., Kawaguchi M., Zen Y., Takahashi K. & Hara N. (2006). Idiopathic retroperitoneal fibrosis associated with IgG4-positive plasmacyte infiltrations and idiopathic chronic pancreatitis. *International Journal of Urology*, Vol.13, No.11, (November 2006), pp. 1442–1444, ISSN 0919-8172

Neild GH., Rodriguez-Justo M., Wall C. & Connolly JO. (2006). Hyper-IgG4 disease: report and characterisation of a new disease. *BMC Medicine*, Vol.4, (October 2006), pp. 23, ISSN 1741-7015

Newman KM., Jean-Claude J., Li H., Ramey WG. & Tilson MD. (1994). Cytokines that activate proteolysis are increased in abdominal aortic aneurysms. *Circulation*, Vol.90, No.5, (November 1994), pp. II224–227, ISSN 0009-7322

Nitecki SS., Hallett JW Jr., Stanson A., Ilstrup DM., Bower TC., Cherry KJ Jr., Gloviczki P. & Pairolero PC. (1996). Inflammatory abdominal aortic aneurysms: a case-control study. *Journal of Vascular Surgery*, Vol.23, No.5, (May 1996), pp. 860–869, ISSN 0741-5214

Okada H., Takahira S., Sugahara S., Nakamoto H. & Suzuki H. (1999). Retroperitoneal fibrosis and systemic lupus erythematosus. *Nephrology, Dialysis, Transplantation*, Vol.14, No.5, (May 1999), pp. 1300–1302, ISSN 0931-0509

Parums DV., Chadwick DR. & Mitchinson MJ. (1986). The localisation of immunoglobulin in chronic periaortitis. *Atherosclerosis*, Vol.61, No.2, (August 1986), pp. 117–125, ISSN 0021-9150

Parums DV. (1990). The spectrum of chronic periaortitis. *Histopathology*, Vol.16, No.6, (December 1990), pp. 423–431, ISSN 0309-0167

Pennell RC., Hollier LH., Lie JT., Bernatz PE., Joyce JW., Pairolero PC., Cherry KJ. & Hallett JW. (1985). Inflammatory abdominal aortic aneurysms: a thirty-year review. *Journal of Vascular Surgery*, Vol.2, No.6, (November 1985), pp. 859-869, ISSN 0741-5214

Petersen E., Gineitis A., Wagberg F. & Angquist KA. (2000). Activity of matrix metalloproteinase-2 and -9 in abdominal aortic aneurysms. Relation to size and rupture. *Eur J Vasc Endovasc Surg,*Vol.20, No.5, (November 2000), pp. 457–461, ISSN 1078-5884

Qian Q., Kashani KB. & Miller DV. Ruptyred abdominal aortic aneurysm related to IgG4 periaortitis. (2009). *New England Journal of Medicine*, Vol.361, No.11, (September 2009), pp. 1121-1123, ISSN 1533-4406

Ramshaw AL. & Parums DV. (1994). The distribution of adhesion molecules in chronic periaortitis. *Histopathology*, Vol.24, No.1, (January 1994), pp. 23–32, ISSN 0309-0167

Ramshaw AL., Roskell DE. & Parums DV. (1994). Cytokine gene expression in aortic adventitial inflammation associated with advanced atherosclerosis (chronic periaortitis). *Journal of Clinical Pathology*, Vol.47, No.8, (August 1994), pp.721–727, ISSN 0021-9746

Rasmussen TE. & Hallett Jr JW. (1997). Inflammatory aortic aneurysms. A clinical review with new perspectives in pathogenesis. *Annals of Surgery*, Vol.225, No.2, (February 1997), pp. 155–164, ISSN 0003-4932

Rasmussen TE., Hallett Jr JW., Metzger RL., Richardson DM., Harmsen WS., Goronzy JJ. & Weyand CM. (1997). Genetic risk factors in inflammatory abdominal aortic aneurysms: polymorphic residue 70 in theHLA-DRB1 gene as a key genetic element. *Journal of Vascular Surgery*, Vol.25, No.2, (February 1997), pp. 356–364, ISSN 0741-5214

Sakata N., Tashiro T., Uesugi N., Kewara T., Furuya K., Hirata Y., Iwasaki H. & Kokima M. (2008). IgG4-positive plasma cells in inflammatory abdominal aortic aneurysm: the possibility of an aortic manifestation of IgG4-related sclerosing disease. *The American Journal of Surgical Pathology*, Vol.32, No.4, (April 2008), pp. 553–559, ISSN 0147-5185

Salvarani C., Pipitone N., Versari A., Vaglio A., Serafini D., Bajocchi G., Slvo D., Buzio C., Greco P. & Boiardi L. (2005). Positron emission tomography (PET): evaluation of chronic periaortitis. *Arthritis Rheumatism*, Vol.53, No.2, (April 2005), pp. 298–303, ISSN 0004-3591

Serra RM., Engle JE., Jones RE. & Schoolwerth AV. (1980). Perianeurysmal retroperitoneal fibrosis. An unusual cause of renal failure. *The American Journal of Medicine*, Vol.68, No.1, (January 1980), pp. 149-153, ISSN 0002-93432

Singh K., Bonaa KH., Jacobsen BK., Bjork L. & Solberg. (2001). Prevalence of and risk factors for abdominal aortic aneurysms in a population-based study: The Tromso Study. *American Journal of Epidemiology*, Vol.154, No.3, (August 2001), pp. 236–244, ISSN 0002-9262

Sterpetti AV., Hunter WJ., Feldhaus RJ., Chansan P., McNamara M., Cisternino S. & Schultz RD. (1989). Inflammatory aneurysms of the abdominal aorta: incidence, pathologic, and etiologic considerations. *Journal of Vascular Surgery*, Vol.9, No.5, (May 1989), pp. 643-650, ISSN 0741-5214

Stone JH., Khosroshahi A., Hilgenberg A., Spooner A., Isselbacher EM. & Stone JR. (2009). IgG4-related systemic disease and lymphoplasmacytic aortitis. *Arthritis Rheumatism*, Vol.60, No.10, (October 2009), pp. 3139-3145, ISSN 1474-547X

Stone JH., Khosroshahi A., Deshpande V. & Stone JR. (2010). IgG4-related systemic disease accounts for a significant proportion of thoracic lymphoplasmacytic aortitis cases. *Arthritis Care Research*, Vol.62, No.3, (March 2010), pp. 316–322, ISSN 2151-4658

Stone JR. (2011). Aortitis, periaortitis, and retroperitoneal fibrosis, as manifestations of IgG4-related systemic disease *Current Opinion in Rheumatology*, Vol.23, No. 1, (January 2011), pp. 88–94, ISSN 1531-6963

Tanaka S., Komori K., Okadome K., Sugimachi K. & Mori R. (1994). Detection of active cytomegalovirus infection in inflammatory aortic aneurysms with RNA polymerase chain reaction. *Journal of Vascular Surgery*, Vol.20, No.2, (August 1994), pp. 235-243, ISSN 0741-5214

Tang T., Boyle JR., Dixon AK. & Varty K. (2005). Inflammatory abdominal aortic aneurysms. *European Journal of Vascular Surgery*, Vol.29, No.4, (April 2005), pp. 353–362, ISSN 1078-5884

Tsai TC., Chang PY., Chen BF., Huang FY. & Shih SL. (1996). Retroperitoneal fibrosis and juvenile rheumatoid arthritis. *Pediatric Nephrology*, Vol.10, No.2, (April 1996), pp. 208-209, ISSN 0931-041X

Uibu T., Oksa P., Auvinen A., Honkanen E., Metsarinne K., Saha H., Uitti J. & Roto P. (2004). Asbestos exposure as a risk factor for retroperitoneal fibrosis. *Lancet*, Vol.363, No.9419, (May 2004), pp. 1422–1426, 1474-547X

Vaglio A., Corradi D., Manenti L., Ferretti L., Garini G. & Buzio C. (2003). Evidence of autoimmunity in chronic periaortitis: a prospective study. *The American Journal of Medicine*, Vol.114, No.6, (April 2003), pp. 454–462, ISSN 0002-9343

Vaglio A. & Buzio C. (2005). Chronic periaortitis: a spectrum of diseases. *Current Opinion in Rheumatology*, Vol.17, No.1, (January 2005), pp. 34–40, ISSN 1531-6963

Vaglio A., Salvarani C. & Buzio C. (2006). Retroperitoneal fibrosis. *Lancet*, Vol.367, No. 9506, (January 2006), pp. 241–251, ISSN 1474-547X

Vaglio A., Greco P., Corradi D., Palmisani A., Martorana D., Ronda N. & Buzio C. (2006). Autoimmune aspects of chronic periaortitis. *Autoimmunity Reviews*, Vol.5, No.7, (August 2006), pp. 458–464, ISSN 1568-9972

Vaglio A., Pipitone N. & Salvarani C. (2011). Chronic periaortitis: a large-vessel vasculitis? *Current Opinion in Rheumatology*, Vol.23, No.1, (January 2011), pp. 1-6, ISSN 1531-6963

van Bommel EF., Siemes C., Hak LE., van der Veer SJ. & Hendriksz TR. (2007). Long-term renal and patient outcome in idiopathic retroperitoneal fibrosis treated with prednisone. *American Journal of Kidney Disease*, Vol.49, No.5, (May 2007), pp. 615–625, ISSN 1523-6838

van Bommel EF., van Tits LJ., van den Berg EA., Prins J. & Stalenhoef AF. (2011). Autoantibodies against oxidized low-density lipoprotein and lipid profile in patients with chronic periaortitis: case–control study. *Rheumatol International*, Vol 31, No.2, (February 2011), pp. 201-208, ISSN 1437-160X

Vanoli M., Daina E., Salvarani C., Sabbadini MG., Rossi C., Bacchiani G., Schieppati A., Baldissera E., Bertolini G. & Itaka Study Group. (2005). Takayasu's arteritis: A study of 104 Italian patients. *Arthritis Rheumatism*, Vol.53, No.1, (February 2005), pp. 100–107, ISSN 0004-3591

von Fritschen U., Malzfeld E., Clasen A. & Kortmann H. (1999). Inflammatory abdominal aortic aneurysm: A postoperative course of retroperitoneal fibrosis. *Journal of Vascular Surgery*, Vol.30, No.6, (December 1999), pp. 1090–1098, ISSN 0741-5214

Warnatz K., Keskin AG., Uhl C., Scholz C., Katzenwadel A., Vaith P., Peter HH. & Walker UA. (2005). Immunosuppressive therapy of chronic periaortitis: a retrospective study of 20 patients with chronic periaortitis and a review of the literature. *Annals of the Rheumatic Disease*, Vol.64, No.6, (June 2005), pp. 828–833, ISSN 0003-4967

Weyand CM., Kurtin PJ. & Goronzy JJ. (2001). Ectopic lymphoid organogenesis: a fast track for autoimmunity. The *American Journal of Pathology*, Vol.159, No.3, (September 2001), pp. 787-793, ISSN 0002-9440

Yusuf K., Murat B., Unal A., Ulku K., Taylan K., Ozerdem O., Erdal Y. & Tahsin Y. (2007). Inflammatory abdominal aortic aneurysm: predictors of long-term outcome in a casecontrol study. *Surgery*, Vol.141, No.1, (January 2007), pp. 83–89, ISSN 0886-0440

Zen Y., Onodera M., Inoue D., Kitao A., Matsui O., Nohara T., Namiki M., Kasashima S., Kawashima A., Matsumoto Y., Katayanagi K., Murata T., Ishizawa S., Hosaka N., Hosaks N., Kuriki K. & Kakanuma Y. (2009). Retroperitoneal fibrosis: a clinicopathologic study with respect to immunoglobulin G4. *The American Journal of Surgical Pathology*, Vol.33, No.12, (December 2009), pp. 1833–1839, ISSN 1532-0979

Subclinical Atherosclerosis in Systemic Autoimmune Disorders

Giannelou M.[1], Gravani F.[1], Papadaki I.[1],
Ioakeimidis D.[1] and Mavragani C.P.[2]

[1]Department of Rheumatology, Athens General Hospital "G.Gennimatas," Athens,
[2]Department of Experimental Physiology, School of Medicine,
University of Athens, Athens,
Greece

1. Introduction

Over the last years, accelerated atherosclerosis with consequent increased prevalence of cardiovascular disease (CV) in autoimmune patients, especially rheumatoid arthritis (RA) and systemic lupus erythematosus (SLE) has been well established (Toloza, Uribe et al. 2004). However, traditional risk factors associated with atherosclerosis including among others smoking, dyslipidemia, diabetes mellitus (DM), hypertension (HT) and increased body mass index (BMI), do not fully account for the high rates of subclinical atherosclerosis in these patients (Meune, Touze et al. 2009). In the present review, traditional and disease related risk factors of CV disease in the setting of chronic autoimmune disorders with special focus in RA, SLE and Sjogren's syndrome (SS) will be discussed.

2. Epidemiology of CV disease in systemic autoimmune disorders

RA

RA, a chronic systemic inflammatory disease affecting 0.5–1% of the adult population is associated with a two fold increase of CV disease. In a recent study by Evans et al, in 636 RA patients, the incidence of acute coronary syndromes (ACS) including myocardial infarction, unstable angina, cardiac arrest or death due to ischemic heart disease was 3.5 per 100 patient-years with the presence of carotid plaque, CV risk factors (particularly diabetes or hypertension), active polyarticular disease, high cumulative dose of glucocorticoids and male sex, being high risk contributors (Evans, Escalante et al. 2011). In patients with early RA, higher intima media thickness (IMT) scores- a surrogate marker of subclinical atherosclerosis- have been detected compared to healthy controls (Sodergren, Karp et al. 2010) (Georgiadis, Voulgari et al. 2008). Of interest, treatment with methotrexate and prednisolone led to significant reduction of IMT scores compared to baseline after one year of treatment. Several studies so far have demonstrated the independent relationship of elevated inflammatory markers (Myasoedova and Gabriel 2010), with the effects of the atherosclerotic process being reversed, after disease activity and chronic inflammation in RA patients are controlled (Bisoendial, Stroes et al. 2011).

SLE

SLE is a highly heterogeneous autoimmune disease, affecting women of childbearing age, with substantial mortality and morbidity. The effect of SLE on atherosclerotic disease has been recognised since the 70s, when Urowitz et al displayed a bimodal mortality peak; the first was attributed to disease activity and infections and the second to CV disease (Urowitz, Bookman et al. 1976). The prevalence of ischemic heart disease in SLE patients is estimated between 8% and 16% (Badui, Garcia-Rubi et al. 1985; Gladman and Urowitz 1987; Petri, Perez-Gutthann et al. 1992; Borchers, Keen et al. 2004) conferring a 50fold risk (Manzi, Meilahn et al. 1997). In regard to subclinical coronary artery disease, the rates seem to be even higher, reaching the percentage of 28%-40% (Manzi, Selzer et al. 1999; Svenungsson, Jensen-Urstad et al. 2001; Asanuma, Oeser et al. 2003; Manger, Kusus et al. 2003; Roman, Shanker et al. 2003; Vlachoyiannopoulos, Kanellopoulos et al. 2003). Esdaile et al revealed that even after statistical correction for the effects of all classical CV risk factors, patients with SLE still had a 7.9-fold increase in the risk of stroke and a 10.1-fold increase in risk of non-fatal myocardial infarction (Esdaile, Abrahamowicz et al. 2001). Given that standard Framingham scores cannot fully account for the rate of ischemic events, lupus is now regarded as an independent risk factor for the development of CV comorbidity (Manzi, Meilahn et al. 1997; Manzi 2000).

SS

SS or autoimmune epithelitis a slowly progressive autoimmune disease is characterized by salivary and lacrimal gland dysfunction and shares many common clinical and serologic features with other immune mediated autoimmune diseases especially SLE (Mavragani and Moutsopoulos 2010). SS has been recently associated with increased rates of subclinical CV disease in a limited number of studies. Vaudo et al, revealed higher carotid and femoral IMT scores in 37 untreated white women with primary SS compared to age and sex matched healthy counterparts, in association with leukopenia and the presence of anti-SSA antibodies (Vaudo, Bocci et al. 2005). In a subsequent study by Satish et al, patients with long standing disease demonstrated abnormal ankle brachial index (ABI) values compared to controls (Rachapalli, Kiely et al. 2009). While endothelium dependent flow mediated vasodilation (FMD) –a marker of endothelial function- did not differ significantly between primary SS patients and controls as a whole, the subset of patients with articular involvement or parotid gland enlargement had lower values of FMV than controls and patients without such characteristics.

On the other hand, nitrate mediated vasodilation (NMV) values -detecting smooth muscle relaxation independently of endothelial contribution- were lower in primary SS patients and particularly in those characterized by leukopenia, rheumatoid factor (RF), anti-SSB antibodies, and articular involvement. Of interest, NMV values, were directly correlated to the number of the circulating white blood cells and inversely correlated to vascular cell adhesion molecule 1 (VCAM-1) levels (Gerli, Vaudo et al. 2010).

3. Traditional CV risk factors in autoimmune diseases

3.1 Metabolic syndrome

The metabolic syndrome (MetS) describes a constellation of major risk factors for CV disease including dyslipidemia, obesity, hypertension and insulin resistance. Several studies so far have documented the increased frequency of MetS in patients with chronic rheumatic diseases compared to healthy control populations; the higher proinflammatory cytokine burden impairs insulin sensitivity and promotes the adverse lipoprotein profile seen in MetS (Pereira, de Carvalho et al. 2009; Santos and Fonseca 2009).

RA

The relationship between the BMI and overall CV mortality in patients with RA is well recognised (Kitas and Gabriel 2011). Quiet unexpectedly, compared to the general population, the risk of CV disease in RA patients is increased in younger females with low body mass index (<20kg/m^2), most likely due to the excess of inflammatory cytokines (Gabriel 2010; Ozbalkan, Efe et al. 2010; Kitas and Gabriel 2011). In accord with the previous observation, obesity is linked to hypertension and dyslipidemia, but with lower RA disease activity and consequently less CV mortality (Summers, Metsios et al. 2010). In contrast, in the study of Kallinoglou et al, multivariate analysis revealed an association of obesity with CV disease in patients with RA mainly due to concomitant presence of risk factors such as HT, high-density lipoprotein (HDL), insulin resistance and Mets (Stavropoulos-Kalinoglou, Metsios et al. 2009). On the other hand, a recent study has shown that in patients with established RA, both very low and very high BMI and BF associate independently with increased disease activity and physical dysfunction but not with the presence of erosions or joint surgery (Stavropoulos-Kalinoglou, Metsios et al. 2009). While the long-term use of glucocorticoids in RA may collectively contribute to the development of Mets syndrome and atherosclerosis, no association with long term low dose glucocorticoid has been detected in this population (Toms, Panoulas et al. 2008). Furthermore, Ku et al showed that RA patients have high basal levels of insulin and increased insulin resistance and that the degree of severity correlates with inflammatory indices (Ku, Imboden et al. 2009). Finally, in a study of a group of 105 Vietnamese women with early RA, a higher prevalence of MetS compared with healthy controls was demonstrated with disease activity, high inflammatory indices, disability score and less use of DMARDs being independent predictors (Dao, Do et al. 2010). The link between obesity and inflammation has recently attracted particular attention. Adipocytokines –a newly identified cytokine subset- have been associated with adipose tissue and include among others leptin, adiponectin, resistin and visfatin. Leptin is essential for the regulation of appetite and body weight, as well as the modulation of immune responses (Rho, Chung et al. 2010). While resistin and visfatin are associated with inflammation, insulin resistance and subclinical atherosclerosis, adiponectin is mainly anti-inflammatory, and inversely associated with obesity, insulin resistance, CRP and CV risk (Fagerer and Kullich 2010; Yoshino, Kusunoki et al. 2011).

In patients with RA, higher levels of adipocytokines have been detected compared to control subjects. In a recent report, leptin and visfatin levels were associated with insulin resistance, but not with the presence of coronary calcification (Ozgen, Koca et al. 2010; Rho, Chung et al. 2010). As expected, in contrast to adiponectin, which was negatively associated with CRP, leptin and resistin levels were positively linked to CRP titers (Yoshino, Kusunoki et al. 2011). While anti-tumor necrosis factor alpha (anti-TNF) treatment in RA patients does not change the levels of circulating visfatin and leptin (Popa, Netea et al. 2009; Gonzalez-Gay, Vazquez-Rodriguez et al. 2010), data on adiponectin is contradictory. In the largest so far study including 97 patients with RA, serum adiponectin was increased after 12 months of anti-TNF treatment (Nishida, Okada et al. 2008), an observation also confirmed in smaller reports with the same follow-up period, implying a potential underlying mechanism for CV risk reduction by anti-TNF agents (Komai, Morita et al. 2007; Serelis, Kontogianni et al. 2008; Engvall, Tengstrand et al. 2010). In contrast, with the exception of the Japanese study by Komai et al who revealed increased adiponectin levels as soon as 2 and 6 weeks, no changes or reduction in adiponectin levels have been reported by studies with a follow-up period of 6 months (Derdemezis, Filippatos et al. 2009; Popa, Netea et al. 2009).

SLE

In a large cohort of 250 patients with SLE and equal number of age-sex matched controls, increased waist-to-hip ratio and sedentary lifestyle in SLE patients was found (Bruce, Urowitz et al. 2003). The prevalence of obesity in SLE has been recently estimated in a cohort of 145 patients by two methods. Using the most common body composition measure (Body mass index, BMI), almost 30% were obese; using a more sensitive measure (by Dual X-ray absorptometry (DXA), the percentage rose to 50% (Katz, Gregorich et al. 2011). A higher prevalence of Mets was found in young lupus patients below 40 years compared to age matched controls (15.8% vs 4.2%) (Sabio, Zamora-Pasadas et al. 2008); the corresponding figures in the study of Chung et al were 32.4% versus 10.9% (using the WHO definition that requires direct determination of insulin resistance) and 29.4% versus 19.8% (using the National Cholesterol Education Program Adult Treatment Panel III definition -NCEP) and found to correlate with higher C-Reactive protein (CRP) levels and endothelial injury. In a subsequent study by Mok et al, the prevalence of Mets was 16.3% in lupus patients and correlated with coronary atherosclerosis (Mok, Poon et al. 2010). In another report, the presence of Mets was associated with higher aortic pulse wave velocity (PWV) –as an indicator of arterial stiffness- and increased biomarkers of subclinical atherosclerosis such as CRP, IL-6, C3, uric acid, homocysteine, fibrinogen and D-dimer (Sabio, Vargas-Hitos et al. 2009). Insulin resistance per se as defined by the WHO criteria was more prevalent in lupus patients compared to controls (44.1% versus 24.8%) (Chung, Avalos et al. 2007).

Similarly to RA, increased levels of adiponectin have been reported in SLE patients (Sada, Yamasaki et al. 2006; Chung, Long et al. 2009; Vadacca, Margiotta et al. 2009) and found to be associated with carotid plaque formation, as a physiologic attempt to limit endothelial damage (Sada, Yamasaki et al. 2006; Vadacca, Margiotta et al. 2009; Clancy and Ginzler 2010; Reynolds, Buyon et al. 2010). Opposite are the findings reported by Chung et al, where lower levels of adiponectin were associated with insulin resistance, BMI and CRP but not with coronary atherosclerosis (Chung, Long et al. 2009). In a murine lupus model, adiponectin has been recently shown to exert protective effects against lupus activity and concomitant atherosclerotic disease. The use of the peroxisome proliferator-activated receptor gamma (PPARgamma) agonist rosiglitazone reduces autoantibody production, renal disease, and atherosclerosis in mouse models of SLE possibly through adiponectin induction. At the same time, lupus mice that lack adiponectin develop more severe disease compared to adiponectin-sufficient lupus mice with the administration of exogenous adiponectin ameliorating disease (Aprahamian, Bonegio et al. 2009). Leptin levels were associated with insulin resistance, BMI and CRP but not with coronary or carotid atherosclerosis (Vadacca, Margiotta et al. 2009). Administration of leptin in lupus prone model led to increased pro-inflammatory HDL scores, atherosclerosis, and accelerated proteinuria, revealing its proatherogenic role (Hahn, Lourencco et al. 2010).

SS

In patients with SS, a higher prevalence of associated dyslipidemia, DM, and hyperuricemia compared to age and sex-matched controls has been observed. Hypercholesterolemia was associated with a lower frequency of immunological markers such as anti-Ro/SSA, anti-La/SSB antibodies, low C3, and C4 levels, while hypertriglyceridemia and DM were positively associated with the presence of extraglandular (renal, liver,vasculitic) involvement. A higher prevalence of DM was found in patients treated with corticosteroids (Ramos-Casals, Brito-Zeron et al. 2007).

3.2 Hypertension (HT)

RA

The prevalence of HT among patients with RA varies between different studies (Panoulas, Metsios et al. 2008). In the largest so far population study by Han et al. prevalence of HT was significantly higher in RA (34% vs 23.4%). However, a recent metaanalysis assessing the effect of traditional risk factors in the pathogenesis of CV disease in RA patients demonstrated similar rates of hypertension in RA patients compared to healthy controls (Gabriel 2010; Boyer, Gourraud et al. 2011).

HT has been found to be associated with subclinical atherosclerosis and CV morbidity in RA patients (Panoulas, Douglas et al. 2007). In a recent Greek cohort study of 325 RA patients, with late disease onset, inadequate early control of disease activity and leflunomide treatment, hypertension was clearly demonstrated to be an important risk factor for CV disease (Serelis, Panagiotakos et al. 2011).

HT and low grade inflammation have been previously linked in general population studies (Panoulas, Douglas et al. 2007; Kitas and Gabriel 2011). High CRP leads to vasoconstriction though reduction of endothelial nitric oxide production, increase in expression of endothelin-1 and upregulation of angiotensin type 1 receptor expression; furthermore, it induces platelet adherence, oxidation and thrombosis. Apart from systemic inflammation, physical inactivity due to articular involvement, genetic predisposition, various medications including NSAIDs, corticosteroids, leflunomide and cyclosporine might account for deregulated arterial pressure in patients with RA (Stavropoulos-Kalinoglou, Metsios et al. 2009; Kitas and Gabriel 2011).

Genetic contribution in occurrence of HT in RA patients was evidenced by the association of previously associated polymorphisms with HT in healthy populations. In RA patients, TGFB1 869T/C and endothelin gene polymorphisms have been shown to be linked with HT, with the latter found to be associated with raised endothelin-1 (ET-1) levels. In contrast to previous studies in healthy subjects, no associations between IL-6-174G/C and HT (Panoulas, Douglas et al. 2009) was detected. Furthermore, a cross-sectional study did not demonstrate significant associations between RA disease activity and hypertension (Panoulas, Metsios et al. 2008; Kitas and Gabriel 2011).

SLE

HT is a well recognised risk factor for CV disease development in SLE patients (Petri, Perez-Gutthann et al. 1992) as evidenced by several studies reporting its contribution in plaque formation (IMT measurement, coronary angiography) and arterial stiffening (Sella, Sato et al. 2003; Selzer, Sutton-Tyrrell et al. 2004; Maksimowicz-McKinnon, Magder et al. 2006; Cypiene, Dadoniene et al. 2010; Gallelli, Burdick et al. 2010). Several studies so far have confirmed the increased prevalence of arterial HT in these patients, ranging from 33% to 56% (de Leeuw, Freire et al. 2006; Bellomio, Spindler et al. 2009; Duarte, Couto et al. 2009; Boucelma, Haddoum et al. 2011; Sabio, Vargas-Hitos et al. 2011). In an effort to investigate the contributors of HT in a cohort of 112 lupus patients, Sabio et al, reported that renal disease, insulin levels and disease activity indices such as Systemic Lupus Erythematosus Disease Activity Index (SLEDAI) were independent predictors of HT in these subjects. Of interest, in the younger age group (<40y), hypertension was also associated with higher non obesity-related insulin levels, while in the older group (>40y), with age and obesity (Sabio, Vargas-Hitos et al. 2011).

Arterial hypertension did not seem to influence subclinical atherosclerotic disease in patients with pSS (Vaudo, Bocci et al. 2005; Rachapalli, Kiely et al. 2009; Gerli, Vaudo et al. 2010).

3.3 Dyslipidemia

Increased levels of total cholesterol (TC), low-density-lipoprotein (LDL) cholesterol and decreased level of HDL cholesterol are associated with increased risk for CV disease in the general population (Nurmohamed 2009). Cholesterol is transported in the blood by LDL which contains esterified cholesterol and triglycerides surrounded by phospholipids, free cholesterol and apolipoprotein B100 (ApoB100). Circulating LDL particles can accumulate in the intima, where ApoB100 binds to proteoglycans of the extracellular matrix, they are oxidised (Hansson and Hermansson 2011) (oxLDLs), become proinflammatory and lead to endothelial activation. Monocytes are stimulated by macrophage colony-stimulating factor produced by activated endothelial cells and differentiate into macrophages. Macrophages upregulate their scavenger receptors that can take up oxLDL (Hahn, Grossman et al. 2008). Cholesterol accumulation in macrophages transforms them into foam cells that are characteristic of the atherosclerotic lesion. Dendritic cells (DCs) may take up LDL for antigen presentation in regional lymph nodes. In the normal artery wall, DCs promote antigen tolerization; however, atherogenesis leads to a switch from tolerance to the activation of adaptive immunity (Hansson and Hermansson 2011). Monocytes attract lymphocytes that recognize antigens and contribute to inflammation by releasing cytokines. As plaque matures, proteases and other proinflammatory molecules are produced, with hypertrophy of smooth muscle, damage to endothelial cells, bulging of plaque into the lumen of the artery, and formation of a fibrous cap over the plaque (Hahn, Grossman et al. 2008).

RA

Lipoprotein (α) (Lp(α)) is a cholesterol-rich modified form of LDL (Van Doornum, McColl et al. 2002) that is transformed in the liver by covalent attachment of ApoB to ApoA, a member of the plasminogen gene family (Tabas, Williams et al. 2007). Lp(α) has been identified as an independent risk factor for coronary heart disease and elevated levels have been demonstrated in RA patients with active disease (Van Doornum, McColl et al. 2002). Several studies suggest that Lp(α) is associated with early atherosclerosis in RA and possibly in other autoimmune disorders (Dursunoglu, Evrengul et al. 2005; Wang, Hu et al. 2008). In recent studies, complexes of β2-glycoprotein I with Lp(α) ((β2)-GPI-Lp(α)) are found in sera of active RA patients and associate with oxLDL, ox-Lpa and CRP levels (Zhang, Li et al. 2011).

On the other hand, low HDL levels have been previously associated with RA related atherosclerosis implying the potential link between HDL and autoimmunity. HDL possesses anti-inflammatory effects and inhibits the ability of antigen-presenting cells (APCs) to stimulate T cells (Yu, Wang et al. 2010). Given that inflammation has been shown to suppress total and LDL cholesterol, active RA patients have lower total cholesterol, low LDL and depressed HDL resulting in a higher atherogenic index (total cholesterol/HDL-cholesterol ratio) (Nurmohamed 2009; Kitas and Gabriel 2011), although such alterations have been also observed 3-5 year prior to RA incidence (Myasoedova, Crowson et al. 2010). In a study of early RA patients higher levels of TC, LDL , triglycerides and very low levels in HDL have been observed compared to healthy controls resulting again in a significantly higher atherogenic ratio of TC/HDL as well as that of LDL/HDL (Georgiadis, Papavasiliou et al. 2006). Raised autoantibody titers against oxLDL and low lipoprotein-associated phospholipase A2 (Lp-PLA2) plasma activity have been also suggested as potential contributors in the pathogenesis of accelerated atherosclerosis in patients with early RA (Lourida, Georgiadis et al. 2007). Of interest, recent findings have revealed the contribution of several known RA susceptible genes such as TRAF1/C5, STAT4 and HLA-DRB1-SE in dyslipidemia observed in these patients (Toms, Panoulas et al. 2011).

Systemic inflammation, drug therapy, lifestyle and genetic factors can result not only in changes of overall lipid levels, but also can modify lipids structure and function (Toms, Symmons et al. 2010). Paraoxonase 1 (PON1) is an antiatherogenic enzyme with the ability to destroy biologically active oxLDL (Hahn, Grossman et al. 2008) and to protect LDL against oxidation (Zhao 2009). PON1 activity in RA patients is inversely related to CRP levels, suggesting that inflammation modulates PON activity (Ku, Imboden et al. 2009).

SLE

The classical pattern of dyslipoproteinemia in SLE is characterized by elevated levels of very-low-density lipoprotein cholesterol (VLDL), triglycerides and LDL and low levels of HDL (Borba, Bonfa et al. 2000), although HDL qualitative abnormalities such as peroxidation have been also described, often in association with active disease. Peroxidised HDLs (piHDLs) are unable to reverse cholesterol transport which normally clears oxLDL from the subendothelial space promoting endothelial injury. piHDLs occur in a larger proportion of patients with SLE compared to RA and are associated with carotid artery plaque formation, documented CV disease and low physical activity (McMahon, Grossman et al. 2006; McMahon, Grossman et al. 2009; Volkmann, Grossman et al. 2010).

Apart from HDL, LDL can be also modified in SLE; Frostergard et al disclosed higher levels of oxidized epitopes on LDL in lupus patients compared to controls, which were associated with arterial disease and renal manifestations (Frostegard, Svenungsson et al. 2005).

In a recent study, circulating lipoprotein remnant particles and the intermediate density lipoprotein (IDL) fraction have been strongly associated with IMT values in lupus patients (Gonzalez, Ribalta et al. 2010). Furthermore, reduced levels of apoA-I -the major apolipoprotein component of HDL- have been found in SLE patients with IgG anticardiolipin antibodies (Delgado Alves, Kumar et al. 2003) while antibodies to apoA-I have been previously documented in 32.5% of patients with SLE and 22.9% of patients with primary antiphospholipid syndrome (Dinu, Merrill et al. 1998).

Anti-HDL, anti-CRP anti-Apo A-I have been detected in SLE patients, with the latter found to be associated with persistent disease activity. In the subset of patients with lupus nephritis, anti-Apo A-I and anti-HDL levels correlated with serum anti-double-stranded DNA levels (O'Neill, Giles et al. 2010). Woo et al evaluated the effects of L-4F, (apolipoprotein A-1 mimetic peptide), alone or with pravastatin, in apoE-/-Fas-/-C57BL/6 female mice that spontaneously develop immunoglobulin G (IgG) autoantibodies, glomerulonephritis, osteopenia, and atherosclerotic lesions. As expected, L-4F treatment, significantly reduced IgG anti-dsDNA and IgG anti-oxPLs (anti-oxidised phospholipids), proteinuria, glomerulonephritis, and osteopenia in a murine lupus model of accelerated atherosclerosis (Woo, Lin et al. 2010).

SS

Low HDL cholesterol levels was a constant finding among SS patients in several studies (Vaudo, Bocci et al. 2005; Lodde, Sankar et al. 2006; Gerli, Vaudo et al. 2010). Of interest, HDL along with total cholesterol were found to be associated with immunoglobulin G levels. In particular, the presence of anti-SSA and anti-SSB antibodies have been linked to lower total cholesterol and reduced HDL cholesterol levels, respectively (Lodde, Sankar et al. 2006). Subsequently, Cruz et al, showed a trend to dyslipidemia defined as total cholesterol >200mg/dL, HDL cholesterol<40mg/dL, LDL cholesterol>130mg/dL or triglycerides > 150mg/dL in patients with pSS compared to controls (Cruz, Fialho et al. 2010).

3.4 Smoking

RA

Smoking is an important risk factor for the development of both RA and CVD. Smoking is associated with severe RA with more erosive disease and extra-articular involvement, as smokers are more likely to have positive RF and anti-CCP antibodies. It is not yet clear if smoking confers the same relative risk for CVD development in RA patients compared to the general population (Ozbalkan, Efe et al. 2010). Cigarette smoking is associated with reduced BMI and body fat (BF) in patients with RA, with heavy smoking particularly linked to lower muscle mass while smoking cessation appears to associate with increased BMI, BF, and waist circumference in these patients (Stavropoulos-Kalinoglou, Metsios et al. 2008). In a recent metaanalysis by Gabriel, the prevalence of smoking, but not of the other traditional CV risk factors appears to be increased in RA compared to non-RA patients, at the time of RA incidence (Gabriel 2010).

SLE

Cigarette smoking along with HT have been identified as the main predictors of extracranial carotid artery atherosclerosis, in an early study including 240 SLE patients (Homer, Ingall et al. 1991). While in the studies conducted by Asanuma and Roman, no association between smoking and carotid or coronary atherosclerosis was detected (Asanuma, Oeser et al. 2003; Roman, Shanker et al. 2003), in a subsequent multiethnic US cohort of 546 SLE patients, the role of smoking in the development of vascular events (cardiovascular, cerebrovascular and peripheral) has been suggested (Toloza, Uribe et al. 2004). Similarly, Selzer et al, compared risk factors for subclinical vascular disease in different vascular beds (carotid and aorta) in SLE female patients. Smoking was identified as a factor correlating with carotid plaque severity, together with older age, systolic hypertension and lower albumin levels. In regard to aortic stiffness, risk factors included older age and higher systolic blood pressure but not smoking (Selzer, Sutton-Tyrrell et al. 2004). Finally, a race-smoking interaction was also identified, as amongst black women with SLE, those with a history of smoking have higher IMT values than non smokers. This effect did not apply to white patients (Scalzi, Bhatt et al. 2009).

Smoking did not seem to influence subclinical atherosclerotic disease in patients with pSS (Vaudo, Bocci et al. 2005; Gerli, Vaudo et al. 2010).

3.5 Hyperomocysteinemia

Hyperhomocysteinemia is a recognised risk factor for arterial and venous disease in the general population. Homocysteine increases oxidative stress on the endothelium and causes modification of LDL, inhibition of nitric oxide synthesis, proliferation of smooth muscle cells, intimal hyperplasia, increased protease activity, activation of proinflammatory mediators and thrombosis (Durga, Verhoef et al. 2004). Hyperhomocysteinemia can originate either from a genetic polymorphism and/or a variety of factors including folic acid or vitamin B12 deficiency, corticosteroid or methotrexate treatment, and renal dysfunction. Hyperhomocysteinemia has been reported in 20%-42% of patients with RA and is related to treatment with antifolate agents and greater disease activity. Genetic investigations identified the C677T polymorphism in the gene coding for the MTHFR enzyme as a new candidate genetic risk factor for CV disease in the general population. The 677TT genotype is associated with higher plasma homocysteine levels than in heterozygotes or in individuals with wild-type C alleles (Palomino-Morales, Gonzalez-Juanatey et al. 2010). The increased levels of homocysteine caused by methotrexate therapy occur more often to patients heterozygous for the C677T mutation. Normal homocysteine levels are restored by folic acid supplementation (El Bouchti, Sordet et al. 2008).

RA

In a recent Spanish study of RA patients, the MTHFR A1298C rather the C677T was associated with increased risk of atherosclerosis, demonstrating that patients homozygous for the MTHFR 1298CC genotype had increased risk of CV events at 5 and 10 years follow up and more severe endothelial dysfunction (lower values of FMD %), when compared with those homozygous for the wild MTHFR 1298AA genotype (Palomino-Morales, Gonzalez-Juanatey et al. 2010). Interestingly an ongoing study from our group indicate that Greek RA patients with carotid or femoral plaque formation have a higher prevalence of MTHFR AC and CC genotypes compared with those without. The so far available results show that MTHFR 1298 A>C gene polymorphism confers an increased risk for plaque formation (Mavragani 2011).

SLE

Attention has been drawn over the past few years to the role of homocysteine concentration in the development of subclinical atherosclerosis in SLE patients. In a prospective study, Petri identified elevated homocysteine levels as a risk factor for the later development of CV disease in SLE patients (Petri 2000).

In the Toronto Risk Factor Study for coronary heart disease, SLE patients had homocysteine values>15μmoles/liter in a larger proportion compared to controls (11.6% versus 0.8%) despite having higher folate blood levels (Bruce, Urowitz et al. 2003). SLE patients with hyperhomocysteinemia have a threefold increase in odds ratio of thrombotic event (Refai, Al-Salem et al. 2002).

Several studies linked hyperhomocysteinemia to subclinical atherosclerosis (Svenungsson, Jensen-Urstad et al. 2001; Von Feldt, Scalzi et al. 2006; Von Feldt 2008). Roman et al prospectively studied a cohort of SLE patients with matched controls and determined carotid IMT scores as well as the presence of plaque. Over a period of approximately 3 years of follow-up, 28% of the patients had progressive atherosclerosis, defined as a higher plaque score (new plaque or more extensive plaque). Determinants of atherosclerotic progression after multivariate analysis were patient age at diagnosis, disease duration, and baseline homocysteine concentration. Lupus patients with stable plaque and progressive plaque were different only in baseline homocysteine concentration (Roman, Crow et al. 2007). A recent study by Perna et al implied a relationship of both asymmetric dimethylarginine and homocysteine to arterial stiffness, but not to the presence or extent of carotid atherosclerosis (Perna, Roman et al. 2010). In the Rho et al study, homocysteine levels in SLE patients were linked to macrophage activation, reflected by increased serum neopterin concentrations. Neopterin (marker of monocyte and macrophage activation associated with atherosclerosis and CV risk in the general population) was associated with atherogenic mediators of inflammation and homocysteine in SLE, but not with coronary atherosclerosis (Rho, Solus et al. 2011).

SS

No data to date regarding the role of homocysteine in the pathogenesis of CV disease in the setting of Sjogren's syndrome is available.

4. Disease related contributors of atherosclerosis in systemic autoimmune diseases

SLE

A number of studies evaluated specific disease parameters and their effect on atherosclerotic disease in SLE patients. Disease duration appears to be an important factor in CVD development. An inverse relationship between SLE activity and plaque size was reported by Manzi et al and longer disease duration was independently associated with carotid plaque (Manzi, Selzer et al. 1999) and coronary calcium scores (Von Feldt, Scalzi et al. 2006). In a cross-sectional and in a longitudinal study, Roman *et al.* found that longer disease duration and higher Systemic Lupus International Collaborative Clinics (SLICC) damage index were independent predictors of carotid plaque formation(Roman, et al. 2003; Roman, et al. 2007). In another report, SLE specific variables were associated with aortic stiffness and included older age, hypertension, higher C3 levels, lower white blood cell count, higher insulin levels, and renal disease (Selzer, Sutton-Tyrrell et al. 2004).

Rua-Figueroa et al who assessed the changes in carotid IMT and the associated risk factors in patients with lupus in a two year period, identified basal measurement IMT, age at diagnosis, homocysteine, C3 and C5a as risk factors for IMT progression (Rua-Figueroa, Arencibia-Mireles et al. 2010). In accord with the previous findings, Haque et al compared SLE patients with verified clinical CV disease (myocardial infarction or angina pectoris) to patients without clinical CV disease. Male sex, older age, increased SLICC damage index, prior use of corticosteroids and azathioprine and more exposure to all classic CV risk factors were positively correlated with clinical CV disease (Haque, Gordon et al. 2010). In our SLE cohort, IMT and the presence of plaque were both statistically significant associated with age, hypertension, triglyceridelevels and SLICC damage index score and only plaque with the levels of C3 and C4 (Giannelou 2011).

The role of SLE activity in the formation of non calcified coronary plaque (NCP) was investigated by Kiani et al.; unlike coronary calcium, which is not associated with SLE activity measures or with active serologies, NCP is more common in patients with active disease (Kiani, Vogel-Claussen et al. 2010). Additionally, the presence of lymphopenia and higher levels of serum creatinine and CRP seem to be disease related risk factors in the progression of carotid IMT in juvenile-onset SLE as demonstrated by Huang et al (Huang, Chung et al. 2009).

Although under normal conditions vascular damage is expected to be coupled by acceleration in repair of the endothelium, SLE patients have decreased numbers of circulating EPCs and aberrant function of cells involved in the vascular repair. In particular, lupus EPCs/CACs (myeloid circulating angiogenic cells) have decreased capacity to differentiate into mature ECs and synthesize decreased amounts of the molecules vascular endothelial growth factor and hepatic growth factor (Rajagopalan, Somers et al. 2004; Denny, Thacker et al. 2007; Lee, Li et al. 2007; Moonen, de Leeuw et al. 2007; Westerweel, Luijten et al. 2007). IFNα -a central mediator in lupus pathogenesis- has been recently suggested as a major player of impaired vasculogenesis and atherogenic risk in lupus patients through transcriptional repression of proangiogenic IL-1 pathways, enhancement of foam cell formation, and platelet activation (Lood, Amisten et al. 2010; Thacker, Berthier et al. 2010; Li, Fu et al. 2011).

Autoantibodies including antiOxLDL, AECAs (anti-endothelial cell antibodies) and antibodies against heat shock proteins and phospholipids (APLs) have been linked to lupus related CV disease. In regard to the role of the latter in the pathogenesis of CV disease in the setting of lupus, current evidence is rather conflicting. While in a multiethnic US cohort of patients with SLE, APLs were identified as an independent predictor of CV, cerebrovascular or peripheral vascular events (Toloza, Uribe et al. 2004), such an association has not been detected in three distinct large SLE cohorts (Manzi, Meilahn et al. 1997; Roman, Shanker et al. 2003; McMahon, Grossman et al. 2009). On the other hand, the presence of positive lupus anticoagulant or anti-β2glycoprotein-I antibodies have been also linked to development of myocardial infarction (Petri 2004). In lupus patients without previous CV history, the occurrence of a first ever CVE (defined as ischemic heart, cerebrovascular peripheral vascular disease or death due to CV disease) was dependent on the presence of positive APLs, markers of endothelial activation/damage advanced age and absence of thrombocytopenia (Gustafsson, Gunnarsson et al. 2009). Proposed mechanisms of APL related CV risk include inhibition of binding of annexin A5 (a protein shown to inhibit to plaque rupture) to the endothelium or reduction of the activity of the atheroprotective enzyme PON1 (Cederholm, Svenungsson et al. 2005) (Delgado Alves, Ames et al. 2002).

The role of anti-OxLDLs has not been yet clarified. In the general population, it is indicated that some aOxLDLs are decreased in the early stage of atherosclerosis development in non autoimmune disease but raised at later stages and in more advanced disease (Lopes-Virella, Virella et al. 1999; Wu, de Faire et al. 1999; Hulthe, Wiklund et al. 2001; Karvonen, Paivansalo et al. 2003). Anti-OxLDL antibodies have been detected in up to 80% of SLE patients with aPS (Vaarala, Alfthan et al. 1993), but no association with thrombosis has been identified (Aho, Vaarala et al. 1996).

In another report by Svenungsson et al anti-OxLDL antibodies were more common in SLE patients with a history of CV disease than in SLE controls or normal subjects (Svenungsson, Jensen-Urstad et al. 2001); titers of anti-OxLDL have been also found to be correlated with anti-double-stranded DNA antibody titres, complement activation and disease activity scores in patients with SLE (Gomez-Zumaquero, Tinahones et al. 2004). Of interest, increased atherosclerotic disease has been attributed to the presence of complexes of oxidized low-density liprotein/beta2 glycoprotein 1 (oxLDL/beta2GPI) and anti-complex IgG as well as IgM often in association with renal involvement and history of previous thromboembolic episodes (Bassi, Zampieri et al. 2009).

Finally, autoantibodies to endothelial cell (AECAs) and heat shock proteins have been proposed as potential mediators of atherosclerotic risk in lupus patients. (George, Harats et al. 1999; Mandal, Foteinos et al. 2005).AECAs are associated with lupus disease activity and vasculitis and can act directly on endothelial cells by promoting their activation (Margutti, Matarrese et al. 2008).

RA

Over the last decade, the inflammatory and immunologic mechanisms in the initiation and progression of atherosclerosis (Van Doornum, McColl et al. 2002) have become the focus of particular research interest. Pro-inflammatory cytokines such as TNF-α and IL-6 are released into the systemic circulation and have multiple effects on distant organs including the endothelium and the formation of the atherosclerotic plaque through upregulation of adhesion molecules such as vascular cellular adhesion molecule (VCAM), inhibiting of endothelial nitric oxide (eNOS) production and induction of formation of oxidized LDL (de Groot, Posthumus et al. 2010). Blockade of TNF-α in RA reduces cytokine levels, leucocyte trafficking and platelet levels which may all promote atherosclerotic complications (Full, Ruisanchez et al. 2009). A recently identified new player in atherosclerosis pathogenesis is the macrophage migration inhibitory factor (MIF) which induces the pro-inflammatory mediators TNF-α, IL-1, IL-6 and metalloproteinases (MMPs), activates T cells and promotes angiogenesis. In mice with advanced atherosclerosis, MIF blockade led to plaque regression and reduced monocyte and T-cell content in the plaques (de Groot, Posthumus et al. 2010). The increased arterial stiffness found in RA patients is significantly correlated with disease duration and inflammatory markers such as CRP and IL-6 (Tabas, Williams et al. 2007). As the atherosclerotic plaque matures, the apoptosis of cells in the plaque leads to extracellular lipid accumulation and cellular debris formation. Under the influence of macrophage proteinases, the fibrous cap of the plaques weakens, ruptures and secondary thrombosis may occur (de Groot, Posthumus et al. 2010).

In RA patients, genetic regulation of inflammation seems to be implicated in pathogenesis of accelerated atherosclerosis. Carriers of the allele IL-6-174 -found to be associated with higher IL-6 levels- demonstrated increased prevalence of CV disease (Panoulas, Douglas et al. 2009). In another study by Gabriel et al, inflammatory indicators such as high erythrocyte sedimentation rate (ESR), swelling of small and large joints, rheumatoid nodules, vasculitis and rheumatoid lung disease were all statistically significantly associated with an increased of CV death after adjusting for the above mentioned traditional CV risk factors (Gabriel 2010). Moreover, in patients with RA, the disease activity scale (DAS) was inversely correlated with the number of circulating EPCs, which are hematopoietic stem cells involved in vascular repair, suggesting an additional mechanism of atherogenesis in these patients (Pakozdi, Besenyei et al. 2009; Szekanecz and Koch 2010). Similarly, in patients with lupus, increased levels of circulating apoptotic ECs were correlated with lupus disease activity and endothelial dysfunction.

Serum concentration of autoantibodies in RA, specifically anti-modified citrullinated vimentin (anti-MCV) and anti-cyclic citrullinated peptide (anti-CCP) were found to be positively correlated with disease activity including hsCRP, IL-6, homeostasis model assessment for insulin resistance (HOMA-IR) index, serum levels of rheumatoid factors and IMT score. While anti-MCV and anti-CCP3 are equally sensitive in diagnosing early RA, the former appears to be very useful for monitoring associated subclinical atherosclerosis in early RA (El-Barbary, Kassem et al. 2011).

SS

Associations between signs of subclinical atherosclerosis with the presence of leukopenia, specific autoantibodies (RF, anti-SSA, anti-SSB), articular involvement and parotid gland enlargement, may suggest that immune dysregulation could contribute to the increased risk for atherosclerosis in pSS patients. In our SS cohort, subclinical atherosclerosis –detected by IMT determination- was associated with higher levels of salivary gland infiltration, reduced salivary flow as well as with the presence of SS specific autoantibodies (unpublished results)(Gravani et al, 2011), implying that SS related poor dental hygiene along with immune hyperactivity could contribute to the higher risk for atherosclerotic disease (Mattila, Nieminen et al. 1989)

Finally, circulating CD4+, CD28- cells –previously associated with atherosclerotic risk- did not differ between pSS patients and controls. However, pSS patients demonstrated higher levels of AECAs, (IgG and IgM), and sTM (soluble thrombomodulin), but lower levels of anti-Hsp60 (IgG and IgM) compared to their healthy counterparts, whereas anti-Hsp65 and anti-oxLDL antibody levels were similar in both groups (Vaudo, Bocci et al. 2005) (Gerli, Vaudo et al. 2010).

5. Conclusion

The increased prevalence of CV disease is well established in autoimmune diseases even after correction of the traditional risk factors. Several associations with disease related clinical or serological features, immunologic profile and proinflammatory cytokines are reported. Further investigation is needed to determine a yet unidentified, possibly disease specific mechanism in autoimmune patients.

6. Acknowledgements

We are indebted to Prof.Moutsopoulos, MD, FRCP, FACP for continuous inspiration, guidance and support.

7. References

Aho, K., O. Vaarala, et al. (1996). "Antibodies binding to anionic phospholipids but not to oxidized low-density lipoprotein are associated with thrombosis in patients with systemic lupus erythematosus." *Clin Exp Rheumatol.* 14(5): 499-506.

Aprahamian, T., R. G. Bonegio, et al. (2009). "The peroxisome proliferator-activated receptor gamma agonist rosiglitazone ameliorates murine lupus by induction of adiponectin." *J Immunol.* 182(1): 340-346.

Asanuma, Y., A. Oeser, et al. (2003). "Premature coronary-artery atherosclerosis in systemic lupus erythematosus." *N Engl J Med.* 349(25): 2407-2415.

Badui, E., D. Garcia-Rubi, et al. (1985). "Cardiovascular manifestations in systemic lupus erythematosus. Prospective study of 100 patients." *Angiology.* 36(7): 431-441.

Bassi, N., S. Zampieri, et al. (2009). "oxLDL/beta2GPI complex and anti-oxLDL/beta2GPI in SLE: prevalence and correlates." *Autoimmunity.* 42(4): 289-291.

Bellomio, V., A. Spindler, et al. (2009). "Metabolic syndrome in Argentinean patients with systemic lupus erythematosus." *Lupus.* 18(11): 1019-1025.

Bisoendial, R. J., E. S. Stroes, et al. (2011). "Critical determinants of cardiovascular risk in rheumatoid arthritis." *Curr Pharm Des.* 17(1): 21-26.

Borba, E. F., E. Bonfa, et al. (2000). "Chylomicron metabolism is markedly altered in systemic lupus erythematosus." *Arthritis Rheum.* 43(5): 1033-1040.

Borchers, A. T., C. L. Keen, et al. (2004). "Surviving the butterfly and the wolf: mortality trends in systemic lupus erythematosus." *Autoimmun Rev.* 3(6): 423-453.

Boucelma, M., F. Haddoum, et al. (2011). "Cardiovascular risk and lupus disease." *Int Angiol.* 30(1): 18-24.

Boyer, J. F., P. A. Gourraud, et al. (2011). "Traditional cardiovascular risk factors in rheumatoid arthritis: a meta-analysis." *Joint Bone Spine.* 78(2): 179-183. Epub 2010 Sep 2017.

Bruce, I. N., M. B. Urowitz, et al. (2003). "Risk factors for coronary heart disease in women with systemic lupus erythematosus: the Toronto Risk Factor Study." *Arthritis Rheum.* 48(11): 3159-3167.

Cederholm, A., E. Svenungsson, et al. (2005). "Decreased binding of annexin v to endothelial cells: a potential mechanism in atherothrombosis of patients with systemic lupus erythematosus." *Arterioscler Thromb Vasc Biol.* 25(1): 198-203. Epub 2004 Nov 2011.

Chung, C. P., I. Avalos, et al. (2007). "High prevalence of the metabolic syndrome in patients with systemic lupus erythematosus: association with disease characteristics and cardiovascular risk factors." *Ann Rheum Dis.* 66(2): 208-214. Epub 2006 Aug 2010.

Chung, C. P., A. G. Long, et al. (2009). "Adipocytokines in systemic lupus erythematosus: relationship to inflammation, insulin resistance and coronary atherosclerosis." *Lupus.* 18(9): 799-806.

Clancy, R. and E. M. Ginzler (2010). "Endothelial function and its implications for cardiovascular and renal disease in systemic lupus erythematosus." *Rheum Dis Clin North Am.* 36(1): 145-160, ix-x.

Cruz, W., S. Fialho, et al. (2010). "Is there a link between inflammation and abnormal lipoprotein profile in Sjogren's syndrome?" *Joint Bone Spine.* 77(3): 229-231. Epub 2010 Apr 2017.

Cypiene, A., J. Dadoniene, et al. (2010). "The influence of mean blood pressure on arterial stiffening and endothelial dysfunction in women with rheumatoid arthritis and systemic lupus erythematosus." *Medicina (Kaunas).* 46(8): 522-530.

Dao, H. H., Q. T. Do, et al. (2010). "Increased frequency of metabolic syndrome among Vietnamese women with early rheumatoid arthritis: a cross-sectional study." *Arthritis Res Ther.* 12(6): R218. Epub 2010 Dec 2023.

de Groot, L., M. D. Posthumus, et al. (2010). "Risk factors and early detection of atherosclerosis in rheumatoid arthritis." *Eur J Clin Invest* 40(9): 835-842.

de Leeuw, K., B. Freire, et al. (2006). "Traditional and non-traditional risk factors contribute to the development of accelerated atherosclerosis in patients with systemic lupus erythematosus." *Lupus.* 15(10): 675-682.

Delgado Alves, J., P. R. Ames, et al. (2002). "Antibodies to high-density lipoprotein and beta2-glycoprotein I are inversely correlated with paraoxonase activity in systemic lupus erythematosus and primary antiphospholipid syndrome." *Arthritis Rheum.* 46(10): 2686-2694.

Delgado Alves, J., S. Kumar, et al. (2003). "Cross-reactivity between anti-cardiolipin, anti-high-density lipoprotein and anti-apolipoprotein A-I IgG antibodies in patients with systemic lupus erythematosus and primary antiphospholipid syndrome." *Rheumatology (Oxford)*. 42(7): 893-899. Epub 2003 Apr 2016.

Denny, M. F., S. Thacker, et al. (2007). "Interferon-alpha promotes abnormal vasculogenesis in lupus: a potential pathway for premature atherosclerosis." *Blood*. 110(8): 2907-2915. Epub 2007 Jul 2916.

Derdemezis, C. S., T. D. Filippatos, et al. (2009). "Effects of a 6-month infliximab treatment on plasma levels of leptin and adiponectin in patients with rheumatoid arthritis." *Fundam Clin Pharmacol*. 23(5): 595-600. Epub 2009 Jun 2025.

Dinu, A. R., J. T. Merrill, et al. (1998). "Frequency of antibodies to the cholesterol transport protein apolipoprotein A1 in patients with SLE." *Lupus*. 7(5): 355-360.

Duarte, C., M. Couto, et al. (2009). "[Cardiovascular risk profile in a Portuguese cohort of SLE Portuguese patients]." *Acta Reumatol Port*. 34(2B): 349-357.

Durga, J., P. Verhoef, et al. (2004). "Homocysteine and carotid intima-media thickness: a critical appraisal of the evidence." *Atherosclerosis*. 176(1): 1-19.

Dursunoglu, D., H. Evrengul, et al. (2005). "Lp(a) lipoprotein and lipids in patients with rheumatoid arthritis: serum levels and relationship to inflammation." *Rheumatol Int*. 25(4): 241-245. Epub 2004 Jul 2031.

El-Barbary, A. M., E. M. Kassem, et al. (2011). "Association of Anti-Modified Citrullinated Vimentin with Subclinical Atherosclerosis in Early Rheumatoid Arthritis Compared with Anti-Cyclic Citrullinated Peptide." *J Rheumatol* 1: 1.

El Bouchti, I., C. Sordet, et al. (2008). "Severe atherosclerosis in rheumatoid arthritis and hyperhomocysteinemia: is there a link?" *Joint Bone Spine*. 75(4): 499-501. Epub 2008 May 2023.

Engvall, I. L., B. Tengstrand, et al. (2010). "Infliximab therapy increases body fat mass in early rheumatoid arthritis independently of changes in disease activity and levels of leptin and adiponectin: a randomised study over 21 months." *Arthritis Res Ther*. 12(5): R197. Epub 2010 Oct 2021.

Esdaile, J. M., M. Abrahamowicz, et al. (2001). "Traditional Framingham risk factors fail to fully account for accelerated atherosclerosis in systemic lupus erythematosus." *Arthritis Rheum*. 44(10): 2331-2337.

Evans, M. R., A. Escalante, et al. (2011). "Carotid atherosclerosis predicts incident acute coronary syndromes in rheumatoid arthritis." *Arthritis Rheum* 28(10): 30265.

Fagerer, N. and W. Kullich (2010). "[Adipocytokines in rheumatoid arthritis and obesity]." *Wien Med Wochenschr*. 160(15-16): 391-398.

Frostegard, J., E. Svenungsson, et al. (2005). "Lipid peroxidation is enhanced in patients with systemic lupus erythematosus and is associated with arterial and renal disease manifestations." *Arthritis Rheum*. 52(1): 192-200.

Full, L. E., C. Ruisanchez, et al. (2009). "The inextricable link between atherosclerosis and prototypical inflammatory diseases rheumatoid arthritis and systemic lupus erythematosus." *Arthritis Res Ther*. 11(2): 217. Epub 2009 Apr 2003.

Gabriel, S. E. (2010). "Heart disease and rheumatoid arthritis: understanding the risks." *Ann Rheum Dis*. 69(Suppl 1): i61-64.

Gallelli, B., L. Burdick, et al. (2010). "Carotid plaques in patients with long-term lupus nephritis." *Clin Exp Rheumatol*. 28(3): 386-392. Epub 2010 Jun 2023.

George, J., D. Harats, et al. (1999). "Atherosclerosis-related markers in systemic lupus erythematosus patients: the role of humoral immunity in enhanced atherogenesis." *Lupus.* 8(3): 220-226.

Georgiadis, A. N., E. C. Papavasiliou, et al. (2006). "Atherogenic lipid profile is a feature characteristic of patients with early rheumatoid arthritis: effect of early treatment--a prospective, controlled study." *Arthritis Res Ther.* 8(3): R82. Epub 2006 Apr 2028.

Georgiadis, A. N., P. V. Voulgari, et al. (2008). "Early treatment reduces the cardiovascular risk factors in newly diagnosed rheumatoid arthritis patients." *Semin Arthritis Rheum.* 38(1): 13-19. Epub 2008 Jan 2014.

Gerli, R., G. Vaudo, et al. (2010). "Functional impairment of the arterial wall in primary Sjogren's syndrome: combined action of immunologic and inflammatory factors." *Arthritis Care Res (Hoboken).* 62(5): 712-718.

Giannelou M, Mavragani C, et al (2011). "Inverse correlation of premature atherosclerosis and bone mass density in patients with systemic lupus erythematosus. EULAR meeting, London.

Gladman, D. D. and M. B. Urowitz (1987). "Morbidity in systemic lupus erythematosus." *J Rheumatol Suppl.* 14(Suppl 13): 223-226.

Gomez-Zumaquero, J. M., F. J. Tinahones, et al. (2004). "Association of biological markers of activity of systemic lupus erythematosus with levels of anti-oxidized low-density lipoprotein antibodies." *Rheumatology (Oxford).* 43(4): 510-513. Epub 2004 Feb 2010.

Gonzalez-Gay, M. A., T. R. Vazquez-Rodriguez, et al. (2010). "Visfatin is not associated with inflammation or metabolic syndrome in patients with severe rheumatoid arthritis undergoing anti-TNF-alpha therapy." *Clin Exp Rheumatol.* 28(1): 56-62.

Gonzalez, M., J. Ribalta, et al. (2010). "Nuclear magnetic resonance lipoprotein subclasses and the APOE genotype influence carotid atherosclerosis in patients with systemic lupus erythematosus." *J Rheumatol.* 37(11): 2259-2267. Epub 2010 Aug 2253.

Gravani F, Mavragani C, et al(2011). "Increased intimal media thickness scores in patients with primary Sjogren's syndrome- association with disease related risk factors. EULAR meeting, London.

Gustafsson, J., I. Gunnarsson, et al. (2009). "Predictors of the first cardiovascular event in patients with systemic lupus erythematosus - a prospective cohort study." *Arthritis Res Ther.* 11(6): R186. Epub 2009 Dec 2010.

Hahn, B. H., J. Grossman, et al. (2008). "Altered lipoprotein metabolism in chronic inflammatory states: proinflammatory high-density lipoprotein and accelerated atherosclerosis in systemic lupus erythematosus and rheumatoid arthritis." *Arthritis Res Ther* 10(4): 213.

Hahn, B. H., E. V. Lourencco, et al. (2010). "Pro-inflammatory high-density lipoproteins and atherosclerosis are induced in lupus-prone mice by a high-fat diet and leptin." *Lupus.* 19(8): 913-917. Epub 2010 Apr 2021.

Hansson, G. K. and A. Hermansson (2011). "The immune system in atherosclerosis." *Nat Immunol.* 12(3): 204-212.

Haque, S., C. Gordon, et al. (2010). "Risk factors for clinical coronary heart disease in systemic lupus erythematosus: the lupus and atherosclerosis evaluation of risk (LASER) study." *J Rheumatol.* 37(2): 322-329. Epub 2009 Dec 2001.

Homer, D., T. J. Ingall, et al. (1991). "Serum lipids and lipoproteins are less powerful predictors of extracranial carotid artery atherosclerosis than are cigarette smoking and hypertension." *Mayo Clin Proc.* 66(3): 259-267.

Huang, Y. L., H. T. Chung, et al. (2009). "Lymphopenia is a risk factor in the progression of carotid intima-media thickness in juvenile-onset systemic lupus erythematosus." *Arthritis Rheum.* 60(12): 3766-3775.

Hulthe, J., O. Wiklund, et al. (2001). "Antibodies to oxidized LDL in relation to carotid atherosclerosis, cell adhesion molecules, and phospholipase A(2)." *Arterioscler Thromb Vasc Biol.* 21(2): 269-274.

Karvonen, J., M. Paivansalo, et al. (2003). "Immunoglobulin M type of autoantibodies to oxidized low-density lipoprotein has an inverse relation to carotid artery atherosclerosis." *Circulation.* 108(17): 2107-2112. Epub 2003 Oct 2106.

Katz, P., S. Gregorich, et al. (2011). "Obesity and its measurement in a community-based sample of women with systemic lupus erythematosus." *Arthritis Care Res (Hoboken).* 63(2): 261-268. doi: 210.1002/acr.20343.

Kiani, A. N., J. Vogel-Claussen, et al. (2010). "Noncalcified coronary plaque in systemic lupus erythematosus." *J Rheumatol.* 37(3): 579-584. Epub 2010 Jan 2028.

Kitas, G. D. and S. E. Gabriel (2011). "Cardiovascular disease in rheumatoid arthritis: state of the art and future perspectives." *Ann Rheum Dis.* 70(1): 8-14. Epub 2010 Nov 2024.

Komai, N., Y. Morita, et al. (2007). "Anti-tumor necrosis factor therapy increases serum adiponectin levels with the improvement of endothelial dysfunction in patients with rheumatoid arthritis." *Mod Rheumatol.* 17(5): 385-390. Epub 2007 Oct 2019.

Ku, I. A., J. B. Imboden, et al. (2009). "Rheumatoid arthritis: model of systemic inflammation driving atherosclerosis." *Circ J* 73(6): 977-985.

Lee, P. Y., Y. Li, et al. (2007). "Type I interferon as a novel risk factor for endothelial progenitor cell depletion and endothelial dysfunction in systemic lupus erythematosus." *Arthritis Rheum.* 56(11): 3759-3769.

Li, J., Q. Fu, et al. (2011). "Interferon-alpha priming promotes lipid uptake and macrophage-derived foam cell formation: a novel link between interferon-alpha and atherosclerosis in lupus." *Arthritis Rheum.* 63(2): 492-502. doi: 410.1002/art.30165.

Lodde, B. M., V. Sankar, et al. (2006). "Serum lipid levels in Sjogren's syndrome." *Rheumatology (Oxford).* 45(4): 481-484. Epub 2005 Nov 2022.

Lood, C., S. Amisten, et al. (2010). "Platelet transcriptional profile and protein expression in patients with systemic lupus erythematosus: up-regulation of the type I interferon system is strongly associated with vascular disease." *Blood.* 116(11): 1951-1957. Epub 2010 Jun 1910.

Lopes-Virella, M. F., G. Virella, et al. (1999). "Antibodies to oxidized LDL and LDL-containing immune complexes as risk factors for coronary artery disease in diabetes mellitus." *Clin Immunol.* 90(2): 165-172.

Lourida, E. S., A. N. Georgiadis, et al. (2007). "Patients with early rheumatoid arthritis exhibit elevated autoantibody titers against mildly oxidized low-density lipoprotein and exhibit decreased activity of the lipoprotein-associated phospholipase A2." *Arthritis Res Ther.* 9(1): R19.

Maksimowicz-McKinnon, K., L. S. Magder, et al. (2006). "Predictors of carotid atherosclerosis in systemic lupus erythematosus." *J Rheumatol.* 33(12): 2458-2463. Epub 2006 Oct 2451.

Mandal, K., G. Foteinos, et al. (2005). "Role of antiheat shock protein 60 autoantibodies in atherosclerosis." *Lupus.* 14(9): 742-746.

Manger, K., M. Kusus, et al. (2003). "Factors associated with coronary artery calcification in young female patients with SLE." *Ann Rheum Dis.* 62(9): 846-850.

Manzi, S. (2000). "Systemic lupus erythematosus: a model for atherogenesis?" *Rheumatology (Oxford).* 39(4): 353-359.

Manzi, S., E. N. Meilahn, et al. (1997). "Age-specific incidence rates of myocardial infarction and angina in women with systemic lupus erythematosus: comparison with the Framingham Study." *Am J Epidemiol.* 145(5): 408-415.

Manzi, S., F. Selzer, et al. (1999). "Prevalence and risk factors of carotid plaque in women with systemic lupus erythematosus." *Arthritis Rheum.* 42(1): 51-60.

Margutti, P., P. Matarrese, et al. (2008). "Autoantibodies to the C-terminal subunit of RLIP76 induce oxidative stress and endothelial cell apoptosis in immune-mediated vascular diseases and atherosclerosis." *Blood.* 111(9): 4559-4570. Epub 2007 Nov 4559.

Mattila, K. J., M. S. Nieminen, et al. (1989). "Association between dental health and acute myocardial infarction." *Bmj.* 298(6676): 779-781.

Mavragani, C. P. and H. M. Moutsopoulos (2010). "The geoepidemiology of Sjogren's syndrome." *Autoimmun Rev.* 9(5): A305-310. Epub 2009 Nov 2010.

Mavragani, C. P., Papadaki I, et al(2011). "Association of subclinical atherosclerosis with disease activity and MTHFR polymorphisms in Greek patients with rheumatoid arthritis, EULAR meeting, London, 2011.

McMahon, M., J. Grossman, et al. (2006). "Proinflammatory high-density lipoprotein as a biomarker for atherosclerosis in patients with systemic lupus erythematosus and rheumatoid arthritis." *Arthritis Rheum.* 54(8): 2541-2549.

McMahon, M., J. Grossman, et al. (2009). "Dysfunctional proinflammatory high-density lipoproteins confer increased risk of atherosclerosis in women with systemic lupus erythematosus." *Arthritis Rheum.* 60(8): 2428-2437.

Meune, C., E. Touze, et al. (2009). "Trends in cardiovascular mortality in patients with rheumatoid arthritis over 50 years: a systematic review and meta-analysis of cohort studies." *Rheumatology (Oxford)* 48(10): 1309-1313.

Mok, C. C., W. L. Poon, et al. (2010). "Metabolic syndrome, endothelial injury, and subclinical atherosclerosis in patients with systemic lupus erythematosus." *Scand J Rheumatol.* 39(1): 42-49.

Moonen, J. R., K. de Leeuw, et al. (2007). "Reduced number and impaired function of circulating progenitor cells in patients with systemic lupus erythematosus." *Arthritis Res Ther.* 9(4): R84.

Myasoedova, E., C. S. Crowson, et al. (2010). "Total cholesterol and LDL levels decrease before rheumatoid arthritis." *Ann Rheum Dis.* 69(7): 1310-1314. Epub 2009 Oct 1323.

Myasoedova, E. and S. E. Gabriel (2010). "Cardiovascular disease in rheumatoid arthritis: a step forward." *Curr Opin Rheumatol* 22(3): 342-347.

Nishida, K., Y. Okada, et al. (2008). "Induction of hyperadiponectinemia following long-term treatment of patients with rheumatoid arthritis with infliximab (IFX), an anti-TNF-alpha antibody." *Endocr J.* 55(1): 213-216. Epub 2008 Feb 2013.

Nurmohamed, M. T. (2009). "Cardiovascular risk in rheumatoid arthritis." *Autoimmun Rev.* 8(8): 663-667. Epub 2009 Feb 2012.

O'Neill, S. G., I. Giles, et al. (2010). "Antibodies to apolipoprotein A-I, high-density lipoprotein, and C-reactive protein are associated with disease activity in patients with systemic lupus erythematosus." *Arthritis Rheum.* 62(3): 845-854.

Ozbalkan, Z., C. Efe, et al. (2010). "An update on the relationships between rheumatoid arthritis and atherosclerosis." *Atherosclerosis* 212(2): 377-382.

Ozgen, M., S. S. Koca, et al. (2010). "Serum adiponectin and vaspin levels in rheumatoid arthritis." *Arch Med Res.* 41(6): 457-463.

Pakozdi, A., T. Besenyei, et al. (2009). "Endothelial progenitor cells in arthritis-associated vasculogenesis and atherosclerosis." *Joint Bone Spine.* 76(6): 581-583. Epub .

Palomino-Morales, R., C. Gonzalez-Juanatey, et al. (2010). "A1298C polymorphism in the MTHFR gene predisposes to cardiovascular risk in rheumatoid arthritis." *Arthritis Res Ther.* 12(2): R71. Epub 2010 Apr 2026.

Panoulas, V. F., K. M. Douglas, et al. (2007). "Prevalence and associations of hypertension and its control in patients with rheumatoid arthritis." *Rheumatology (Oxford).* 46(9): 1477-1482. Epub 2007 Aug 1417.

Panoulas, V. F., K. M. Douglas, et al. (2009). "Transforming growth factor-beta1 869T/C, but not interleukin-6 -174G/C, polymorphism associates with hypertension in rheumatoid arthritis." *Rheumatology (Oxford).* 48(2): 113-118. Epub 2008 Dec 2023.

Panoulas, V. F., G. S. Metsios, et al. (2008). "Hypertension in rheumatoid arthritis." *Rheumatology (Oxford).* 47(9): 1286-1298. Epub 2008 May 1288.

Pereira, R. M., J. F. de Carvalho, et al. (2009). "Metabolic syndrome in rheumatological diseases." *Autoimmun Rev.* 8(5): 415-419. Epub 2009 Jan 2023.

Perna, M., M. J. Roman, et al. (2010). "Relationship of asymmetric dimethylarginine and homocysteine to vascular aging in systemic lupus erythematosus patients." *Arthritis Rheum.* 62(6): 1718-1722.

Petri, M. (2000). "Detection of coronary artery disease and the role of traditional risk factors in the Hopkins Lupus Cohort." *Lupus.* 9(3): 170-175.

Petri, M. (2004). "The lupus anticoagulant is a risk factor for myocardial infarction (but not atherosclerosis): Hopkins Lupus Cohort." *Thromb Res.* 114(5-6): 593-595.

Petri, M., S. Perez-Gutthann, et al. (1992). "Risk factors for coronary artery disease in patients with systemic lupus erythematosus." *Am J Med.* 93(5): 513-519.

Popa, C., M. G. Netea, et al. (2009). "Circulating leptin and adiponectin concentrations during tumor necrosis factor blockade in patients with active rheumatoid arthritis." *J Rheumatol.* 36(4): 724-730. Epub 2009 Feb 2027.

Rachapalli, S. M., P. D. Kiely, et al. (2009). "Prevalence of abnormal ankle brachial index in patients with primary Sjogren's syndrome." *Clin Rheumatol.* 28(5): 587-590. Epub 2009 Feb 2010.

Rajagopalan, S., E. C. Somers, et al. (2004). "Endothelial cell apoptosis in systemic lupus erythematosus: a common pathway for abnormal vascular function and thrombosis propensity." *Blood.* 103(10): 3677-3683. Epub 2004 Jan 3615.

Ramos-Casals, M., P. Brito-Zeron, et al. (2007). "High prevalence of serum metabolic alterations in primary Sjogren's syndrome: influence on clinical and immunological expression." *J Rheumatol.* 34(4): 754-761. Epub 2007 Feb 2015.

Refai, T. M., I. H. Al-Salem, et al. (2002). "Hyperhomocysteinaemia and risk of thrombosis in systemic lupus erythematosus patients." *Clin Rheumatol.* 21(6): 457-461.

Reynolds, H. R., J. Buyon, et al. (2010). "Association of plasma soluble E-selectin and adiponectin with carotid plaque in patients with systemic lupus erythematosus." *Atherosclerosis*. 210(2): 569-574. Epub 2009 Dec 2016.

Rho, Y. H., C. P. Chung, et al. (2010). "Adipocytokines, insulin resistance, and coronary atherosclerosis in rheumatoid arthritis." *Arthritis Rheum*. 62(5): 1259-1264.

Rho, Y. H., J. Solus, et al. (2011). "Macrophage activation and coronary atherosclerosis in systemic lupus erythematosus and rheumatoid arthritis." *Arthritis Care Res (Hoboken)*. 63(4): 535-541. doi: 510.1002/acr.20365.

Roman, M. J., M. K. Crow, et al. (2007). "Rate and determinants of progression of atherosclerosis in systemic lupus erythematosus." *Arthritis Rheum*. 56(10): 3412-3419.

Roman, M. J., B. A. Shanker, et al. (2003). "Prevalence and correlates of accelerated atherosclerosis in systemic lupus erythematosus." *N Engl J Med*. 349(25): 2399-2406.

Rua-Figueroa, I., O. Arencibia-Mireles, et al. (2010). "Factors involved in the progress of preclinical atherosclerosis associated with systemic lupus erythematosus: a 2-year longitudinal study." *Ann Rheum Dis*. 69(6): 1136-1139. Epub 2009 Aug 1116.

Sabio, J. M., J. Vargas-Hitos, et al. (2009). "Metabolic syndrome is associated with increased arterial stiffness and biomarkers of subclinical atherosclerosis in patients with systemic lupus erythematosus." *J Rheumatol*. 36(10): 2204-2211. Epub 2009 Sep 2201.

Sabio, J. M., J. A. Vargas-Hitos, et al. (2011). "Prevalence of and Factors Associated with Hypertension in Young and Old Women with Systemic Lupus Erythematosus." *J Rheumatol* 16: 16.

Sabio, J. M., M. Zamora-Pasadas, et al. (2008). "Metabolic syndrome in patients with systemic lupus erythematosus from Southern Spain." *Lupus*. 17(9): 849-859.

Sada, K. E., Y. Yamasaki, et al. (2006). "Altered levels of adipocytokines in association with insulin resistance in patients with systemic lupus erythematosus." *J Rheumatol*. 33(8): 1545-1552.

Santos, M. J. and J. E. Fonseca (2009). "Metabolic syndrome, inflammation and atherosclerosis - the role of adipokines in health and in systemic inflammatory rheumatic diseases." *Acta Reumatol Port*. 34(4): 590-598.

Scalzi, L. V., S. Bhatt, et al. (2009). "The relationship between race, cigarette smoking and carotid intimal medial thickness in systemic lupus erythematosus." *Lupus*. 18(14): 1289-1297. Epub 2009 Oct 1227.

Sella, E. M., E. I. Sato, et al. (2003). "Coronary artery angiography in systemic lupus erythematosus patients with abnormal myocardial perfusion scintigraphy." *Arthritis Rheum*. 48(11): 3168-3175.

Selzer, F., K. Sutton-Tyrrell, et al. (2004). "Comparison of risk factors for vascular disease in the carotid artery and aorta in women with systemic lupus erythematosus." *Arthritis Rheum*. 50(1): 151-159.

Serelis, J., M. D. Kontogianni, et al. (2008). "Effect of anti-TNF treatment on body composition and serum adiponectin levels of women with rheumatoid arthritis." *Clin Rheumatol*. 27(6): 795-797. Epub 2008 Feb 2028.

Serelis, J., D. B. Panagiotakos, et al. (2011). "Cardiovascular disease is related to hypertension in patients with rheumatoid arthritis: a greek cohort study." *J Rheumatol*. 38(2): 236-241. Epub 2010 Nov 2015.

Sodergren, A., K. Karp, et al. (2010). "Atherosclerosis in early rheumatoid arthritis: very early endothelial activation and rapid progression of intima media thickness." *Arthritis Res Ther.* 12(4): R158. Epub 2010 Aug 2016.

Stavropoulos-Kalinoglou, A., G. S. Metsios, et al. (2008). "Cigarette smoking associates with body weight and muscle mass of patients with rheumatoid arthritis: a cross-sectional, observational study." *Arthritis Res Ther.* 10(3): R59. Epub 2008 May 2020.

Stavropoulos-Kalinoglou, A., G. S. Metsios, et al. (2009). "Underweight and obese states both associate with worse disease activity and physical function in patients with established rheumatoid arthritis." *Clin Rheumatol.* 28(4): 439-444. Epub 2008 Dec 2019.

Summers, G. D., G. S. Metsios, et al. (2010). "Rheumatoid cachexia and cardiovascular disease." *Nat Rev Rheumatol.* 6(8): 445-451. Epub 2010 Jul 2020.

Svenungsson, E., K. Jensen-Urstad, et al. (2001). "Risk factors for cardiovascular disease in systemic lupus erythematosus." *Circulation.* 104(16): 1887-1893.

Szekanecz, Z. and A. E. Koch (2010). "Vasculogenesis in rheumatoid arthritis." *Arthritis Res Ther.* 12(2): 110. Epub 2010 Mar 2018.

Tabas, I., K. J. Williams, et al. (2007). "Subendothelial lipoprotein retention as the initiating process in atherosclerosis: update and therapeutic implications." *Circulation.* 116(16): 1832-1844.

Thacker, S. G., C. C. Berthier, et al. (2010). "The detrimental effects of IFN-alpha on vasculogenesis in lupus are mediated by repression of IL-1 pathways: potential role in atherogenesis and renal vascular rarefaction." *J Immunol.* 185(7): 4457-4469. Epub 2010 Aug 4430.

Toloza, S. M., A. G. Uribe, et al. (2004). "Systemic lupus erythematosus in a multiethnic US cohort (LUMINA). XXIII. Baseline predictors of vascular events." *Arthritis Rheum.* 50(12): 3947-3957.

Toms, T. E., V. F. Panoulas, et al. (2008). "Lack of association between glucocorticoid use and presence of the metabolic syndrome in patients with rheumatoid arthritis: a cross-sectional study." *Arthritis Res Ther.* 10(6): R145. Epub 2008 Dec 2017.

Toms, T. E., V. F. Panoulas, et al. (2011). "Rheumatoid arthritis susceptibility genes associate with lipid levels in patients with rheumatoid arthritis." *Ann Rheum Dis* 11: 11.

Toms, T. E., D. P. Symmons, et al. (2010). "Dyslipidaemia in rheumatoid arthritis: the role of inflammation, drugs, lifestyle and genetic factors." *Curr Vasc Pharmacol.* 8(3): 301-326.

Urowitz, M. B., A. A. Bookman, et al. (1976). "The bimodal mortality pattern of systemic lupus erythematosus." *Am J Med.* 60(2): 221-225.

Vaarala, O., G. Alfthan, et al. (1993). "Crossreaction between antibodies to oxidised low-density lipoprotein and to cardiolipin in systemic lupus erythematosus." *Lancet.* 341(8850): 923-925.

Vadacca, M., D. Margiotta, et al. (2009). "Adipokines and systemic lupus erythematosus: relationship with metabolic syndrome and cardiovascular disease risk factors." *J Rheumatol.* 36(2): 295-297.

Van Doornum, S., G. McColl, et al. (2002). "Accelerated atherosclerosis: an extraarticular feature of rheumatoid arthritis?" *Arthritis Rheum.* 46(4): 862-873.

Vaudo, G., E. B. Bocci, et al. (2005). "Precocious intima-media thickening in patients with primary Sjogren's syndrome." *Arthritis Rheum.* 52(12): 3890-3897.

Vlachoyiannopoulos, P. G., P. G. Kanellopoulos, et al. (2003). "Atherosclerosis in premenopausal women with antiphospholipid syndrome and systemic lupus erythematosus: a controlled study." *Rheumatology (Oxford)*. 42(5): 645-651.

Volkmann, E. R., J. M. Grossman, et al. (2010). "Low physical activity is associated with proinflammatory high-density lipoprotein and increased subclinical atherosclerosis in women with systemic lupus erythematosus." *Arthritis Care Res (Hoboken)*. 62(2): 258-265.

Von Feldt, J. M. (2008). "Premature atherosclerotic cardiovascular disease and systemic lupus erythematosus from bedside to bench." *Bull NYU Hosp Jt Dis*. 66(3): 184-187.

Von Feldt, J. M., L. V. Scalzi, et al. (2006). "Homocysteine levels and disease duration independently correlate with coronary artery calcification in patients with systemic lupus erythematosus." *Arthritis Rheum*. 54(7): 2220-2227.

Wang, J., B. Hu, et al. (2008). "Native, oxidized lipoprotein(a) and lipoprotein(a) immune complex in patients with active and inactive rheumatoid arthritis: plasma concentrations and relationship to inflammation." *Clin Chim Acta*. 390(1-2): 67-71. Epub 2008 Jan 2011.

Westerweel, P. E., R. K. Luijten, et al. (2007). "Haematopoietic and endothelial progenitor cells are deficient in quiescent systemic lupus erythematosus." *Ann Rheum Dis*. 66(7): 865-870. Epub 2007 Feb 2028.

Woo, J. M., Z. Lin, et al. (2010). "Treatment with apolipoprotein A-1 mimetic peptide reduces lupus-like manifestations in a murine lupus model of accelerated atherosclerosis." *Arthritis Res Ther*. 12(3): R93. Epub 2010 May 2018.

Wu, R., U. de Faire, et al. (1999). "Autoantibodies to OxLDL are decreased in individuals with borderline hypertension." *Hypertension*. 33(1): 53-59.

Yoshino, T., N. Kusunoki, et al. (2011). "Elevated serum levels of resistin, leptin, and adiponectin are associated with C-reactive protein and also other clinical conditions in rheumatoid arthritis." *Intern Med*. 50(4): 269-275. Epub 2011 Feb 2015.

Yu, B. L., S. H. Wang, et al. (2010). "HDL and immunomodulation: an emerging role of HDL against atherosclerosis." *Immunol Cell Biol*. 88(3): 285-290. Epub 2010 Jan 2012.

Zhang, C., X. Li, et al. (2011). "Increased serum levels of beta(2)-GPI-Lp(a) complexes and their association with premature atherosclerosis in patients with rheumatoid arthritis." *Clin Chim Acta* 4: 4.

Zhao, Q. (2009). "Inflammation, autoimmunity, and atherosclerosis." *Discov Med*. 8(40): 7-12.

3

Endothelial Progenitor Cells: New Targets to Control Autoimmune Disorders

Sarah L. Brice, Andrew J. Sakko, Pravin Hissaria and Claudine S. Bonder
Human Immunology, Centre for Cancer Biology, SA Pathology,
Co-operative Research Centre for Biomarker Translation, LaTrobe University,
Australia

1. Introduction

The formation of blood vessels is essential for preparing a closed circulatory system in the body, and for supply of oxygen and nutrients to all tissues and organs. One of the key mechanisms behind many autoimmune diseases is abnormal blood vessel structure and function. This dysfunction is reflected in some of the serious manifestations of rheumatoid arthritis (RA), type 1 diabetes mellitus (T1DM) and systemic sclerosis (SSc) that are currently difficult to treat, such as loss of fingers due to reduced blood flow, kidney failure due to renal hypertensive crisis and heart failure due to pulmonary arterial hypertension. The cells that line blood vessels (endothelial cells) not only confine blood to the vessels but actively participate in the recruitment of circulating cell subsets to sites of inflammation and vascular permeability for the exchange of solutes and gases. Collectively, endothelial cells play many roles in the development and maintenance of blood vessels. Blood vessel development occurs primarily via one of two mechanisms, angiogenesis (the generation of blood vessels from pre-existing vasculature) and vasculogenesis (the recruitment of endothelial progenitor cells from the bone marrow to sites of vascularisation). In recent decades, extensive studies have revealed that a variety of factors and their receptors regulate angiogenesis in vertebrates, including vascular endothelial growth factor (VEGF)-VEGFRs, angiopoietin-Tie, Ephrins-EphRs and Delta-Notch (reviewed by Karamysheva (Karamysheva, 2008)). Indeed, targeting these molecules has resulted in significant advances in the treatment of cancer and cardiovascular disease. However, the burden of diseases that involve vascular dysfunction is immense and continues to rise with drug resistance, intolerance and ineffectiveness being significant contributors. Less is known about the mechanisms underpinning vasculogenesis and despite an explosion of research in this area over the past decade we are yet to fully exploit these cells for therapeutic benefit (Sen et al., 2011, Sieveking and Ng, 2009). This chapter discusses whether the endothelial progenitor cells (EPCs) from patients with autoimmune diseases, such as RA, T1DM and SSc, behave differently from normal EPCs and whether there are factors in the serum of these patients that may be responsible for this abnormal behaviour. The altered behaviour of EPCs in patients with autoimmune disease is poorly understood, based on limited studies to date. This chapter addresses whether EPCs would be a prime target for therapeutic intervention in the serious complications of autoimmune disease.

2. Vascular dysfunction in autoimmune disease

2.1 Rheumatoid arthritis

RA is a chronic and debilitating autoimmune disease that affects the joints. The disease is characterised by inflammation of the synovial tissue, which lines the joints and tendons. In healthy tissue, the synovium is made up of synovial cells, a network of capillaries and lymphatic vessels, and a well-organized matrix containing proteoglycan aggregates. Between the cartilage and synovium is the synovial fluid, which nourishes and lubricates the joint. In RA, cells of lympho-haematopoietic origin, e.g. T-helper cells, B cells and macrophages, infiltrate the synovium. The synovium also becomes thickened, from a layer of 1–2 cells to approximately 6–8 cells, and becomes locally invasive at the interface with the cartilage and the bone or tendon. The volume of the synovial fluid eventually increases in volume as a result of oedema, which causes swelling of the joints and pain.

Several lines of evidence indicate that RA is associated with aberrant and severe vasculogenesis (i.e. the de novo formation of blood vessels) within the inflamed joints (Paleolog, 2009, Grisar et al., 2007, Grisar et al., 2005, Herbrig et al., 2006, Hirohata et al., 2004, Jodon de Villeroche et al., 2010, Ruger et al., 2004, Silverman et al., 2007). One of the first observations of vasculogenesis in RA was the discovery that the synovial fluids from patients with RA contained a low molecular weight vasculogenesis factor apparently identical to that derived from tumours (Brown et al., 1980). Subsequent studies revealed that synovial fluid from patients with RA stimulated proliferation of human endothelial cells (Kumar et al., 1985) and the formation of tubular networks (Semble et al., 1985). A study of synovial tissue histology from patients with RA revealed that there is a significant correlation between the number of synovial blood vessels and vessel proliferation, mononuclear cell infiltration, fibrosis and clinical measurements of joint tenderness (Rooney et al., 1988). Capillaries are distributed more deeply in the synovium from patients with RA (Stevens et al., 1991). The different stages of rheumatoid arthritis are shown in Figure 1 (upper panel). Although perivascular mononuclear cell infiltration and increased thickness of the synovial lining layer are observed in tissue from both inflamed and non-inflamed joints of RA patients, vascular proliferation is seen only in tissues from inflamed joints (FitzGerald et al., 1991). In addition, endothelial cells lining blood vessels within RA synovium have been shown to express cell cycle-associated antigens such as proliferating cell nuclear antigen and Ki67, and integrin alpha 5 beta 3, which is associated with vascular proliferation (Ceponis et al., 1998). Hypoxia, which can activate vasculogenesis factors and cause further invasion of the synovium, is another common event that occurs within the synovial joints in RA (FitzGerald et al., 1991, Muz et al., 2009). Taken together, these studies indicate that vascular dysfunction in synovial tissue is a likely therapeutic target in RA.

2.2 Type 1 diabetes mellitus

T1DM is a life-long autoimmune disease characterised by hyperglycaemia. Hyperglycaemia in T1DM occurs when the number of insulin-producing ß-cells in the pancreatic Islets of Langerhans drops below the number required to control glycaemia. Hyperglycaemia leads to macrovascular complications, such as coronary artery disease, peripheral arterial disease, and stroke, and microvascular complications, such as diabetic nephropathy, neuropathy, and retinopathy. Onset is early in life and patients exhibit increased risks of renal failure, blindness, amputation, stroke and heart attack (Shapiro et al., 2006). Best available practice with insulin therapy is not a cure as it does not protect the remaining islets from inflammatory attack or the patient from long-term complications.

Insulin-producing ß-cells, which comprise 60-80% of islet mass, are crucial for the maintenance of normal blood sugar. Pancreatic islets are highly metabolically active and densely vascularised with specialized endothelium – they receive 10% of pancreatic blood flow despite comprising only 1% of tissue mass. Pancreatic islets come under a myriad of cellular assaults during isolation including ischemia, enzymatic damage and physical stress. Dysfunction of the endothelium plays a critical role in the development of vascular complications in T1DM (Stehouwer et al., 1997, Flyvbjerg, 2000). Clinical trials have shown that hyperglycaemia leads to changes in the proliferation of endothelial cells, barrier function and the adhesion of other circulating cells to endothelial cells (Schalkwijk and Stehouwer, 2005). This vascular dysfunction may be mediated by several distinct mechanisms and different stages of diabetic retinopathy are shown in Figure 1 (middle panel). Hyperglycaemia results in an increase in intracellular glucose, which leads to an increase in the conversion of glucose to sorbitol via the polyol pathway. This increase in sorbitol can cause osmotic stress, tissue hypoxia and oxidative stress (Williamson et al., 1993, Schalkwijk and Stehouwer, 2005). Hyperglycaemia also results in activation of protein kinase C, which can cause dysregulation of vascular permeability and blood flow, basement membrane thickening and impaired fibrinolysis (Williamson et al., 1993, Chen et al., 2000). In addition, hyperglycaemia causes increased glucosamine-6-phosphate and consequently increased transcription of cytokines such as transforming growth factor beta, which can regulate the proliferation and apoptosis of endothelial cells (Nerlich et al., 1998, Ziyadeh, 2004). Greater insight into the mechanisms underlying endothelial dysfunction may lead to important treatment strategies which can reduce the morbidity and mortality rate caused by endothelial dysfunction in patients with T1DM.

2.3 Systemic sclerosis

SSc is a heterogeneous disease in which vascular dysfunction, extensive fibrosis and autoimmunity are the hallmark characteristics. The aetiology of SSc is unknown as there are many unresolved questions as to both cause and initiating factors (Geyer and Muller-Ladner, 2011). Multiple genetic and environmental factors, combined with other specific factors (e.g. alterations to the immune system, vasculature and extracellular matrix) are the most likely causes of this insidious disorder. The pathophysiology of SSc is diverse and includes abnormal immunologic processes such as cytokine and chemokine dysregulation, abnormal T cell signalling, B cell dysfunction, endothelial injury, aberrant wound healing due to dysregulation of matrix homeostasis, abnormalities in the fibrinolytic system, polymorphisms in critical molecules of the immune system and matrix homeostasis, and microchimerism due to foetal/maternal placental exchange of HLA compatible cells (Gabrielli et al., 2009).

Vascular dysfunction is an early event in SSc (Kahaleh, 2008) and the different stages of SSc are shown in Figure 1 (lower panel). The preferred site of early lesions in SSc is the perivascular space. Progressive wall thickening and perivascular infiltrates are features of the vascular lesions in this compartment, indicating the involvement of vascular smooth-muscle cells and pericytes. Endothelial cells are the only type of mesodermal cell that

Rheumatoid arthritis

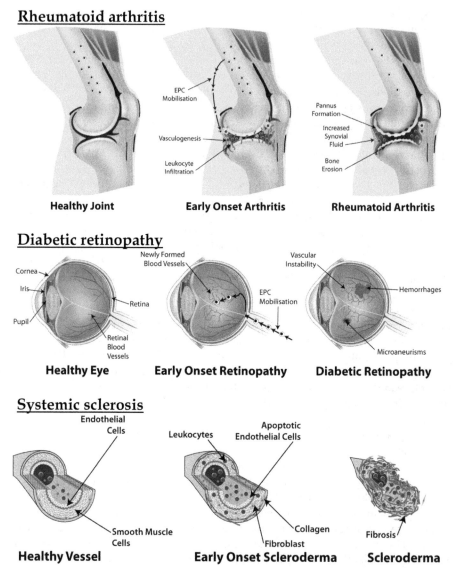

In rheumatoid arthritis (upper panel), circulating endothelial progenitor cells (EPCs) and vasculogenesis are causally linked to the influx of pro-inflammatory **leukocytes** and increased capillary beds contribute to thickening of the synovial lining and joint pain. In diabetic patients with proliferative retinopathy (middle panel), infiltrating EPCs contribute to the dense vascularisation in the eye and reduced vascular stability associated with blindness. Vascular injury is one of the early events in the pathogenesis of systemic sclerosis (lower panel) and is characterized by endothelial-cell damage and apoptosis, the proliferation of fibroblasts, production of collagen and **infiltration** of circulating leukocytes. Despite the increased number of circulating EPCs in these patients, the endothelial layer of the vasculature remains denuded and is ultimately obliterated.

Fig. 1. Vascular dysfunction in autoimmune disease.

undergo apoptosis in early SSc, whereas vascular smooth-muscle cells and pericytes proliferate vigorously. This vascular damage, which eventually occurs in almost all organs (Harrison et al., 1993), presents as large gaps between endothelial cells, loss of integrity of the endothelial lining, and the formation of vacuoles in the endothelial cell cytoplasm. In addition, several basal lamina-like layers build up, mononuclear immune cells infiltrate the vessel walls, obliterative microvascular lesions occur, and the capillaries rarefy (Prescott et al., 1992, Fleming et al., 2008). In the later stages of SSc, relatively few small blood vessels remain. Serum levels of VEGF are high in SSc despite the progressive loss of blood vessels (Distler et al., 2004, Davies et al., 2006), possibly as a result of an adaptive response to hypoxia (Fleming et al., 2008, Kuwana et al., 2004, Cipriani et al., 2007). The molecular mechanisms underlying this defect in vasculogenesis are unknown and both vasculogenic (Davies et al., 2006, Distler et al., 2004) and anti-vasculogenic (Fleming et al., 2008, Hebbar et al., 2000, Scheja et al., 2000) factors have been detected in early SSc. Inflammatory cytokines, such as tumour necrosis factor (TNF), can stimulate or inhibit angiogenesis depending on the duration of the stimulus (Sainson et al., 2008). Collectively, these data indicate that vascular dysfunction is a common event in SSc and an important therapeutic target.

3. Endothelial progenitor cells

EPCs were first discovered in peripheral blood by Asahara and colleagues in 1997 (Asahara et al., 1997). This discovery revealed that vasculogenesis occurs after post-natal development. Vascular insult or disease causes the upregulation of cytokines such as VEGF, stromal cell-derived factor-1 (SDF-1) matrix metalloproteinase 9 (MMP9), hypoxia inducible factor 1α (HIF-1α) and erythropoietin (EPO) at the site of injury and this stimulates the release of EPCs from the stem cell niche in the bone marrow into the circulation (Aicher et al., 2005). EPCs then follow the cytokine gradient to the site of vascular trauma where they contribute to vasculogenesis either by (1) paracrine assistance (via production of VEGF and endothelial nitric oxide synthase (eNOS)) (2) integration or (3) new vessel formation (Figure 2).

There are currently two distinct ways in which EPCs are identified, i.e. (1) they are directly identified in the peripheral blood by the surface antigen expression of any combination of CD133, CD34 and VEGR2 or (2) they are isolated from either peripheral blood (Asahara et al., 1997), umbilical cord blood (Asahara et al., 1997, Shi et al., 1998) or bone marrow (Shi et al., 1998) and cultured ex vivo. The complication associated with using the cell surface markers CD133, CD34 and VEGFR2 to identify EPCs is that these markers are not exclusively expressed on EPCs and can be found on many other cell types including the closely related haematopoietic progenitors and mature endothelial cells as well as fibroblasts, epithelial cells and cancer stem cells (Hirschi et al., 2008, Kumar and Caplice, 2010). Further evidence of a need to standardise the isolation technique, culture conditions and phenotyping strategy is exemplified by Case et al., who suggest that it is not possible to culture EPCs from a CD133+ CD34+ VEGFR2+-sorted population (Case et al., 2007).

Currently, the term 'EPC' is used to describe two populations of cells cultured in vitro, both of which show vascular potential, but differ in both phenotype and function. The first EPC population to be characterised in vitro were the early-outgrowth EPCs, or colony forming unit-endothelial cells (CFU-ECs). Early-outgrowth EPCs form colonies after 3-5 days in culture on fibronectin-coated wells, consist of multiple thin, flat cells emanating from a

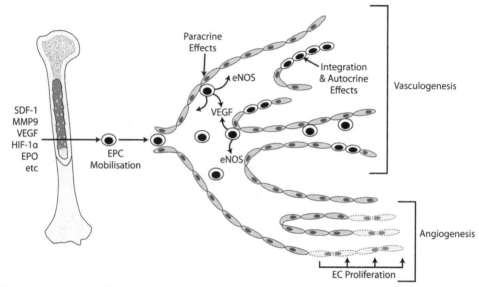

Recruitment of endothelial cells from pre-existing vessel walls or circulating endothelial progenitor cells (EPCs) play a critical role in blood vessel development and repair during disease states. Mobilised bone-marrow derived EPCs with high proliferative capacity may have the potential to home to a site for vascularisation and act in a paracrine or autocrine way to promote vessel wall development.
Abbreviations: SDF-1, stromal derived factor -1; MMP9, matrix metalloproteinase 9; VEGF, vascular endothelial growth factor; HIF-1α, hypoxia inducible factor 1α; EPO, erythropoietin; eNOS, endothelial nitric oxide.

Fig. 2. Model of postnatal angiogenesis and vasculogenesis.

central cluster of round cells and express CD133, VEGFR2 and CD34 (Hur et al., 2004). Early-outgrowth EPCs secrete pro-angiogenic factors (Hur et al., 2004, Rehman et al., 2003, Yoon et al., 2005), but are not able to form tubes when seeded alone in Matrigel (Rehman et al., 2003, Timmermans et al., 2007, Yoder et al., 2007, Yoon et al., 2005). When transplanted into mice, they are able to increase capillary density in a model of limb ischemia (Hur et al., 2004, Yoon et al., 2005), suggesting that they contribute to tube formation through paracrine mechanisms. Early-outgrowth EPCs express the pan-leukocyte marker CD45 and the myeloid marker CD14 and have been shown to be of monocyte origin (Medina et al., 2010) and are thus not considered true endothelial cell progeny.

The second EPC population to be characterised are the late-outgrowth EPCs, which as also referred to as outgrowth endothelial cells (OECs) and endothelial colony forming cells (ECFCs). Late-outgrowth EPCs can be isolated from bone marrow, cord blood and peripheral blood and form colonies with distinct cobblestone morphology, similar to that of endothelial cells within 2-4 weeks when cultured on either collagen or gelatin (Lin et al., 2000, Shi et al., 1998). Late-outgrowth EPCs have 10 times the proliferative capacity of mature ECs, they express mature endothelial cell markers including von Willebrand factor (vWF), CD31 and VEGFR2, but not the progenitor marker CD133 and they are able to form tubes in Matrigel (Bompais et al., 2004, Ingram et al., 2004, Lin et al., 2000, Rehman et al., 2003, Timmermans et al., 2007, Yoder et al., 2007, Yoon et al., 2005). Late-outgrowth EPCs have been shown to increase neovascularisation in a mouse limb ischemic model (Hur et al., 2004, Yoon et al., 2005) and are haemangioblastic in origin (Medina et al., 2010) and are thus considered to be true endothelial cell progeny.

Whilst the monocytic early-outgrowth EPCs and the haemangioblastic late-outgrowth EPCs are distinct EPC populations, the combined therapeutic potential of these two EPC populations is greater than either of the EPC populations when delivered individually in a mouse model of limb ischemia (Yoon et al., 2005), suggesting that these EPC populations may function synergistically during vasculogenesis.

4. Endothelial progenitor cells in autoimmune disease

4.1 Endothelial progenitor cells in rheumatoid arthritis

The association between EPC numbers and RA has brought about conflicting results (Table 1). Some studies have reported a lower circulating EPC number in RA patients compared with controls (Grisar et al., 2005, Herbrig et al., 2006), whilst others report higher numbers (Jodon de Villeroche et al., 2010) and a few report no differences (Egan et al., 2008, Kuwana et al., 2004). A schematic of a potential role for EPCs in RA is depicted in Figure 1 (upper panel).

In the studies that reported lower circulating EPC numbers in patients with active RA compared to healthy controls (Grisar et al., 2005, Herbrig et al., 2006), the circulating EPCs were identified through the expression of CD133, CD34 and VEGFR2 and the formation of early-outgrowth EPC colonies. It is highly likely that these studies were not specifically identifying a pure EPC population, but rather a mixed population consisting of both early-outgrowth EPCs, late-outgrowth EPCs and haematopoietic progenitors, as the biomarkers used to identify EPCs are not specific for any one cell type.

In contrast, Jodan de Villeroche et al used a method to exclusively identify haemangioblastic late-outgrowth EPCs distinct from monocytic early-outgrowth EPCs (Jodon de Villeroche et al., 2010). Jodan de Villeroche et al exclusively monitored the number of late-outgrowth EPCs by detecting Lin-/7-aminoactinomycin (7-AAD)-/CD34+/CD133+/VEGFR2+ cells from CD14 depleted peripheral blood. This detection panel eliminated apoptotic cells (using 7-AAD) and early-outgrowth EPCs (through CD14 depletion). Using these methods this study revealed that RA patients with active RA had significantly higher levels of circulating late-outgrowth EPCs compared with controls. To complement these findings, this study also investigated the formation of late-outgrowth EPC colonies and found that RA patients had a higher number of late-outgrowth colonies compared to controls. This study was the first to implement a method that made a distinction between the two EPC populations.

4.2 Endothelial progenitor cells in type 1 diabetes mellitus

A decrease in EPC number and function has been associated with T1DM and has been reported by several groups (Table 2). However before comparisons can be made between studies, it is important to consider the methods used to quantify EPC numbers in these studies. Circulating EPC numbers were quantified either by surface antigen expression on peripheral blood mononuclear cells (PBMNCs) (Brunner et al., 2009, Sibal et al., 2009), through the culture of early-outgrowth EPC colonies (Asnaghi et al., 2006) or through the uptake of acetylated LDL and binding of UEA-l to cultured PBMNCs (Loomans et al., 2004). To the best of our knowledge, there are currently no reports on the correlation between T1DM and the growth of late-outgrowth EPCs.

Reference	Method of EPC identification	Comments
Grisar et al., 2005	Expression of CD133/CD34/VEGFR2 from PBMNC using flow cytometry.	EPCs were lower in active RA patients compared to healthy controls when assessing surface antigen expression.
	In vitro culture of PBMNCs and detection of early-outgrowth EPCs colonies.	Reduced number of early-outgrowth EPC colonies in active RA patients compared to healthy controls.
Grisar et al., 2007	Expression of CD133/CD34/VEGFR2 from PBMNC using flow cytometry.	TNF may be partly responsible for the reduction of circulating EPCs seen in RA patients.
Egan et al., 2008	Expression of CD133/CD117/CD34/CD31 from PBMNCs using flow cytometry.	No difference in the number of EPCs in RA patients and healthy controls when assessing surface antigen expression.
	In vitro culture of PBMNCs and detection of early-outgrowth EPCs colonies.	Reduced number of early-outgrowth EPCs in active RA patients compared to healthy controls.
		Early-outgrowth EPC colony numbers were associated with cardiovascular risk.
Jodon de Villeroche et al., 2010	Surface antigen profile Lin-/7AAD-/CD34+/CD133+/VEGFR2+ from CD14-depleted PBMNCs using flow cytometry.	RA patients had higher numbers of circulating EPCs than healthy controls.
	In vitro culture PBMNCs and detection of late-outgrowth colonies.	Circulating EPCs correlated with disease activity.
Herbrig et al., 2006	In vitro culture of PMNCs and assessment of Ac-LDL uptake, UEA-1 lectin binding and the surface antigen profile VE-cadherin+/CD31+/VEGFR2+/CD146-.	EPCs from RA patients showed reduced migratory activity in response to VEGF.

Abbreviations: RA, rheumatoid arthritis; PBMNCs, peripheral blood mononuclear cells; EPCs, endothelial progenitor cells; Ac-LDL, acetylated-low density lipoprotein; UEA-1 lectin, *Ulex Europaeus* Lectin; TNF, tumour necrosis factor; VEGF, vascular endothelial growth factor.

Table 1. Studies that have reported aberrant EPC numbers in patients with RA.

EPC dysfunction has been seen in patients with T1DM, as shown by Loomans et al. when conditioned media from EPCs isolated from T1DM patients impaired in vitro tube formation of HUVEC (Loomans et al., 2004). An inverse relationship between the number of

EPCs and HbA1C in patients has also been identified (Loomans et al., 2004). Moreover, there appears to be an association between the progression of diabetic retinopathy and the level of circulating EPCs. In patients with T1DM and proliferative retinopathy a marked increase in circulating EPCs has been reported (Asnaghi et al., 2006, Brunner et al., 2009). Conversely, circulating EPC numbers have been identified as being lower in patients with T1DM and non-proliferative retinopathy (Brunner et al., 2009). These studies highlight how atypical EPC numbers and function are associated with T1DM pathology and a schematic of a potential role for EPCs in diabetic retinopathy is depicted in Figure 1 (middle panel).

Reference	Method of EPC identification	Comments
Loomans et al., 2004	In vitro culture of PMNCs and assessment of Ac-LDL uptake, UEA-1 lectin binding and CD31 expression.	T1DM patients had lower EPC levels compared to healthy controls.
Sibal et al., 2009	Expression of CD133/CD34/VEGFR2/VE-cadherin from PBMNC using flow cytometry.	EPC counts were lower in patients with T1DM compared to healthy controls.
Asnaghi et al., 2006	Immunostaining with CD133 and CD31	Patients with T1DM and retinopathy had higher EPC levels than healthy controls and patients with T1DM and no retinopathy.
	In vitro culture of PBMNCs and detection of early-outgrowth EPCs colonies.	Patients with T1DM and no retinopathy had lower EPC levels than healthy controls and patients with T1DM and retinopathy.
Brunner et al., 2008	CPC surface antigen profile CD133+/CD34+	Patients with T1DM and proliferative retinopathy had increased levels of mature EPCs.
	EPCs surface antigen profile CD133+/CD34+/VEGFR2+	Patients with T1DM and nonproliferative retinopathy had decreased levels of EPCs.
	Mature surface antigen profile CD133+/CD34+/VEGFR2+/CD31+	
	Nonmature surface antigen profile CD133+/CD34+/VEGFR2+/CD31-	

Abbreviations: T1DM, type 1 diabetes mellitus; PBMNCs, peripheral blood mononuclear cells; EPCs, endothelial progenitor cells; CPC, circulating progenitor cells; Ac-LDL, acetylated-low density lipoprotein; UEA-1 lectin, *Ulex Europaeus* Lectin

Table 2. Studies that have reported aberrant EPC numbers in patients with T1DM.

4.3 Endothelial progenitor cells in systemic sclerosis

Aberrant EPC numbers within the circulation of patients with SSc has been described extensively (Table 3). The majority of these studies used flow cytometry to assess EPC numbers using various combinations of the markers CD133, CD34 and VEGFR2. As mentioned previously, the use of these markers does not unambiguously identify circulating EPCs as they are expressed by other progenitor cells and mature endothelial cells. Avouac et al describe the most stringent method of EPC identification, which involved culturing the PBMNCs from both SSc patients and healthy controls and assessing late-outgrowth EPC colony formation. This study showed that the number of late-outgrowth EPC colonies correlated with the number of circulating EPCs detected using the surface antigen profile Lin-/7AAD-/CD34+/CD133+/VEGFR2+ (Avouac et al., 2008).

Reference	Method of EPC identification	Comments
Allanore et al., 2007	Expression of CD133/CD34 from PBMNC using flow cytometry.	SSc patients had higher numbers of EPCs than osteoarthritis patients, but lower than RA patients.
Yamaguchi et al., 2010	In vitro culture of PBMNCs depleted for platelets. Expression of CD34/VEGFR1/CD1a/CD83/CD80 using flow cytometry and CD31/CD144 by immunohistochemistry.	The number of early-outgrowth EPCs was higher in SSc patients compared to RA patients and healthy controls. Early-outgrowth EPCs derived from SSc patients showed greater vascular potential in vitro and in vivo than early-outgrowth EPCs derived from healthy controls.
Kuwana et al., 2004	Expression of CD133/CD34/VEGR2 from CD34-enriched PBMNC using flow cytometry.	EPCs were lower in SSc patients compared to RA patients and healthy controls. Levels of angiogenic factors within the circulation were higher in SSc patients than in health controls.
Kuwana et al., 2006	Expression of CD133/CD34/VEGR2 from CD34-enriched PBMNC using flow cytometry.	Atorvastatin treatment resulted in an increase in circulating EPCs from baseline, however levels did not reach those of healthy controls.
Del Papa et al., 2004	Surface antigen profile CD133+/CD34+ from PBMNC using flow cytometry.	High levels of EPCs in patients with SSc and counts were higher in early stages of disease.
Del Papa et al., 2006	Surface antigen profile CD133+/CD45- from PBMNC and BM using flow cytometry.	Circulating EPCs were higher in patients with early stage disease, but not in those with late stage disease. BM EPCs were reduced and functionally impaired.
Avouac et al., 2008	Surface antigen profile Lin-/7AAD-/CD34+/CD133+/VEGFR2+ from PBMNCs detected using flow cytometry. In vitro culture of PBMNCs and detection of late-outgrowth colonies.	Circulating EPC levels were higher in SSc patients than in healthy controls. Positive correlation between the number of late-outgrowth EPC colonies and the level of circulating EPCs detected by flow cytometry in patients with SSc.

Abbreviations: SSc, systemic sclerosis; PBMNCs, peripheral blood mononuclear cells; EPCs, endothelial progenitor cells; BM, bone marrow.

Table 3. Studies that have reported aberrant EPC numbers in patients with SSc.

It has been well documented that circulating EPC numbers are elevated in patients with SSc (Allanore et al., 2007, Avouac et al., 2008, Del Papa et al., 2004, Del Papa et al., 2006, Yamaguchi et al., 2010). However, two studies by Kuwana and colleagues have reported reduced EPC numbers in SSc patients (Kuwana et al., 2006, Kuwana et al., 2004). Del Papa et al showed that in early stage SSc (3-5 years) there appears to be an increase in circulating EPCs and post 5 years, there appears to be either a normal or decreased number of circulating EPCs (Del Papa et al., 2006). A schematic of a potential role for EPCs in SSc is depicted in Figure 1 (lower panel). There is also evidence to suggest that the vascular function of EPCs from SSc patients is actually higher than that of healthy controls as early-outgrowth EPCs from SSc patients are able to promote tube formation of HUVEC in vitro as well as enhance tumour growth and blood vessel formation in vivo (Yamaguchi et al., 2010).

5. Therapeutic intervention targeting EPCs in autoimmune diseases

There have been rapid advances in the field of therapeutic angiogenesis since the original description of bone marrow derived EPCs in 1997 (Asahara et al., 1997). Most of these bench-to-bed-side studies have been done in models of atherosclerosis and acute ischemic events such as myocardial infarction (MI) and critical limb ischemia. The first pre-clinical studies in these diseases were executed (within four years of their initial discovery) in a MI model in mice (Kocher et al., 2001) and demonstrated improvement in angiogenesis and cardiac function. This was followed by a series of publications showing the effectiveness of EPCs in preventing the extent of damage (Orlic et al., 2001) after MI as well as effectiveness in the large vessel occlusive damage (Griese et al., 2003) and prevention of atherosclerosis in a highly prone mouse model (Rausher et al, 2003). However, the exact mechanism of action of these interventions, in particular whether the benefit was due to neo-angiogenesis modulated by EPCs or due to paracrine mechanisms that improved the survival of resident endothelial cells, is not entirely clear.

There was a rapid transition of these studies to humans as autologous marrow transplantation became a relatively safe and well established procedure in haematological malignancies and non-invasive methods to mobilise bone marrow progenitors became well established. In 2002, there were two studies published reporting the benefit of locally injecting ex-vivo expanded autologous bone marrow derived mononuclear cells in MI critical lower limb ischemia (Strauer et al., 2002, Tateishi-Yuyama et al., 2002). Furthermore, there have been multiple randomised controlled trials looking at the effectiveness of bone marrow derived cell therapies, which have been reviewed in a recent meta-analysis (Martin-Rendon et al., 2008).

The therapeutic use of EPCs in inflammatory diseases is more complicated as they have been implicated in pathogenesis of the inflammatory process as well as being an important cause of long term morbidity. There have been no studies of direct intervention with EPCs in autoimmune diseases. This is mainly due to their differential effects on the immunopathogenesis of these diseases. Attempts to understand this field are further bedevilled by observations of patients with systemic lupus erythematosus (SLE) who exhibit a significant decrease in circulating EPCs as well as a striking increase in premature atherosclerosis of unclear aetiology (de Leeuw et al., 2005, Westerweel et al., 2007) demonstrating no significant difference in EPC number between SLE patients without and with advanced coronary artery calcification (Baker et al., 2011). As detailed above, the inflammatory milieu in autoimmune diseases is characterized by neo-angiogenesis and as such it would seem that increased EPCs might contribute to inflammation. On the other hand, the most common cause of long term morbidity and mortality in these diseases is attributed to atherosclerosis and its complications where EPCs might have beneficial effect. There have been numerous studies looking at the effect of various disease modifying therapies in patients with autoimmune diseases on the circulating EPCs (both monocytic and haemangioblastic) reviewed in a recent article (Westerweel and Verhaar, 2009). These studies show an increase in the levels of circulating haemangioblastic EPCs after various immunosuppressive therapies including anti-TNF drugs, corticosteroids and hydroxychloroquine in these patients. However, the association of these changes with long term clinically useful outcome, such as incidence of atherosclerosis and coronary artery disease, has not been demonstrated. This finding is intriguing as it is well known from long term clinical studies that corticosteroids are known to promote atherosclerosis and anti-TNF medications reduce long term morbidity and mortality due to this complication (Kaplan, 2010). Moreover, methotrexate, a commonly used disease modifying agent in various autoimmune diseases is known to induce EPC apoptosis in vitro (Herbrig et al., 2006) but has beneficial effects in patients.

There needs to be better understanding of the role of EPCs in the different stages of the disease, i.e. early active versus long standing, and its pathophysiological implications relating to long term outcome of patients to be able to design studies with intervention directed at EPCs. The knowledge of various paracrine mechanisms involved in the beneficial effects of EPCs in atherosclerosis models might help to dissect the pathways involved in neo-angiogenesis versus survival of resident endothelial cells. This knowledge can then be exploited to design intervention at various stages of autoimmune diseases.

6. Conclusions

Faced with an ever-increasing burden of autoimmune diseases such as RA, T1DM and SSc, modern medicine is confronted with the need to provide new therapies that not only mitigate the symptoms of these diseases but may also facilitate regeneration of organ function. Given their role in development and in maintaining and repairing injured vessels, stem and progenitor cells represent an exciting alternative for regenerative medicine. Since their first identification over a decade ago, the use of EPCs as a diagnostic tool or therapeutic was greeted with great enthusiasm. However, progress in their clinical application remains limited by identification and *ex vivo* expansion factors, and as a result, variable functional attributes. It can be seen from the aforementioned examples that the timing and methods used to detect EPCs can greatly affect the outcome of studies. The major issues associated with EPC identification within the circulation are (1) identifying the bone marrow progenitors from the circulating mature endothelial cells and (2) defining the distinction between haemangioblastic late-outgrowth EPCs and monocytic early-outgrowth EPCs. These matters are the focus of ongoing research, especially the search for a unique EPC marker. Nevertheless, EPCs are a robust biomarker of vascular dysfunction (based on their direct interaction and influence on endothelial function), and the unique ability to monitor their peripheral number or function as a marker of response to therapy. Notwithstanding the current knowledge regarding EPC cell signalling, activation and migration, the precise mechanisms of activation of these cells and their functional significance is not known. In the research setting, continued understanding of EPC function improves insight into vasculogenesis, and the pathology of vascular dysfunction in autoimmune disease.

7. Acknowledgements

This work was supported by the Co-operative Research Centre for Biomarker Translation (Transbio Ltd) and Arthritis Australia. CSB is a Heart Foundation Research Fellow and we thank P. Dunne for preparation of the figures.

8. References

Aicher, A., Zeiher, A. M. & Dimmeler, S. 2005. Mobilizing endothelial progenitor cells. *Hypertension*, 45, 321-5.

Allanore, Y., Batteux, F., Avouac, J., Assous, N., Weill, B. & Kahan, A. 2007. Levels of circulating endothelial progenitor cells in systemic sclerosis. *Clin Exp Rheumatol*, 25, 60-6.

Asahara, T., Murohara, T., Sullivan, A., Silver, M., Van Der Zee, R., Li, T., Witzenbichler, B., Schatteman, G. & Isner, J. M. 1997. Isolation of putative progenitor endothelial cells for angiogenesis. *Science*, 275, 964-7.

Asnaghi, V., Lattanzio, R., Mazzolari, G., Pastore, M. R., Ramoni, A., Maestroni, A., Ruggieri, D., Luzi, L., Brancato, R. & Zerbini, G. 2006. Increased clonogenic potential of circulating endothelial progenitor cells in patients with type 1 diabetes and proliferative retinopathy. *Diabetologia*, 49, 1109-11.

Avouac, J., Juin, F., Wipff, J., Couraud, P. O., Chiocchia, G., Kahan, A., Boileau, C., Uzan, G. & Allanore, Y. 2008. Circulating endothelial progenitor cells in systemic sclerosis: association with disease severity. *Ann Rheum Dis*, 67, 1455-60.

Baker, J. F., Zhang, L., Imadojemu, S., Sharpe, A., Patil, S., Moore, J. S., Mohler, E. R., 3rd & Von Feldt, J. 2011. Circulating endothelial progenitor cells are reduced in SLE in the absence of coronary artery calcification. *Rheumatol Int*.

Bompais, H., Chagraoui, J., Canron, X., Crisan, M., Liu, X. H., Anjo, A., Tolla-Le Port, C., Leboeuf, M., Charbord, P., Bikfalvi, A. & Uzan, G. 2004. Human endothelial cells derived from circulating progenitors display specific functional properties compared with mature vessel wall endothelial cells. *Blood*, 103, 2577-84.

Brown, R. A., Weiss, J. B., Tomlinson, I. W., Phillips, P. & Kumar, S. 1980. Angiogenic factor from synovial fluid resembling that from tumours. *Lancet*, 1, 682-5.

Brunner, S., Schernthaner, G. H., Satler, M., Elhenicky, M., Hoellerl, F., Schmid-Kubista, K. E., Zeiler, F., Binder, S. & Schernthaner, G. 2009. Correlation of different circulating endothelial progenitor cells to stages of diabetic retinopathy: first in vivo data. *Invest Ophthalmol Vis Sci*, 50, 392-8.

Case, J., Mead, L. E., Bessler, W. K., Prater, D., White, H. A., Saadatzadeh, M. R., Bhavsar, J. R., Yoder, M. C., Haneline, L. S. & Ingram, D. A. 2007. Human CD34+AC133+VEGFR-2+ cells are not endothelial progenitor cells but distinct, primitive hematopoietic progenitors. *Exp Hematol*, 35, 1109-18.

Ceponis, A., Konttinen, Y. T., Imai, S., Tamulaitiene, M., Li, T. F., Xu, J. W., Hietanen, J., Santavirta, S. & Fassbender, H. G. 1998. Synovial lining, endothelial and inflammatory mononuclear cell proliferation in synovial membranes in psoriatic and reactive arthritis: a comparative quantitative morphometric study. *Br J Rheumatol*, 37, 170-8.

Chen, S., Apostolova, M. D., Cherian, M. G. & Chakrabarti, S. 2000. Interaction of endothelin-1 with vasoactive factors in mediating glucose-induced increased permeability in endothelial cells. *Lab Invest*, 80, 1311-21.

Cipriani, P., Guiducci, S., Miniati, I., Cinelli, M., Urbani, S., Marrelli, A., Dolo, V., Pavan, A., Saccardi, R., Tyndall, A., Giacomelli, R. & Cerinic, M. M. 2007. Impairment of endothelial cell differentiation from bone marrow-derived mesenchymal stem cells: new insight into the pathogenesis of systemic sclerosis. *Arthritis Rheum*, 56, 1994-2004.

Davies, C. A., Jeziorska, M., Freemont, A. J. & Herrick, A. L. 2006. The differential expression of VEGF, VEGFR-2, and GLUT-1 proteins in disease subtypes of systemic sclerosis. *Hum Pathol*, 37, 190-7.

De Leeuw, K., Kallenberg, C. & Bijl, M. 2005. Accelerated atherosclerosis in patients with systemic autoimmune diseases. *Ann N Y Acad Sci*, 1051, 362-71.

Del Papa, N., Colombo, G., Fracchiolla, N., Moronetti, L. M., Ingegnoli, F., Maglione, W., Comina, D. P., Vitali, C., Fantini, F. & Cortelezzi, A. 2004. Circulating endothelial cells as a marker of ongoing vascular disease in systemic sclerosis. *Arthritis Rheum*, 50, 1296-304.

Del Papa, N., Quirici, N., Soligo, D., Scavullo, C., Cortiana, M., Borsotti, C., Maglione, W., Comina, D. P., Vitali, C., Fraticelli, P., Gabrielli, A., Cortelezzi, A. & Lambertenghi-Deliliers, G. 2006. Bone marrow endothelial progenitors are defective in systemic sclerosis. *Arthritis Rheum*, 54, 2605-15.

Distler, O., Distler, J. H., Scheid, A., Acker, T., Hirth, A., Rethage, J., Michel, B. A., Gay, R. E., Muller-Ladner, U., Matucci-Cerinic, M., Plate, K. H., Gassmann, M. & Gay, S. 2004. Uncontrolled expression of vascular endothelial growth factor and its receptors leads to insufficient skin angiogenesis in patients with systemic sclerosis. *Circ Res*, 95, 109-16.

Egan, C. G., Caporali, F., Garcia-Gonzalez, E., Galeazzi, M. & Sorrentino, V. 2008. Endothelial progenitor cells and colony-forming units in rheumatoid arthritis: association with clinical characteristics. *Rheumatology (Oxford)*, 47, 1484-8.

Fitzgerald, O., Soden, M., Yanni, G., Robinson, R. & Bresnihan, B. 1991. Morphometric analysis of blood vessels in synovial membranes obtained from clinically affected and unaffected knee joints of patients with rheumatoid arthritis. *Ann Rheum Dis*, 50, 792-6.

Fleming, J. N., Nash, R. A., Mcleod, D. O., Fiorentino, D. F., Shulman, H. M., Connolly, M. K., Molitor, J. A., Henstorf, G., Lafyatis, R., Pritchard, D. K., Adams, L. D., Furst, D. E. & Schwartz, S. M. 2008. Capillary regeneration in scleroderma: stem cell therapy reverses phenotype? *PLoS One*, 3, e1452.

Flyvbjerg, A. 2000. Putative pathophysiological role of growth factors and cytokines in experimental diabetic kidney disease. *Diabetologia*, 43, 1205-23.

Gabrielli, A., Avvedimento, E. V. & Krieg, T. 2009. Scleroderma. *N Engl J Med*, 360, 1989-2003.

Geyer, M. & Muller-Ladner, U. 2011. The pathogenesis of systemic sclerosis revisited. *Clin Rev Allergy Immunol*, 40, 92-103.

Griese, D. P., Ehsan, A., Melo, L. G., Kong, D., Zhang, L., Mann, M. J., Pratt, R. E., Mulligan, R. C. & Dzau, V. J. 2003. Isolation and transplantation of autologous circulating endothelial cells into denuded vessels and prosthetic grafts: implications for cell-based vascular therapy. *Circulation,* 108, 2710-5.

Grisar, J., Aletaha, D., Steiner, C. W., Kapral, T., Steiner, S., Saemann, M., Schwarzinger, I., Buranyi, B., Steiner, G. & Smolen, J. S. 2007. Endothelial progenitor cells in active rheumatoid arthritis: effects of tumour necrosis factor and glucocorticoid therapy. *Ann Rheum Dis,* 66, 1284-8.

Grisar, J., Aletaha, D., Steiner, C. W., Kapral, T., Steiner, S., Seidinger, D., Weigel, G., Schwarzinger, I., Wolozcszuk, W., Steiner, G. & Smolen, J. S. 2005. Depletion of endothelial progenitor cells in the peripheral blood of patients with rheumatoid arthritis. *Circulation,* 111, 204-11.

Harrison, A., Lusk, J. & Corkill, M. 1993. Reliability of skin score in scleroderma. *Br J Rheumatol,* 32, 170.

Hebbar, M., Peyrat, J. P., Hornez, L., Hatron, P. Y., Hachulla, E. & Devulder, B. 2000. Increased concentrations of the circulating angiogenesis inhibitor endostatin in patients with systemic sclerosis. *Arthritis Rheum,* 43, 889-93.

Herbrig, K., Haensel, S., Oelschlaegel, U., Pistrosch, F., Foerster, S. & Passauer, J. 2006. Endothelial dysfunction in patients with rheumatoid arthritis is associated with a reduced number and impaired function of endothelial progenitor cells. *Ann Rheum Dis,* 65, 157-63.

Hirohata, S., Yanagida, T., Nampei, A., Kunugiza, Y., Hashimoto, H., Tomita, T., Yoshikawa, H. & Ochi, T. 2004. Enhanced generation of endothelial cells from CD34+ cells of the bone marrow in rheumatoid arthritis: possible role in synovial neovascularization. *Arthritis Rheum,* 50, 3888-96.

Hirschi, K. K., Ingram, D. A. & Yoder, M. C. 2008. Assessing identity, phenotype, and fate of endothelial progenitor cells. *Arterioscler Thromb Vasc Biol,* 28, 1584-95.

Hur, J., Yoon, C. H., Kim, H. S., Choi, J. H., Kang, H. J., Hwang, K. K., Oh, B. H., Lee, M. M. & Park, Y. B. 2004. Characterization of two types of endothelial progenitor cells and their different contributions to neovasculogenesis. *Arterioscler Thromb Vasc Biol,* 24, 288-93.

Ingram, D. A., Mead, L. E., Tanaka, H., Meade, V., Fenoglio, A., Mortell, K., Pollok, K., Ferkowicz, M. J., Gilley, D. & Yoder, M. C. 2004. Identification of a novel hierarchy of endothelial progenitor cells using human peripheral and umbilical cord blood. *Blood,* 104, 2752-60.

Jodon De Villeroche, V., Avouac, J., Ponceau, A., Ruiz, B., Kahan, A., Boileau, C., Uzan, G. & Allanore, Y. 2010. Enhanced late-outgrowth circulating endothelial progenitor cell levels in rheumatoid arthritis and correlation with disease activity. *Arthritis Res Ther,* 12, R27.

Kahaleh, B. 2008. Vascular disease in scleroderma: mechanisms of vascular injury. *Rheum Dis Clin North Am,* 34, 57-71; vi.

Kaplan, M. J. 2010. Cardiovascular complications of rheumatoid arthritis: assessment, prevention, and treatment. *Rheum Dis Clin North Am,* 36, 405-26.

Karamysheva, A. F. 2008. Mechanisms of angiogenesis. *Biochemistry (Mosc),* 73, 751-62.

Kocher, A. A., Schuster, M. D., Szabolcs, M. J., Takuma, S., Burkhoff, D., Wang, J., Homma, S., Edwards, N. M. & Itescu, S. 2001. Neovascularization of ischemic myocardium by human bone-marrow-derived angioblasts prevents cardiomyocyte apoptosis, reduces remodeling and improves cardiac function. *Nat Med,* 7, 430-6.

Kumar, A. H. & Caplice, N. M. 2010. Clinical potential of adult vascular progenitor cells. *Arterioscler Thromb Vasc Biol*, 30, 1080-7.

Kumar, P., Erroi, A., Sattar, A. & Kumar, S. 1985. Weibel-Palade bodies as a marker for neovascularization induced by tumor and rheumatoid angiogenesis factors. *Cancer Res*, 45, 4339-48.

Kuwana, M., Kaburaki, J., Okazaki, Y., Yasuoka, H., Kawakami, Y. & Ikeda, Y. 2006. Increase in circulating endothelial precursors by atorvastatin in patients with systemic sclerosis. *Arthritis Rheum*, 54, 1946-51.

Kuwana, M., Okazaki, Y., Yasuoka, H., Kawakami, Y. & Ikeda, Y. 2004. Defective vasculogenesis in systemic sclerosis. *Lancet*, 364, 603-10.

Lin, Y., Weisdorf, D. J., Solovey, A. & Hebbel, R. P. 2000. Origins of circulating endothelial cells and endothelial outgrowth from blood. *J Clin Invest*, 105, 71-7.

Loomans, C. J., De Koning, E. J., Staal, F. J., Rookmaaker, M. B., Verseyden, C., De Boer, H. C., Verhaar, M. C., Braam, B., Rabelink, T. J. & Van Zonneveld, A. J. 2004. Endothelial progenitor cell dysfunction: a novel concept in the pathogenesis of vascular complications of type 1 diabetes. *Diabetes*, 53, 195-9.

Martin-Rendon, E., Brunskill, S. J., Hyde, C. J., Stanworth, S. J., Mathur, A. & Watt, S. M. 2008. Autologous bone marrow stem cells to treat acute myocardial infarction: a systematic review. *Eur Heart J*, 29, 1807-18.

Medina, R. J., O'neill, C. L., Sweeney, M., Guduric-Fuchs, J., Gardiner, T. A., Simpson, D. A. & Stitt, A. W. 2010. Molecular analysis of endothelial progenitor cell (EPC) subtypes reveals two distinct cell populations with different identities. *BMC Med Genomics*, 3, 18.

Muz, B., Khan, M. N., Kiriakidis, S. & Paleolog, E. M. 2009. Hypoxia. The role of hypoxia and HIF-dependent signalling events in rheumatoid arthritis. *Arthritis Res Ther*, 11, 201.

Nerlich, A. G., Sauer, U., Kolm-Litty, V., Wagner, E., Koch, M. & Schleicher, E. D. 1998. Expression of glutamine:fructose-6-phosphate amidotransferase in human tissues: evidence for high variability and distinct regulation in diabetes. *Diabetes*, 47, 170-8.

Orlic, D., Kajstura, J., Chimenti, S., Limana, F., Jakoniuk, I., Quaini, F., Nadal-Ginard, B., Bodine, D. M., Leri, A. & Anversa, P. 2001. Mobilized bone marrow cells repair the infarcted heart, improving function and survival. *Proc Natl Acad Sci U S A*, 98, 10344-9.

Paleolog, E. M. 2009. The vasculature in rheumatoid arthritis: cause or consequence? *Int J Exp Pathol*, 90, 249-61.

Prescott, R. J., Freemont, A. J., Jones, C. J., Hoyland, J. & Fielding, P. 1992. Sequential dermal microvascular and perivascular changes in the development of scleroderma. *J Pathol*, 166, 255-63.

Rehman, J., Li, J., Orschell, C. M. & March, K. L. 2003. Peripheral blood "endothelial progenitor cells" are derived from monocyte/macrophages and secrete angiogenic growth factors. *Circulation*, 107, 1164-9.

Rooney, M., Condell, D., Quinlan, W., Daly, L., Whelan, A., Feighery, C. & Bresnihan, B. 1988. Analysis of the histologic variation of synovitis in rheumatoid arthritis. *Arthritis Rheum*, 31, 956-63.

Ruger, B., Giurea, A., Wanivenhaus, A. H., Zehetgruber, H., Hollemann, D., Yanagida, G., Groger, M., Petzelbauer, P., Smolen, J. S., Hoecker, P. & Fischer, M. B. 2004.

Endothelial precursor cells in the synovial tissue of patients with rheumatoid arthritis and osteoarthritis. *Arthritis Rheum,* 50, 2157-66.

Sainson, R. C., Johnston, D. A., Chu, H. C., Holderfield, M. T., Nakatsu, M. N., Crampton, S. P., Davis, J., Conn, E. & Hughes, C. C. 2008. TNF primes endothelial cells for angiogenic sprouting by inducing a tip cell phenotype. *Blood,* 111, 4997-5007.

Schalkwijk, C. G. & Stehouwer, C. D. 2005. Vascular complications in diabetes mellitus: the role of endothelial dysfunction. *Clin Sci (Lond),* 109, 143-59.

Scheja, A., Wildt, M., Wollheim, F. A., Akesson, A. & Saxne, T. 2000. Circulating collagen metabolites in systemic sclerosis. Differences between limited and diffuse form and relationship with pulmonary involvement. *Rheumatology (Oxford),* 39, 1110-3.

Semble, E. L., Turner, R. A. & Mccrickard, E. L. 1985. Rheumatoid arthritis and osteoarthritis synovial fluid effects on primary human endothelial cell cultures. *J Rheumatol,* 12, 237-41.

Sen, S., Mcdonald, S. P., Coates, P. T. & Bonder, C. S. 2011. Endothelial progenitor cells: novel biomarker and promising cell therapy for cardiovascular disease. *Clin Sci (Lond),* 120, 263-83.

Shapiro, A. M., Ricordi, C., Hering, B. J., Auchincloss, H., Lindblad, R., Robertson, R. P., Secchi, A., Brendel, M. D., Berney, T., Brennan, D. C., Cagliero, E., Alejandro, R., Ryan, E. A., Dimercurio, B., Morel, P., Polonsky, K. S., Reems, J. A., Bretzel, R. G., Bertuzzi, F., Froud, T., Kandaswamy, R., Sutherland, D. E., Eisenbarth, G., Segal, M., Preiksaitis, J., Korbutt, G. S., Barton, F. B., Viviano, L., Seyfert-Margolis, V., Bluestone, J. & Lakey, J. R. 2006. International trial of the Edmonton protocol for islet transplantation. *N Engl J Med,* 355, 1318-30.

Shi, Q., Rafii, S., Wu, M. H., Wijelath, E. S., Yu, C., Ishida, A., Fujita, Y., Kothari, S., Mohle, R., Sauvage, L. R., Moore, M. A., Storb, R. F. & Hammond, W. P. 1998. Evidence for circulating bone marrow-derived endothelial cells. *Blood,* 92, 362-7.

Sibal, L., Aldibbiat, A., Agarwal, S. C., Mitchell, G., Oates, C., Razvi, S., Weaver, J. U., Shaw, J. A. & Home, P. D. 2009. Circulating endothelial progenitor cells, endothelial function, carotid intima-media thickness and circulating markers of endothelial dysfunction in people with type 1 diabetes without macrovascular disease or microalbuminuria. *Diabetologia,* 52, 1464-73.

Sieveking, D. P. & Ng, M. K. 2009. Cell therapies for therapeutic angiogenesis: back to the bench. *Vasc Med,* 14, 153-66.

Silverman, M. D., Haas, C. S., Rad, A. M., Arbab, A. S. & Koch, A. E. 2007. The role of vascular cell adhesion molecule 1/ very late activation antigen 4 in endothelial progenitor cell recruitment to rheumatoid arthritis synovium. *Arthritis Rheum,* 56, 1817-26.

Stehouwer, C. D., Lambert, J., Donker, A. J. & Van Hinsbergh, V. W. 1997. Endothelial dysfunction and pathogenesis of diabetic angiopathy. *Cardiovasc Res,* 34, 55-68.

Stevens, C. R., Blake, D. R., Merry, P., Revell, P. A. & Levick, J. R. 1991. A comparative study by morphometry of the microvasculature in normal and rheumatoid synovium. *Arthritis Rheum,* 34, 1508-13.

Strauer, B. E., Brehm, M., Zeus, T., Kostering, M., Hernandez, A., Sorg, R. V., Kogler, G. & Wernet, P. 2002. Repair of infarcted myocardium by autologous intracoronary mononuclear bone marrow cell transplantation in humans. *Circulation,* 106, 1913-8.

Tateishi-Yuyama, E., Matsubara, H., Murohara, T., Ikeda, U., Shintani, S., Masaki, H., Amano, K., Kishimoto, Y., Yoshimoto, K., Akashi, H., Shimada, K., Iwasaka, T. & Imaizumi, T. 2002. Therapeutic angiogenesis for patients with limb ischaemia by autologous transplantation of bone-marrow cells: a pilot study and a randomised controlled trial. *Lancet*, 360, 427-35.

Timmermans, F., Van Hauwermeiren, F., De Smedt, M., Raedt, R., Plasschaert, F., De Buyzere, M. L., Gillebert, T. C., Plum, J. & Vandekerckhove, B. 2007. Endothelial outgrowth cells are not derived from CD133+ cells or CD45+ hematopoietic precursors. *Arterioscler Thromb Vasc Biol*, 27, 1572-9.

Westerweel, P. E., Luijten, R. K., Hoefer, I. E., Koomans, H. A., Derksen, R. H. & Verhaar, M. C. 2007. Haematopoietic and endothelial progenitor cells are deficient in quiescent systemic lupus erythematosus. *Ann Rheum Dis*, 66, 865-70.

Westerweel, P. E. & Verhaar, M. C. 2009. Endothelial progenitor cell dysfunction in rheumatic disease. *Nat Rev Rheumatol*, 5, 332-40.

Williamson, J. R., Chang, K., Frangos, M., Hasan, K. S., Ido, Y., Kawamura, T., Nyengaard, J. R., Van Den Enden, M., Kilo, C. & Tilton, R. G. 1993. Hyperglycemic pseudohypoxia and diabetic complications. *Diabetes*, 42, 801-13.

Yamaguchi, Y., Okazaki, Y., Seta, N., Satoh, T., Takahashi, K., Ikezawa, Z. & Kuwana, M. 2010. Enhanced angiogenic potency of monocytic endothelial progenitor cells in patients with systemic sclerosis. *Arthritis Res Ther*, 12, R205.

Yoder, M. C., Mead, L. E., Prater, D., Krier, T. R., Mroueh, K. N., Li, F., Krasich, R., Temm, C. J., Prchal, J. T. & Ingram, D. A. 2007. Redefining endothelial progenitor cells via clonal analysis and hematopoietic stem/progenitor cell principals. *Blood,* 109, 1801-9.

Yoon, C. H., Hur, J., Park, K. W., Kim, J. H., Lee, C. S., Oh, I. Y., Kim, T. Y., Cho, H. J., Kang, H. J., Chae, I. H., Yang, H. K., Oh, B. H., Park, Y. B. & Kim, H. S. 2005. Synergistic neovascularization by mixed transplantation of early endothelial progenitor cells and late outgrowth endothelial cells: the role of angiogenic cytokines and matrix metalloproteinases. *Circulation,* 112, 1618-27.

Ziyadeh, F. N. 2004. Mediators of diabetic renal disease: the case for tgf-Beta as the major mediator. *J Am Soc Nephrol*, 15 Suppl 1, S55-7.

4

A Possible Link Between Autoimmunity and Cancer

Erika Cristaldi, Giulia Malaguarnera,
Alessandra Rando and Mariano Malaguarnera
University of Catania
Italy

1. Introduction

The most important cause of mortality after cardiovascular diseases is due to cancer, that affects both young and elderly people. The increasing incidence of tumour discovery is a consequence of improving diagnosis techniques and sensitization acts, thus facilitating a precocious identification and consequently an immediate therapeutic approach (Malaguarnera et al., 2010).

Autoimmune diseases represent one of the main growing health problem worldwide with wide variations in incidence and severity (Silink, 2002). Autoimmune diseases arise from an overactive immune response of the body against substances and tissues normally present in the body and they are due to the breakdown of immune tolerance to specific self-antigens.

Cancers and autoimmunity are often coincident—more coincident than is generally appreciated; thereby it has been raised more interest the relationship and the possible temporal consequence between autoimmune disease and cancer onset. Particularly, since a high level of autoimmunity is unhealthy, a low level of autoimmunity may actually be beneficial, thereby autoimmune reactions may be considered as a defence processes played by the host against tumour, or it may be possible that the anti-tumour immune response may result in elicitation of auto-antibodies against various auto-antigens, including self antigens expressed in tumour cells.

Some autoimmune diseases, such as Sjögren's syndrome, rheumatoid arthritis and systemic lupus erythematosus have been associated with the development of lymphoproliferative malignancies (Kiss et al., 2010), and a pleyade of autoantibodies have been found in patients with solid tumours (Bei et al., 2009). In addition, patients with dermatomyositis have a greater risk of developing solid-organ malignancies than the general population. In these patients, cancer can precede, parallel or follow myositis diagnosis (Zampieri et al., 2010).

The mechanism behind disease etiology remains unknown for most autoimmune diseases. This situation is distinct from cancer where our understanding of how genetic mutations lead to disease, is increasing. These advancements in cancer biology may have provided a very important piece to the autoimmunity puzzle. However, the relationship between cancer and autoimmunity is not well known. Despite minimal supporting evidence, the standard model for explaining this coincidence is that autoimmunity leads to cancer due to the rapid cell division associated with the regeneration of damaged tissues at the site of inflammation (Coussens & Werb, 2002). The relationship between autoimmunity and cancer was investigated, focusing on implication of immune system, apoptosis and new therapeutic agents for autoimmune diseases.

2. Break tolerance mechanisms in autoimmune diseases

The clinical signs and symptoms of different autoimmune diseases overlap, and individual patients often present with syndromes that combine features of more than one disease. Different autoimmune diseases share some genetic predisposing factors, including human leukocyte antigen (HLA) alleles (SLEGEN et al., 2008) or the T-cell regulatory gene CTLA-4 (Ueda et al., 2003). Our current knowledge suggests that multiple mutation might be needed before a self-reactive clone bypasses sequential tolerance-checkpoints and gives rise to an autoimmune disease (Baechler et al., 2003). The development of autoantibodies reflects a loss of B- and T- cell tolerance, which might result from a combination of genetic predisposition, persistent inflammatory responses, abnormal handling of apoptotic material and immune complexes, abnormal presentation of self-antigens and other events. As a high level of autoimmunity is unhealthy, a low level of autoimmunity may actually be beneficial. First, low-level autoimmunity might aid in the recognition of neoplastic cells by CD8+ T cells, and thus reducing the incidence of cancer. Second, autoimmunity may have an important role, allowing a rapid immune response in the early stages of an infection when the availability of foreign antigens limits the response (i.e., when there are few pathogens present).

Diseases such as rheumatoid arthritis and tireotoxicosis are associated with the loss of immunological tolerance, which is the ability of an individual to ignore self, while reacting to non-self. This breakage leads to the immune system mounting an effective and specific immune response against self determinants. The exact genesis of immunological tolerance is still unclear, but several theories have been proposed to explain its origin. Two hypotheses have gained widespread attention among immunologists:

- Clonal Deletion theory, proposed by Burnet (1988), according to which self-reactive lymphoid cells are destroyed during their development. The extent to which the thymus can mediate tolerance to tissue-specific proteins and how organ specific tolerance is mediated remains an open question. While some tissue-specific proteins might reach the thymus through the circulation, this mechanism may be unnecessary due to expression within the thymus of the autoimmune regulator protein AIRE, which acts as a promiscuous ubiquitin ligase with the potential function of controlling transcription of a broad array of tissue-specific target genes in thymic epithelial cells (Nagamine et al., 1997).

- Clonal Anergy theory, proposed by Nossal et al. (1982), in which self-reactive T- or B-cells become inactivated in the normal individual and cannot amplify the immune response. This process is based upon the requirement of two signals for T-cell activation. The first is provided by the recognition of MHC-complexes and the second is due to the interaction between CD28 on T cells and B7 on activated antigen presenting cell (APC), that are induced by pro-inflammatory factors, such as bacterial products, pro-inflammatory cytokines, and other signals.

Previously, conditions such as cancer could not stimulate immune responses due to lack of co-stimulatory signals. However, this notion was based on cancers at late or advanced stages of disease, when tumour-induced immunosuppression may be at its highest degree (e.g. through production of the regulatory cytokines, transforming growth factor (TGF)-β and IL-10); in fact there is a considerable potential for newly transformed cells to evoke danger signals through the engagement of pro-inflammatory signaling pathways (Eisenlohr & Rothstein, 2006).

3. Autoimmune diseases and cancer - pathogenetic aspects

Positive associations have been reported between certain lymphomas and inflammation, autoimmune disease and infectious agents (Rosenquist, 2008).

Normally, tolerance checkpoints silence self-reactive T and B cells by preventing uncontrolled stimulation through self-antigens exposure. Several observations suggest that lymphocyte clones having bypassed tolerance mechanisms may be involved both in autoimmunity and malignancy (Goodnow, 2007). There are epidemiological observations of autoimmunity and lymphoma occurring simultaneously in diseases like systemic lupus erythematosus, rheumatoid arthritis and Sjögren's syndrome regardless of the use of immunosuppressive therapy (Bernatsky et al., 2007).

Infectious agents causing lymphomas can be classified according to several mechanisms. First, some viruses can directly transform lymphocytes as for Burkitt's lymphomas that may occur following infection with HIV; as well as T-cell lymphomas may occur following chronic antigen challenge with wheat in celiac disease (Cellier et al., 2000). Second, some infections increase lymphoma risk through chronic immune stimulation (Engels, 2007), which is also present in autoimmune diseases. Since uncontrolled stimulation of antigen receptors and lymphocyte proliferation triggered by chronic infection (e.g. Helicobacter pylori) may result in mucosa-associated lymphoid- tissue B-cell lymphomas (Suarez et al.,2006), it may be supposed that chronic stimulation of autoreactive cells paired with somatic hypermutation and recombinase activator gene (RAG) activity directed at non-antigen receptor loci may underlie lymphoma in systemic lupus erythematosus, rheumatoid arthritis and Sjögren's syndrome (Schuetz et al., 2010).

Treatments for autoimmune and chronic inflammatory disorders could also affect the risk of lymphoproliferative malignancies. Another reason for the association could be shared environmental risk factors (Landgren et al., 2006), and in some autoimmune diseases genetic mutations are discovered, leading to lymphoproliferation (Turbyville & Rao, 2010). Somatic mutations in lymphocytes may additionally contribute to the pathogenesis of autoimmunity and lymphoid malignancies as observed in patients with autoimmune lymphoproliferative syndrome carrying a mutated FAS gene in a single hematopoietic stem cell that contributes to a small fraction of blood cells. These patients may present with autoimmune symptoms and lymphoma formation just like patients with inherited FAS mutations (Holzelova et al., 2004).

4. The role of adaptive immunity

4.1 Treg cells

Regulatory T (Treg) cells are currently considered as key players in the mechanisms of peripheral immune tolerance. They are classified in natural and inducible CD4+CD25+ FOXP3+ Treg cells. The transcription regulator FOXP3 (Forkhead box P3) appears to be required for the development, maintenance, and suppressor function of Treg cells (Hori et al., 2003), and the loss of FOXP3 in Treg cells - or its reduced expression - leads to the acquisition of effector T-cell properties including the production of non-Treg cell specific cytokines (Wan & Flavell, 2007). Treg cells are engaged in the control of immune self-tolerance, allograft rejection, allergy, and are also important for inhibiting the effector functions during infection and tumours development. In addition, the removal or a functional defect of Treg cells from normal rodents leads to the development of various autoimmune diseases (Weiner, 2001), because these cells actively suppress the activation and expansion of autoreactive immune cells.

Sometimes the studies investigating the role of Treg cells in SLE, have given controversial results (Khun et al., 2009). Most studies have found a reduced or normal frequency of Treg cells in SLE (La Cava, 2008), although other studies may have shown increased number. It has been observed a decreased number of Treg cells, during active disease flares (Miyara et al., 2005) and active SLE pediatric patients, thereby showing a poor suppressive capacity and an inverse correlation between Treg cells and disease activity as well as autoantibody levels (Lee et al., 2006). However, treatment with corticosteroids and/or immunosuppressive agents has been found to promote an increase in the number of Treg cells, particularly of peripheral Treg cells. Also, increased mRNA levels of CD25, FOXP3, and GITR have been found in B-cell depleted patients treated with rituximab at the time of B cell repopulation (Cepika et al., 2007).

In the collagen-induced arthritis model of systemic joint inflammation, the adoptive transfer of Treg cells protects from disease, whereas a depletion of Treg cells accelerates it (Morgan et al., 2005). Furthermore, in patients with early rheumatoid arthritis (RA), a reduced number of peripheral Treg cells is observed (Lawson et al., 2006), although the synovial fluid can often contain increased numbers of Treg cells (Cao et al., 2003).

Furthermore, increased frequency of Foxp3+ Treg cells has been documented in tumour tissues and peripheral blood of patients with several types of cancer consistent with a role in tumour escape from immunological control. And also, not only the quantitative aspect of Treg cells, but also their functions are different between tumour patients and healthy control. Treg cells are considered inhibitors of anti-tumour immunity and CD4+CD25+Foxp3+ regulatory T cells have been considered as a candidate for cancer immunotherapy for over a decade. Attempts to block or eliminate Treg cells have been made by the use of chemotherapy; these strategies, aimed at block Treg cells induction and migration, may be clinically useful, as suggested by experimental evidences in tumour models (Langier et al., 2010).

Data concerning the role of CD4+CD25+ regulatory T cells in human cancer derived from a work, which showed that the presence of such Treg cells in advanced ovarian cancer correlated with reduced survival (Curiel et al., 2004). In addition, TGF-β is a cytokine produced by Treg and Type 1 T regulatory cells, that is involved in the suppression of T cell proliferation and function (M.L. Chen et al., 2005). The experimental results supplied by other researchs indicate that TGF-β, secreted by ovarian carcinoma cells, owns vital function in the process of converting peripheral CD4+CD25- T cells into CD4+CD25+ regulatory T cells, likely providing a possible immunotherapeutic target for ovarian cancer (Zheng et al., 2004).

One of the new therapeutic approach to cancer is based on the adoptive transfer of tumour-specific cytotoxic T cells and anti-CD25 antibodies. A combination of Treg cell-depletion, using anti-CD25 monoclonal antibodies, and cytotoxic T lymphocytes administration is a possible approach for treatment of cancers which enable further exploration in the clinical setting (Ohmura et al., 2008), though these future approaches suggest a possible development of autoimmune diseases, due to decreased Treg cells occurrence.

4.2 Dendritic cells

Dendritic cells have been recognized as the most efficient antigen presenting cells that have the capacity to initiate naïve T-cell response *in vitro* and *in vivo*. During their differentiation and maturation pathways, DCs can efficiently capture, process and present antigens for T-cell activation. The functional activities of DCs mainly depend on their state of activation and differentiation: iDC are involved in the maintenance of peripheral tolerance whereas mature DC can efficiently induce the development of effector T cells. Thereby, accumulated iDCs, which are educated at the tumour site, act as functional inhibitors of a tumour-specific immune response in cancer, immature pDCs are activated by Toll-like receptors, which lead to B- and T-cell immune responses in autoimmune disease (Lang et al., 2005). The immunological tolerance is produced by tumour-derived soluble factors (TDSFs) and immature dendritic cells (iDCs), which inhibit DC and T-cell activation, and exclusively inhibit the DNA–IgG immune complex, inducing pro-inflammatory responses needed for an immune response. Immunological ignorance is produced by reduced levels of tumour antigens. Dendritic cells not only initiate T-cell responses, but are also involved in silencing T-cell immune response. DC can play a central role in the development of T-cell tolerance, and its maintenance in the periphery is critical for the prevention of autoimmunity.

4.3 T helper 17 cells (Th17)

T helper 17 cells constitute a third subset of T helper cells that are important in the development of autoimmune diseases and in the immune response against infections. These cells are characterized as preferential producers of IL-17A, IL-17F, IL-21, IL-22 and IL-26 in humans. The IL-17 production is required to differentiate Th17 cells, from IFN-γ producing Th1 cells, or IL-4 producing Th2 cells. IL-17 (A and F) induces production of a broad range of pro-inflammatory cytokines and chemokines, including IL-6, colony-stimulating factors, chemokines (CCL2, CCL7, CXCL1, and CCL20), human β-defensin-2 and matrix metalloproteinases (MMP-3 and MMP-13), by a variety of cells (Weaver et al., 2007). Conversely, inhibition of IL-17 signaling leads to impaired host defence against bacterial infection (Ye et al., 2001) and resistance to autoimmune diseases (Yang et al., 2008). IL-17 regulates host defence against infectious organisms through promoting granulopoiesis and neutrophil trafficking (Linden et al., 2005).

Although FOXP3+ Treg cells are critical for control of autoimmunity and inflammation (Sakaguchi, 2004), Th17 cells have been implicated in mediating inflammation and autoimmune diseases (Weaver et al., 2007). It has been shown that the balance between Treg and Th17 cells is a key factor which regulates T-helper cell function relating to the Th1 / Th2 shift in autoimmune disease and graft versus host disease (GVHD) (Afzali et al., 2007). In fact, elevated levels of IL-17 have been associated with inflammatory diseases in humans, including rheumatoid arthritis, scleritis, uveitis, asthma, systemic lupus erythematosus, and allograft rejection (Kolls & Linden, 2004).

However, there are limited information on the balance between Treg and Th17 cells in cancer patients and on the active role played by Th 17 in anti-tumour immunity (Kryczek et al., 2009). The function of IL-17 in tumour immunity is a controversial subject. The effects of IL-17 on tumour development are directly influenced by the existence of an adaptive immune system. In the presence of lymphocytes, IL-17 promotes tumour rejection, whereas in the absence of those, IL-17 favours tumour growth and angiogenesis (Martin-Orozco & Chen Dong, 2009a). By using IL-17-deficient mice in a model of lung melanoma, it has been provided direct evidence for a protective role of IL-17 in anti tumour responses (Martin-

Orozco et al., 2009b). It has also found that Th17 cells provided better protection to tumours than Th1 cells, and this difference was largely due to their unique ability to promote CD8+ T cell priming. In Th17- but not Th1-treated tumour-bearing mice, it has been observed increased numbers of CD8+ T cells in the lung, suggesting that Th17 cells may promote the activation or recruitment of tumour antigen-specific CD8+ T cells (Martin-Orozco et al., 2009 b). There are data supporting the existence of IL17-producing effector CD8+ T cells (Tc17) which are also induced by IL23 and may play a role in cancer development as well as in autoimmunity (Ciric et al., 2009). Thereby, the protective role of Th 17 cells, inhibiting tumour growth, may influence the onset of autoimmune diseases.

5. Apoptosis mechanism

Apoptosis is an active, genetically controlled process of cell death required to ensure that the rate of cell division were balanced by the rate of cell death in multicellular organisms. The control of apoptosis is critical for the homeostasis of the immune system as it happens during infections, where antigen specific lymphocytes need to rapidly proliferate. After clearance of the infectious microbe lymphocytes need to die in order to prevent dysregulated proliferation with the consequence of leukemia or lymphoma (Lorenz et al., 2000). Importantly, as explained below, during apoptotic breakdown many nuclear constituents are post-translation modified, possibly altering antigenicity. Therefore it is not surprising that failure to achieve programmed cell death and to clear apoptotic cell fragments may be discussed as a key pathogenetic factor leading to autoimmunity. This could be explained by a failure to kill an autoreactive cell or by inducing autoantibodies against apoptotically modified cellular constituents. If the preload is excessive, as in massive cell death (e.g. upon infection), regulatory clearance mechanisms cannot effectively remove apoptotic residuals and thereby allowing the persistence of antigens for stimulation of the immune system. During apoptosis, the cellular contents of the nucleus, cytosol and membrane are brought together in close proximity, a mechanism that could lead to epitope spreading (Vidalino et al., 2009). Altered structures of intracellular proteins produced during cleavage events in apoptosis could also be a source of immunogenic antigens. Altered apoptosis mechanism is associated with the pathogenesis of a wide array of diseases: cancer, neurodegeneration, autoimmunity, heart disease and others.

5.1 Phases of apoptotic death

Apoptotic cell death can be divided into a "triggering phase" (e.g., ligation of "dedicated death receptor" such as Fas, or withdrawal of growth/survival factors), a "signaling phase" (e.g., protein kinase cascades that include MAPK family, JNK and p38), an "execution phase" (e.g., activation of caspases and nucleases), and a "burial phase" (e.g. phagocytosis of dying cells by neighboring cells) (Utz & Anderson, 1998).

5.1.1 Triggering phase

Fas ligand (FasL) and tumor necrosis factor α (TNF-α) are the prototypical inducers of apoptosis. These ligands induce clustering of their respective receptors (Fas, TNFR-I or TNFR-II), which leads to recruitment of the early signal-transducing molecules. The Fas/FasL system is the most studied receptor mediated apoptotic pathway. Fas/Apo-1/CD95 is a type I trans membrane protein with a cysteine-rich extracellular domain and is a member of the tumor necrosis factor receptor (TNFR) superfamily (Itoh & Nagata, 1993). A variety of cell types express Fas, but differing between tissues for the expression levels. Its ligand, FasL, is a type II transmembrane protein that can also exist as a soluble factor in a stable trimer configuration (Mountz et al.,1994). On ligation of FasL, Fas trimerizes and recruits an adaptor protein known as Fas-associated protein with death domain (FADD, also called MORT-1) through its intracellular death domain (Chinnaiyan et al., 1995). The cytotoxic signal is further propagated as FADD recruits and interacts with another adapter protein as FADD-like interleukin-1β converting enzyme (FLICE), also known as caspase-8 (Muzio et al., 1997). Formation of the Fas-FADD-FLICE/ caspase-8 complex, known as death-inducing signal complex (DISC), facilitates the autocleavage and activation of caspase- 8 (Kischkel et al., 1995). A protein known as inhibitor of FLICE (I-FLICE) and FLICE-inhibitory protein (FLIP) can prevent the formation of DISC required for further apoptotic signaling (Irmler et al., 1997).

5.1.2 Signaling phase
Apoptosis is a multistep process and protein kinases have been implicated both in the upstream induction phase of apoptosis and in the downstream execution stage, as the direct targets for caspases. The serine/threonine protein kinases that have been suggested to play a role in apoptosis are the mitogen- activated protein kinase (MAPK) family, specifically, p42/ 44 ERK, p38 MAPK and c-Jun N-terminal kinase (JNK), cyclic AMP-dependent protein kinase A (PKA), protein kinase B (PKB), or Akt and protein kinase C (PKC). The activation of JNK/SAPK and p38 MAP kinases is generally associated with the promotion of apoptosis, while p42/44 ERK activity inhibits apoptosis (Mc Cubrey et al., 2000).

5.1.3 Execution phase
In mammalian cells, activation of caspases is achieved through at least two independent mechanisms which are initiated by distinct caspases, but results in activation of common executioner caspases. Once activated, caspase-8 can induce either directly or indirectly the activation of a number of distal caspases such as caspase-3, -6 and -7 (CD95 type I cells) (Muzio et al., 1997). Another pathway for caspase activation involves cytochrome c, which in mammalian cells is often released from the mitochondria into the cytosol during apoptosis (CD95 type II cells) (Scaffidi et al., 1999) (fig.1).

5.2 The cell death regulator: Bcl-2 and TNF-R
The B cell leukemia-2 (Bcl-2) was the first mammalian cell death regulator identified. Bcl-2 and the tumor necrosis factor receptor (TNF-R) family contribute to the regulation of apoptosis with their corresponding ligands. The proto-oncogene Bcl-2 has been cloned from the t(14:18) chromosomal translocation breakpoint in human follicular centre B lymphoma (Korsmeyer, 1995) and its function was first discovered when it was over-expressed in cytokine-dependent haematopoietic cell lines. Upon removal of the growth factor, Bcl-2 promoted survival of these cells in the quiescent state (Gerl & Vaux, 2005). An important discovery from the studies in lymphocytes was that Bcl-2 did not only promote survival of growth factor-deprived cells but could inhibit apoptosis triggered by a broad range of physiological or experimentally applied cytotoxic stimuli (Sentman et al., 1991). Bcl-2 family can be divided into two groups according to their function: those which are structurally most similar to Bcl-2 and inhibit apoptosis, on the other side there are the members of the Bcl-2 family that enhance cell death. The mitochondrial pathway, is triggered by

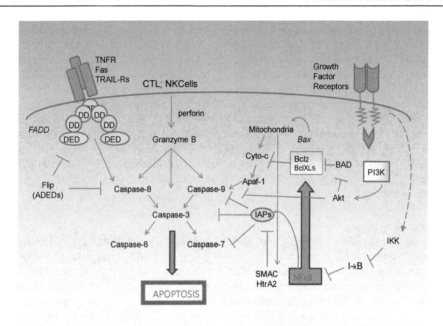

Fig. 1. ADEDs: Anti-apoptotic Death Effector Domain proteins; Akt: serine/threonine
protein kinase ; Apaf-1: Apoptotic protease activating factors-1; BAD: Bcl-2-associated death
promoter protein; Bax: Bcl-2–associated X protein; Bcl-2: B-cell lymphoma 2; Bcl-xl: B-cell
lymphoma-extra large; CTL: Cytolytic T-cells; Cyto-c: Cytochrome-c; DED: Death Effector
Domains; FADD: Fas-associated death domain; Flip: FLICE (Fadd-Like Interleukin-1β
Converting Enzyme) inhibitory protein; HTRA2/Omi: mammalian homolog of the bacterial
high temperature requirement protein (HTRA); IAPs: Inhibitor of apoptosis protein; IKK:
IκB kinase ; IκB: Inhibitor of κB ; NFkB: nuclear factor kappa-B; NK: Natural Killer; PI3K:
phosphatidylinositol 3-kinase ; SMAC: Second Mitocondrial-derived Activator of Caspase ;
TNFR: Tumor Necrosis Factor Receptors; TRAIL-Rs: TNF-related apoptosis inducing ligand-
Receptors.

proapoptotic members of the Bcl-2 family. In response to environmental cues these proteins
engage another set of proapoptotic Bcl-2 members, the Bax sub family residing on the
mitochondrial outer membranes or in the cytosol. The interaction induces the latter to
oligomerize and insert into the mitochondrial membrane (Eskes et al., 2000). Here the
complex acts to trigger the sudden and complete release of cytochrome c and other proteins
from all of the mitochondria in the cell. Bcl-2 block death by preventing the mitochondrial
release of the intermembrane proteins, including cytochrome c (Moriishi et al., 1999). A
protein with the dual name of Smac/DIABLO is released from the mitochondria along with
cytochrome c during apoptosis, and this protein functions to promote caspase activation by
associating with the Apaf- 1 apoptosome and inhibiting inhibitor of apoptosis proteins.
Members of the tumour necrosis factor (TNF) receptor family and their corresponding
ligands are critical regulators of apoptosis, and also control other cellular processes
(Wallach, 1997). CD95 (also called Fas or APO-1) and p55 TNF-RI receptors, and a few other
members of the family, contain a cytoplasmic region, called "death domain" (DD), which is

essential for inducing apoptosis (Tartaglia et al., 1993). Upon receptor activation, the death domain undergoes interaction with a death domain in the adaptor proteins FADD (Fas-Associated protein with Death Domain)/Mort-1 or TRADD (Tumor necrosis factor receptor type 1-associated DEATH domain protein) (Hsu et al., 1996). FADD/MORT 1 binds directly to CD95 and indirectly to p55 TNF-R I via TRADD, and it is essential for cell death signaling from both receptors. This complex binds caspase-8, therefore inducing its self-processing (Boldin et al., 1996). The members of the TNF receptor family (death receptors) bearing death domain can also activate signaling pathways that promote survival, proliferation, and differentiation of cells. Signaling via TRADD is essential for TNF-induced activation of Jun kinase and its absence renders cells less susceptible to the pro-apoptotic activity of TNF (Yeh et al., 1997). Death domain RIP (receptor-interacting protein) kinase is required for TNF-receptor transduced activation of NF-kB and its absence also sensitizes cells to TNF-induced apoptosis (Kelliher 1998). This indicates that Jun kinase and NF-kB elicit signals that protect cells against death receptor-induced apoptosis. Moreover, FADD/MORT1, which was originally thought to transducing only a death signal (Hsu et al., 1996), it is now known to be also essential for mitogen-induced proliferation of T lymphocytes (Zhang et al., 1998).

5.3 The role of apoptosis in development, function and homeostasis of lymphocytes

Apoptosis plays a critical role in the immune system, both during the development of B and T cells in primary lymphoid organs as well as during immune responses of mature lymphocytes (Strasser et al., 1995). Programmed cell death is thought to be responsible for the elimination of immature B and T cells that failed to receive a survival signal due to both the lack of growth factors, and either to the failure to productively rearrange antigen receptor genes, or failure of the T cell antigen receptor on thymocytes to bind to MHC molecules on stromal cells (lack of positive selection) (Lu & Osmond, 1997). The effector functions of activated lymphocytes (i.e. secretion of antibodies, production of cytokines or cytotoxicity) are potentially hazardous and it is therefore beneficial to delete these cells when an infection has been overcome (Strasser et al., 1995). The survival of T lymphoblasts is controlled by two distinct mechanisms, both availability of growth factors (e.g. IL-2) and exposure to death ligands (e.g. Fas ligand), which are produced by T cells themselves as a consequence of repeated TCR stimulation (Brunner et al., 1995). The lack of IL-2 triggers a death pathway that can be inhibited by Bcl-2, instead the pathway triggered by Fas ligand is insensitive to Bcl-2 and its homologues (Newton et al., 1998). The death pathway controlled by growth factors and Bcl-2 is thought to be responsible for removing T cells activated by foreign, non-persisting antigens, while death receptor-signaling is critical for removal of activated T cells specific to self-antigens or persistent foreign antigens (Van Parijs et al., 1998).

6. Apoptosis in autoimmune disease

The association between autoimmunity and apoptotic cell death is under extensive investigation. The process of apoptosis defines a series of biochemical and morphologic events that contribute to the normal homeostasis and regulation of immune autoreactivity (Mevorach et al., 1998). During apoptosis, the cellular components as the nucleus, cytosol and, membrane are brought together in close proximity, a mechanism that could lead to epitopes spreading. Altered structures of intracellular proteins produced during cleavage events in apoptosis could also be a source of immunogenic antigens, as cleavage by granzyme B is a common phenomenon for the release of autoantigens. If cell death is excessive, regulatory clearance mechanisms may not effectively remove apoptotic debris, thereby leading to the persistence of antigens for immune system stimulation. Also, the resistance to clearance by defective proteins may lead to autoimmune phenomenon. Furthermore, the rapid clearance of apoptotic cells by macrophages is important to inhibit inflammation and autoimmune responses against intracellular antigens. Mice deficient in receptor tyrosine kinases, such as Tyro 3, Axl, and Mer, have defective clearance of apoptotic cells, lymphadenopathy, and features of autoimmunity (Scott et al., 2001). A common feature of autoimmune diseases such as systemic lupus erythematosus, systemic sclerosis, Sjogren's syndrome, and mixed connective tissue disease is the breakdown of tolerance to self antigens, which induces the production of antibodies reactive with multiple self proteins (Von Muhlen & Tan, 1995). Accumulating evidences show that modifications of autoantigens during apoptosis lead to the development of autoantibodies, thus bypassing normal mechanisms of tolerance (Amoura et al., 1999). Furthermore, direct evidence exists associating faulty apoptotic machinery with the development of autoimmune disease in experimental models and in human disease. Genetic evidences have shown that defects in individual cell-death genes can lead to autoimmune disease. In humans, direct evidence was found in deficient Fas patients, leading to the development of the autoimmune lymphoproliferative syndrome, manifested by lymphadenopathy, renal disease and hemolytic anemia. This syndrome parallels the autoimmune phenomena found in mrl/lpr mice that lack the Fas protein (Straus et al., 1999). In addition, expression of a bcl-2 transgene in mouse B lymphocytes causes extended survival of B lineage cells, sustained humoral immune responses and consequently accumulation of non-transformed B cells and plasma cells and increased levels of serum Ig (O'Reilly et al.,1997). Auto-antibody-secreting plasma cells have been found in normal individuals, but they had no detrimental effect since they were relatively infrequent and short-lived. Expression of a bcl-2 transgene prolongs the survival of such cells and consequently auto-antibodies reach pathogenic levels.

6.1 Apoptosis and systemic lupus erythematosus

Systemic lupus erythematosus (SLE) is an autoimmune disease clinically characterized by a broad variety of symptoms, mostly affecting the joints. In Europe the incidence of this disease is about 1/10,000. Based on new therapeutic approaches, most of the patients will experience a remission and about 90% of SLE patients are still alive after a five year follow-up (Pons-Estel, et al., 2010). The etiopathogenesis of SLE, although partially understood, is due to multifactorial process. Genetic predisposition in association with environmental factors, including infectious agents, drugs, occupational factors, and food may lead to profound alterations in immune system (Love,1994). These changes include the appearance of autoantibodies with different specificity, altered T cell function, as well as a defective phagocytosis and changes in oncogenes (Kalden et al., 1991). In the pathogenesis of systemic lupus erythematosus an important role is due to a dysregulated apoptosis, which may contribute to development of the disease, regulating the induction of nuclear antibodies frequently found in SLE. This hypothesis is partly based on experiments with an animal model used for SLE (i.e. MRL/lpr mice). Mutational inactivation of the genes encoding CD95 (lpr) or its ligand, Fas ligand (gld), cause lymphadenopathy and SLE-like autoimmune disease in mice (Adachi et al., 1995). Two spontaneous mutations found in the CD95 gene have been considered the cause of deficient expression of a membrane molecule Fas/Apo-1 (CD95). Animals with a deficient expression of Fas/Apo 1 molecule showed an insufficient elimination of lymphocytes, leading to the assumption that autoreactive lymphocytes could survive and consequently cause autoimmune phenomena (Watson et al., 1992). However, in all humans with SLE the Fas/Apo-1 dependent apoptosis pathway was unaffected (Mysler et al., 1994), and patients with a defect in the Fas/Apo-1 molecule develop a non malignant lymphoproliferation (Rieux-Laucat, 1995). Although this, it has been reported in patients with SLE increased numbers of apoptotic lymphocytes and macrophages (Emlen et al., 1994). Likely, this could be the result of both a fail during the apoptosis phase and an increased triggering of apoptosis, thus delaying the end of programmed cell death process. A sustained apoptotic activity, due to continuous stimuli, is responsible of producing autoantigens, which may lead to the development of autoantibodies directed against macromolecular complex, thereby acting some pathologic effects. In summary, SLE is a complex disorder in which defects in apoptosis and impaired clearance are strong contributing factors for susceptibility, onset and severity of the disease.

6.2 Apoptosis in rheumatoid arthritis

Rheumatoid arthritis (RA) is a chronic inflammatory disease, characterized by chronic synovial inflammation and synovial cell proliferation, both responsible of "pannus" production. Its development is related to mononuclear cell infiltration, neoangiogenesis, and abnormal proliferation of fibroblast-like synoviocytes (FLS). The pathogenesis of the rheumatoid pannus, has been partly explained by a study on FLS biology (Pap et al., 2000). Two general mechanisms contribute to synovial hyperplasia: increased FLS proliferation and decreased synoviocyte apoptosis. However, apoptotis of synovial cells has been also identified in histologic sections, suggesting that the relative rate of apoptotic cells to proliferating cells is suppressed in proliferating tissues such as in the synovium of RA patients (Sekine et al., 1996). Several studies have examined the mechanisms that could contribute to the resistance against Fas-mediated apoptosis in RA, demonstrating that though Fas is normally expressed by the cells of the pannus both *in vivo* and *in vitro*, the persistence of synovial proliferation in RA patients may lead to bone damage and cartilage erosion (Kawakami et al., 1999). The function of the Fas/FasL system seems to be inadequate to eliminate the cells in the proliferating RA synovium suggesting a strong anti-apoptotic effect in the RA joint.

FLICE inhibitory protein (Flip) is highly expressed at sites of erosion, in the pannus, in the lining, and in the areas of the synovial tissue where apoptosis has not been observed (Perlman et al., 2001). This prospect was supported by the fact that, when synovial tissues were examined by immunohistochemistry, high levels of Flip were associated with low levels of apoptosis in early RA. In contrast, decreased Flip was detected later in the disease course, and this was related with increased apoptosis and decreased numbers of macrophages (Catrina et al., 2002). In addition, it has been supposed that the potential beneficial effects of TNF-α antagonist therapy might be related to the reduction of Flip, which would permit Fas/FasL-mediated apoptosis and result in subsequent clinical improvement.

In the antigen-induced arthritis model of RA, Bcl-2 was present at sites of early erosion and correlated with levels for erosion and inflammation, thus supporting the importance of this factor. Since either the presence of Bcl-2 or anti-apoptotic Bcl-2 family members (Bcl-2, Bcl-xL, A1 and myeloid-cell leukaemia sequence 1) at sites of early erosion in antigen-induced model of arthritis was greatly expressed on synovial fibroblasts, in the synovial lining and in the sublining region from RA patients, it has been largely examined the potential mechanisms that may contribute to the augmented expression of Bcl-2 (Perlman et al., 2001). Activated   NF-kB, has been implicated in the regulation of gene transcription that contributes to cytokine generation, expression of cell surface adhesion epitopes, lymphocyte maturation, protection from TNF-α induced apoptosis, and antigen processing and presentation by MHC class I molecules. NF-kB is expressed in almost all cell types, and plays a significant role in regulating the production of inflammatory cytokines, such as TNF-α, IL-1 and IL-6, as well as anti-apoptotic molecules such as Flip (Pope & Perlman, 2000). Different cytokines such as IL-lβ, platelet-derived growth factor (PDGF), basic fibroblast growth factor (bFGF), transforming growth factor β (TGF-β) and TNF-α are present in synovial tissues of RA patients, promoting the proliferation of human synovial cells. Fas antigen expression on synovial cells is inhibited by the addition of TGF-βl with up-regulation of Bcl-2, Bcl-xL and XIAP. The expression of FLIP, is increased in bFGF-treated synovial cells. These results show that bFGF treatment augmented the expression of FLIP, resulting in resistance toward Fas-mediated apoptosis. The tumour suppressor gene p53 regulates cell cycle, DNA repair, and inhibits angiogenesis. Although, early study reported an upregulation of p53 expression in RA joints (Firestein et al., 1996), a more recent interesting study about the role of several genes, involved in apoptosis mechanisms, reported that p53 gene was deeply reduced in peripheral blood mononuclear cells from patients with RA, SLE, insulin-dependent diabetes mellitus and multiple sclerosis compared with that in normal controls; thus suggesting, that the decreased expression of p53, might contribute to the development of autoimmune disease, possibly by failing to eliminate potentially pathogenetic cells (Maas et al., 2002). Its increase is due to DNA damage, thus permitting DNA repair through cell cycle prolongation, or leading to apoptosis in more severe cases. Deletions, mutations or other mechanisms leading to its lost are often associated with tumour growth.

Although Fas and FasL are greatly expressed on synovial lining macrophages, paucity of apoptosis within the joint might be the result of a variety of mechanisms. An improved understanding of the mechanisms regulating apoptosis will provide insights to aid with a more effective therapy patients with RA.

6.3 Apoptosis and Sjögren's syndrome

Sjögren's syndrome (SS) is a chronic autoimmune disorder, occurring primarily in women, affecting the salivary and lacrimal glands. The histopathological changes in the minor salivary gland biopsy are characterized by the infiltration of these glands by mononuclear cells with secondary destruction of the parenchymal tissue, resulting in oral and ocular dryness (Moutsopoulos et al., 1980). The pathogenesis of glandular damage in Sjögren's syndrome is currently poorly understood; however, the predominance among the infiltrating mononuclear cells of activated CD4+ T cells suggests that cell-mediated immunity plays an important role in tissue destruction (Skopouli et al., 1991). In recent years, it has been reported that the expression of the apoptosis regulating-proteins in salivary glands of Sjögren's syndrome patients suggests a role for apoptotic cell death in the pathogenesis of glandular damage (Patel & McHugh, 2000). The resistance of infiltrating mononuclear cells to apoptosis may result in longer survival that might also increase the production of pro-inflammatory cytokines and autoantibodies, or predispose to the late development of lymphoma in some Sjögren's syndrome patients. T lymphocytes induce apoptotic cell death through either the release of proteases, such as perforin and granzymes, or the interaction of FasL, expressed by activated CD4+ T cells, with Fas on target cells (Russell & Ley, 2002). In murine models, defective signaling and blocked apoptosis caused by mutations in Fas or FasL resulted in autoimmune disease as well as lymphadenopathy (Skarstein et al., 1997). Corresponding mutations were not found in genes encoding Fas and FasL in primary Sjögren's syndrome patients (Bolstad et al., 2000). However, it has been suggested that increased levels of Fas induced apoptosis among epithelial cells explaining the damage of the glands. On the other hand, increased expression of intracellular anti-apoptotic molecules could lead to dysregulation of apoptosis and the formation of large foci of infiltrating mononuclear cells. In the field of autoimmune disease, a common feature is the lack of specific serum markers of disease. Among the most widely used serological markers in confirming the diagnosis of Sjögren's syndrome (SS), there are anti-SSB/La and SSA / Ro antibodies, with a prevalence between 70 and 80% . Although this prevalence is high, they are not specific for Sjögren's syndrome, but also found patients with other autoimmune diseases: anti-SSA / Ro in 35% of patients with systemic lupus erythematosus and 85% of patients with congenital heart block (BCC), and anti-SSB / La in 15% of patients with systemic lupus erythematosus. SSA and SSB are two ribonucleoproteins, located mainly in the nucleus and in the cytoplasm. In patients with Sjögren's syndrome it has been recently studied a new autoantibody that recognizes a structural protein, bound to actin, and that is part of the cytoplasmic skeleton: the α-fodrin (Ulbricht et al., 2003). The fodrin has a localization predominantly near the inner surface of the cell membrane and physiologically it participates in the process of cellular secretion. When antibodies directed against the α-fodrin are present, the cellular mechanism of secretion is impaired. Since the salivary glands are rich in α-fodrin, their secretory mechanism is inhibited, resulting in xerostomia and keratoconjunctivitis sicca. Therefore α-fodrin antibodies would more precocious than those commonly used in the diagnosis of SS (anti-Ro and anti-La), especially in the early stages of the disease. The cleaved α-fodrin fragment has been shown to be a marker of apoptosis (Janicke et al., 1998). Furthermore, a monospecific antibody recognizing the cleaved α-fodrin is available. In Sjögren's syndrome, cleaved α-fodrin autoantigen is greatly expressed on ductal epithelium, on sporadic acinar cells and strongly associated with infiltrating mononuclear cells, however it is rarely detected in normal salivary glands. Further studies are required to verify the specific association of cleaved α-fodrin with primary and secondary Sjögren's syndrome. Therefore based on results of studies of SS-like disease in mice, there may be 2 distinct phases in the pathogenesis of SS (Humphreys-Beher et al., 1999). The first, a lymphocyte-independent step may be characterized by a genetically determined anomaly responsible for epithelial cell apoptosis, resulting in either the production of nucleosomes or the exposure on the cell membrane of autoantigens, such as α-fodrin, SS-A (Ro), and SS-B (La) ribonucleoproteins. In fact, apoptosis allows the translocation either of the ribonucleoproteins SS-A (Ro) and SS-B (La) or the cytoplasmic protein α-fodrin on epithelial cell membranes, where they may be exposed to antigen-presenting cells such as macrophages, and thus generate an autoimmune response (McArthur et al., 2002). After this phase, an elevated expression of proinflammatory cytokines and metalloproteases also may occur, with consequent degradation of epithelial basal membranes (Pérez et al., 2000). The second phase is characterized by mononuclear cells (MNC) infiltration, lymphocyte mediated apoptosis through Fas/FasL interaction, perforin and granzyme B release and production of cytokines

(IFN-γ, TNF-α, and TGF-β1) leading to glandular damage and secretory flow injury (Perez et al., 2000). Improved understanding of the primary cellular events responsible for the glandular damage occurring in SS may allow the discovery of new therapeutic strategies able to interfere with the mediators of apoptosis and thus prevent epithelial cell death and consequent impairment of secretory function.

7. Apoptosis and malignancies

Altered function of apoptosis mechanism occurs frequently in cancers and has been implicated in many events relevant for the pathogenesis and progression of tumours, including cell accumulation caused by failure of programmed cell death (Reed, 1999). Thereby, it may be induce a permissive environment for genetic instability and oncogene activation, promote resistance to immune cell attack, and contribute to resist to the cytotoxic effects of chemotherapy and radiation, allowing tumour cell survival. In the same way, defects in DNA repair and chromosome segregation normally trigger cell suicide as a defence mechanism for eradicating genetically unstable cells. Apoptosis defects permit the survival of the genetically unstable cells, and thus provide opportunities of selection of progressively aggressive clones (Anthoney et al., 1996). In addition, apoptosis defects play a role in tumour resistance to hypoxia, growth factor deprivation, immune surveillance mechanisms, chemotherapy, and radiation (Medh & Thompson, 2000). Tumour immunosuppression that favours tumour progression and metastasis is the consequence of the activation of an immunosuppressive network, mediated by several tumour-derived soluble factors, such as interleukin- 10 (IL-10), transforming growth factor (TGF)- β and vascular endothelial growth factor (VEGF), and which involves the primary tumour site, secondary lymphoid organs and peripheral vessels (Zou, 2005). There are different pathways leading to dysregulated immune responses in cancer and autoimmune disease, such as the impaired clearance of apoptotic cells, played by macrophages. Although the fact that tumour cells generate pro-inflammatory conditions, the immune cells induce an anti-inflammatory environment , due to impaired clearance of apoptotic cells by macrophages during the turnover of tumour cells. The impaired clearance of apoptotic cells induces anti-DNA antibodies to self-antigens that lead to a pseudo-autoimmune status, which, provoking a pro-inflammatory response, allows tumour progression (Kim et al., 2005). The increased concentration of autoantibodies and dendritic cells can induce the production of CD4+ CD25+ regulatory T cells (Tregs) that inhibit T-cell function, causing immunological tolerance (Ward et al., 2004). Thus, it is likely that cancer immunosuppression is produced by tumour-derived soluble factors, due to an anti-inflammatory response to immune cells triggered by a defective apoptotic cell clearance, and increased concentration of Treg cells.

There are significant differences in immunological dysregulation between cancer and autoimmune disease. In the first case, the impaired clearance of apoptotic cells causes accumulation of autoantibodies, which is attributed to the inhibition of T-cell function through increased Treg cells, which play a crucial role in immunological tolerance in cancer cells. In autoimmune diseases, defective apoptotic cell clearance causes accumulation of DNA–IgG immune complexes, which provokes an immune response through Toll-like receptor 9 (TLR9), leading to tissue injury. Unfortunately, the Treg cells are decreased and dysregulated, in this case (Lang et al., 2005).

7.1 Apoptosis and the genes that control it - effect on the malignant phenotype

Elucidation of the genetic alterations of molecules with a central role in apoptosis pathway has provided new insights into tumour biology, revealing novel strategies for combating cancer. More weight has been placed on core apoptosis components such as, Bcl-2 family proteins, death receptor signaling, endogenous inhibitors of caspases, transcriptional control of apoptosis, apoptosis regulation by oncogenes and tumour suppressor genes. The proteins of Bcl-2 family play a key role in the normal regulation of apoptosis and aberrant expression of members of this family has been associated with several tumours. The anti-apoptotic members include Bcl-2 and Bcl-xl and the pro-apoptotic members include Bax, Bad, Bim, Bid (Chang et al., 2003). Experiments involving knockout mice have contributed to our understanding of the role of Bcl-2 family members in tumourigenesis. Bad-knockout mice develop B-cell lymphomas and are less able to hold-out with sub-lethal doses of γ-irradiation (Ranger et al., 2003), while Bid-knockout mice develop myelomonocytic leukemia (Zinkel et al., 2005). Interesting results, involving tumours and Bcl-2, derive from studies undergone on human beings. Over-expression of Bcl-2 has been observed in both B-cell lymphomas (where it was originally discovered) as well as in non-Hodgkin's lymphomas. Furthermore, over-expression of Bcl-2 has been observed in solid tumours such as lung, renal, stomach, and brain cancer. Instead, lower levels of Bcl-2 have been observed in breast cancers. However, either over-expression of Bcl-2 in some subtypes of lymphoma or low levels in breast cancer correlate with poor prognosis (Gascoyne et al., 1997; Chang et al.,2003). It seems that the prognostic value of Bcl-2 expression differs between tumour types and in some cases there may be no correlation with disease progression. The importance of p53 in maintaining genome stability is exemplified by the finding that approximately half of all human tumours carry mutant p53. At present, there are > 10 million people with tumours that contain inactivated p53, while a similar number have tumours in which the p53 pathway is in part blocked by inactivation of other signaling components (Brown et al., 2009). It is well confirmed that the p53 response is defective in most cancers, either by mutations or deletions in the p53 gene, or by alterations in the p53 pathway caused by other oncogenic events. These observations have raised a wide range of clinical possibilities both for diagnosis and treatment, rendering p53 an ideal target for anti-cancer drug design. p53 mutations, the first tumour suppressor gene linked to apoptosis, occur in the most of human tumours and are often associated with advanced tumour stage and poor patient prognosis. Studies using p53 knockout mice demonstrated that endogenous p53 could play a part in apoptosis, in fact p53 has been required for radiation-induced cell death in the thymus, but not cell death induced by glucocorticoids or other apoptotic stimuli (Lowe et al., 1993). p53 can exhibits different and global functions (e.g. promote apoptosis, cell-cycle arrest and senescence). Evidences indicate that p53 apoptotic activity is important in tumour suppression. Therefore, the occurrence of p53 mutations correlates with a decreased apoptosis in some transgenic mice (Attardi & Jacks, 1999) and in clonal progression of tumour cells (Bardeesy et al., 1995). Furthermore alterations of several p53 effectors in apoptosis (e.g. Bax, apaf-1 and casp-9) can promote oncogenic transformation and tumour development in mouse model systems (Soengas et al., 1999). Activation of p53 is sufficient to directly or indirectly trigger apoptosis by inducing pro-apoptotic Bcl-2 family members (Schuler et al., 2000). In addition, alterations in genes encoding various modulators of NF-kB can occur in several types of B-cell malignancies, including non-Hodgkin lymphomas, B-chronic lymphocytic leukemia, and multiple myeloma (Rayet & Gelinas, 1999).

8. The role of TNF-α antagonist therapy in cancer onset

As biologic therapy becomes more common in treating a spectrum of conditions, awareness of side-effects is becoming more important. Mouse models and in vitro experiences indicate that TNF-α plays an important role in tumour growth control. Thus, anti- TNF-α agents might influence the risk of malignancy.

TNF-α is one of main regulator of chronic inflammation and contributes to tumour development, therefore suggesting a role in the progression of solid tumours. However, therapy with TNF-blockers, such as infliximab or etanercept, in patients with advanced cancer was well tolerated, with no evidence of disease acceleration (E.R. Brown et al., 2008). Nevertheless, a systematic review and metanalysis of data from randomized controlled trials of monoclonal antibodies against TNF-α in patients with rheumatoid arthritis showed that there were 29 case of cancers in patients with infliximab group compared to 3 in the control group (Bongartz et al., 2006). In a study of 404 patients with Crohn's disease and 404 matched controls, there were 3 cases of breast cancer in the infliximab-exposed group compared to 1 case in the other group (Biancone et al., 2006). In the Swedish nationwide cancer registry, 4160 patients exposed to TNF-α antagonists (etanercept, infliximab, or adalimumab) were identified (Askling et al., 2005a). Although it has been reported 67 solid cancers, including 8 cases of breast cancer, it has not been found excess risk of solid cancer in this cohort.

TNF-α generates a variety of cellular responses that may either promote or inhibit tumourigenesis. This variability may explain the discrepancies in study results. Some studies on experimental models suggest increased tumour progression with TNF-α blockade. Clinical trials, in contrast, suggest that TNF-α blockade may decrease the activity of solid cancers (kidney and breast). These discordant data generate uncertainty about the potential effects of TNF-α antagonists on the risk of human malignancies in general and on male breast cancer in particular (Williams, 2008). Infliximab is a chimeric mouse-human monoclonal antibody targeting TNF-α. Blocking the actions of tumour necrosis factor-alpha is highly effective in treating several inflammatory disorders. Although safety data have been encouraging, there are reports of immunosuppressive sequelae resulting from the use of the drug.

The soluble dimeric form of p75 TNF receptor, etanercept, binds free TNF in the circulation and cell-bound TNF, thus acting as a competitive inhibitor, blocking TNF interaction with TNF receptors on cell surface (Tsimberidou & Giles, 2002). It inhibits binding of both TNF and lymphotoxin (LT)-a (also known as TNF-β) to cell surface TNF receptors, rendering TNF biologically inactive. It has been postulated that etanercept acts both as a cytokine carrier and TNF antagonist, and can modulate biological responses that are induced or regulated by TNF, such as expression of adhesion molecules responsible for leukocyte migration (Tsimberidou & Giles, 2002). Etanercept has shown activity and is currently indicated in patients with moderately to severely active rheumatoid arthritis; moderately to severely active polyarticular-course juvenile rheumatoid arthritis with inadequate response to disease-modifying antirheumatic drugs; or psoriatic arthritis (Lovell et al., 2000; Mease et al., 2000). In a pilot study, it was given Etanercept to 13 patients affected by cutaneous T-cell lymphoma (CTCL), because of the role played by TNF in tumour progression. An improvement was observed in patients with early disease, and a larger cohort of patients with early disease merits investigation, while it is unlikely that it will be effective in patients with advanced CTCL (Tsimberidou et al., 2004).

Adalimumab is a fully human recombinant IgG1 monoclonal antibody with specificity for human TNF-α. Bongartz et al. (2006) conducted a systematic review and meta-analysis that included 9 trials employing either infliximab or adalimumab in 3493 patients with RA versus 1512 patients taking placebo to further elucidate the carcinogenic potential of TNF-α blockers. The odds ratio for malignancy was found to be 3.3, and the incidence of cancer was associated with higher doses of the biologic. For patients treated with anti-TNF-α antibodies included in these trials, the number needed to harm was 154 within the 6- to 12-month follow-up period. But the study failed to give some adjustments.

The relationship between lymphoma and TNF-α blockers has been documented in a few case reports focusing on psoriasis patients. One report reviewed relevant data in the MedWatch postmarketing adverse event surveillance system run by the Food and Drug Administration and discovered 26 cases of lymphoma following treatment with either etanercept (18 cases) or infliximab (8 cases) (S.L. Brown, 2002). Frequently, those receiving etanercept were reported to be taking MTX concurrently (5 of 18) or had a history of prior exposure to MTX (4 of 18), or a history of exposure to another immunosuppressive agent (4 of 18). Another noteworthy clinical feature of the lymphomas observed was the very short latent period of only few weeks between the initiation of anti-TNF therapy and the development of malignancy.

In two instances (one etanercept, one infliximab), lymphoma regression was observed following discontinuation of the TNF-α -blocker in the absence of specific cytotoxic therapy directed toward the lymphoma.

The association between lymphoma and biologic therapy was weakened by data reported by Askling et al. (2005b) who epidemiologically studied cohorts of RA patients with either long-standing disease, incident disease, or TNF-α -antagonist treated disease linked with the Swedish Cancer Registry. The lymphoma risk in those treated with TNF-blockers was no higher versus the other RA cohorts, given that the standardized incidence ratio (SIR) for RA patients on TNF blockers was 2.9 and not statistically significant after adjustment for sex, age, and disease duration from the SIR of 2.0 in control subjects with RA.

A study reviewed 1440 patients having psoriasis treated with etanercept for more than 5 years, without founding any increase of malignancies (Burge, 2003). However, a multitude of recent case reports have begun to strengthen the link between anti-TNF-α therapy and induction or rapid reactivation of latent malignancies.

In the literature many case-reports were found about the cancer onset after anti-TNF-α therapy, such as anorectal carcinoma (Melichar et al.,_2006) and non-Hodgkin Lymphoma (Bickston et al., 1999) after infliximab therapy in Crohn's disease, cutaneous and systemic T-cell lymphoma after treatment with infliximab and also with etanercept (Adams et al., 2004). One reason for the safety concerns surrounding anti-TNF-α therapy is the role of the members of the TNF family in normal immune system development and function (Bazzoni & Beutler, 1996). However, "knock-out" mutations of the TNF gene complex in mouse models of disease cause an increased susceptibility to certain infections, but not autoimmunity or malignancy (Erickson et al., 1994). In addition, it is noteworthy the absence of a clear immunosuppressive effects of TNF antagonism in preclinical and human studies. Thus, in contrast to the pleiotropic effects of TNF with the immune system, blockade of TNF with infliximab does not suppress global immune function in the manner of drugs such as azathioprine (Meenan et al., 1997). Therapy with infliximab has not been associated with decreases in absolute lymphocyte counts (Meenan et al., 1997), development of anergy (Feldmann et al., 1997), or emergence of opportunistic viral and fungal infections. Together, these data suggest that blockade of TNF with a drug such as infliximab may lead to limited and selective rather than broad-spectrum immune suppression.

Also for adalimumab therapy carried on patients affected by rheumatoid arthritis it was observed the incidence of cancer, especially the onset of melanoma in two patients, after two years from the start of therapy with adalimumab (Dewan et al., 2009).

However, it is not easy to establish clearly the real risk associated with anti- TNF-α therapies because of various confounding factors including possible increased predisposition to cancer due to the underlying disorder and the concomitant or prior use of other potentially cancer-promoting therapies.

9. Possible link between autoimmune diseases and cancer

In many systemic autoimmune diseases, where disproportional humoral autoimmune responses are pivotal in the pathogenesis (e.g. systemic lupus erythematosus and Sjögren's syndrome), exaggerated B-cell processes exist, resembling B-cell malignancies (Illes et al., 2009). Both conditions are characterized by cell-cycle regulation abnormalities, which affect lymphocyte survival, proliferation and differentiation, as well.

9.1 Systemic lupus erythematosus

Systemic lupus erythematosus (SLE) is a systemic autoimmune disease, characterized by a wide array of symptoms and organ involvements, leading to varying disease courses and outcome. In patients with SLE, the incidence and risk of malignancy development is increased. The malignancies occurred frequently in SLE patients are Non-Hodgkin's Lymphoma, Hodgkin's Lymphoma, as well as solid tumours, as lung, cervical and breast cancer (Kiss et al., 2010).

The frequent occurrence of malignancies can be associated with the common pathogenetic pathways for cancer and autoimmune disease development. This phenomenon is reinforced by the following notions: generally, in autoimmune diseases malignancies occur with high frequency; in neoplastic disorders, autoimmune diseases can develop, as part of the paraneoplastic syndrome; also, immunosuppressive treatment in autoimmune diseases increases the development of malignancies (Zintzaras et al., 2005).

The long-term, in many instances aggressive immunosuppressive treatment in lupus is evidently related to the development of malignant transformations and manifest tumours. Besides these common extrinsic etiological factors, the intrinsic errors of the immune system contribute to the development of both disease entities (Bernatsky et al., 2002).

9.1.1 Cancer before systemic lupus erythematosus

Since the clinical appearance of Non-Hodgkin's Lymphoma and systemic lupus erythematosus is similar, and it is sometimes difficult to distinguish the two disease entities in the initial phases, these raise the possibility that SLE might be a paraneoplastic syndrome and appears on the grounds of the lymphoid malignancy (Kiss et al., 2010).

9.1.2 Cancer after systemic lupus erythematosus

The pathogenic background behind the more frequent presence of NHL in SLE can be due to the chronic, persistent antigen-stimulus, chronic inflammation, uncontrolled B cell proliferation, defected apoptosis, and the increased risk of oncogene translocation. Common environmental and genetic factors, linked with major histocompatibility complex (MHC)-associated genes, further contribute to lymphomagenesis in lupus. Also, treatment with immunomodulating and immunosuppressive drugs, commonly used in SLE can contribute to the development of lymphomagenesis, either by directly causing mutagenesis, or by weakening the immune surveillance, which can lead to uncontrolled B cell proliferation (Kiss et al., 2010).

In 9% of SLE patients may occur some inflammatory diseases, such as pneumonitis-fibrosis or bronchiolitis obliterans organizing pneumonia, that may lead to a chronic stimulation and extensive DNA damage which underlie lung cancer.

Moreover, in female affected by SLE it has been reported a higher risk of breast cancer, without any family history or exogenous hormonal exposure (Ramsey-Goldman et al., 1998). Thereby, likely the pathological immune responses triggered by the autoimmune disease can lead to uncontrolled cell proliferation and decreased apoptosis, and breast cancer development, indeed (Kiss et al.,2010).

9.1.3 Antiphospholipid antibodies

Another link between lupus and malignant diseases can be served by antiphospholipid antibodies (aPL), frequently present in SLE and cancer as well.

Patients with cancer are at higher risk of thromboembolic complications than healthy people for many reasons. It is known that an important thrombogenic mechanism is mediated by antiphospholipid antibodies (aPL). Although the evidence on their association, the relationship between aPL presence and cancer is contradictory. It is unclear whether aPL antibody positivity has a pathogenetic role in the development of thromboses or whether, in contrast, these antibodies are an epiphenomenon in cancer patients (Reinstein & Shoenfeld, 2007).

In the last years a higher prevalence of aPL antibodies was observed in patients with solid tumours compared to controls (Zuckerman et al., 1995) and in patients with haematological malignancies (Pusterla et al., 2004). The reasons of this increased antibody production are only partially clarified: their production may be induced by particular immunotherapy of cancer such as interferon α (Becker et al., 1994) or started by immune system response to new tumour antigens (Sawamura et al., 1994).

In particular it is possible that autoantibodies to malignant cells arise secondary to changes in the cell membrane that induce exposure of certain antigens that are normally facing the intracellular compartment (Reinstein & Shoenfeld, 2007), then activating pathogenetic autoreactive human T cells (Yamaguchi et al., 2007). In this context, it has been reported that viable tumour cells (Fernandes et al., 2006) as well as tumour blood vessels (Ran et al., 2002) showed increased exposure of anionic phospholipids on the outer layer of their membranes, directly triggering coagulation cascade by providing a procoagulatory surface (Vogt et al., 1997). Therefore, tumour microenvironment may be a source of anionic lipid surfaces that facilitate aPL antibodies production. It is also possible that tumoural cells directly synthetize antibodies as in the case of multiple myeloma or Waldenstrom's macroglobulinemia (Tincani et al., 2010).

Moreover, an interesting study carried on aPL antibodies healthy carriers, reported that the major cause of morbidity and mortality was the occurrence of malignancies, in particular non-Hodgkin's lymphoma seemed to affect this group with an higher incidence than the general population (Finazzi, 1997).

9.2 Rheumatic arthritis

The link between autoimmune phenomena, particularly rheumatic arthritis, and cancers has been suggested in several studies. It may be due to the generation of autoantibodies against self and non-self antigens, paraneoplastic syndromes or by chemotherapy.

As the presence of autoantibodies has been identified in the sera of patients both with solid tumours and haematological malignancies, it may be considered as the consequence of the immune response against the tumour (Conrad, 2000).

The natural autoantibodies (NAA), frequently occurring in high titres in the sera of patients with multiple myeloma, Waldenstrom's macroglobulinemia, chronic lymphocytic leukaemia, and B cell lymphoma, are generated by CD5+ B cells. They are mainly IgM, which bind with low affinity self and non-self antigens, and they also have rheumatoid factor activity (Abu-Shakra et al., 2001). This autoantibody activity is the result of malignant transformation of B cells, that produce autoantibodies (Dighiero, 1998).

9.2.1 Cancer after rheumatic arthritis

An increased occurrence of malignancies in patients with established rheumatoid arthritis (RA) has been found by several studies (Bernatsky et al., 2006). In most cases, the higher rate of cancer is linked to the use of immunosuppressive therapy, and the tumour generally takes several years to develop.

9.2.2 Cancer before rheumatic arthritis

However, the early manifestation of an occult malignancy may be a rapid-onset arthritis mimicking rheumatoid arthritis. More often, the rheumatoid arthritis-like syndrome precedes the development of cancer by 6–12 months. (Racanelli et al., 2008)

Rheumatoid arthritis-like syndromes have been associated with malignancies of the lung, colon, breast, ovary, stomach and oropharynx cancer and with haematopoietic malignancies. (Andrai et al., 2006)

Patients with paraneoplastic rheumatic disease generally exhibit a form of asymmetric polyarthritis that may be confused with seronegative rheumatoid arthritis or spondyloarthropathy.

The paraneoplastic disorders disappear after surgical removal or pharmacological treatment of the cancer, otherwise these treatments have any influence on rheumatic symptoms that are tumour-associated (Naschitz, 2001).

9.3 Polymyositis and dermatomyositis

The association between malignancy and autoimmune myositis, in particular polymyositis (PM) and dermatomyositis (DM), has been largely described (Briani et al., 2006). The diagnosis of tumour can precede, parallel or follow myositis diagnosis. Most commonly cancer is diagnosed after the onset of myositis, but in many cases the course of the myopathy paralleled the course of the tumour (Zampieri et al., 2010). The incidence of cancer in patients with an established autoimmune myopathies was estimated ranging from 6% to 60% (Hill et al., 2001). In contrast, the incidence of myopathies as an early manifestation of an occult malignancies is undefined.

9.3.1 Cancer before autoimmune myositis

The malignancies more frequently associated with PM and DM are ovarian, colorectal, breast, and lung cancer (Wakata et al., 2002). The so called "paraneoplastic" inflammatory myopathies are autoimmune myositis, that develop in patients with primary cancer as the consequence of its presence. In the paraneoplastic syndromes the surgical removal or pharmacological treatment of cancer results in the disappearance of the clinical symptoms of the paraneoplastic disease (Raccanelli et al., 2008). Some myopathies can develop also in response to chemotherapeutic agents used to treat cancer (Chakravarty & Genovese, 2003). The paraneoplastic myositis show different clinical features and laboratory data, as well as a later onset and a lower or absent response to immunosuppressive drugs (Buchbinder et al., 2001).

9.3.2 Cancer after autoimmune myositis

Patients with DM have a greater risk of developing malignancy than the general population, while PM patients seem to be associated to a lesser extent to an increased risk. Also the drugs used to treat autoimmune myositis can be responsible for cancer onset in these patients. These drugs are administered in order to modulate the response of immune system and therefore their use can induce an altered state of immune surveillance which can be responsible for the consequent development of tumour (Szekanecz et al., 2006).

The pathogenetic molecular mechanisms underlying the association between cancer and myositis are still unknown, even though some hypotheses have been purposed (Eisenlohr & Rothstein, 2006). It is possible that an immune response directed against cancer cells in both breast and lung adenocarcinoma, as well as hepatocellular carcinoma, cross-reacts with regenerating muscle cells (Casciola-Rosen et al., 2005). These regenerating muscle fibers and tumour cells expressing myositis specific autoantigens, may be responsible for the induction of autoimmune response in those patients with a predisposing genetic background to autoimmunity. Casciola-Rosen et al. (2005) have been demonstrated that some tumours (e.g. breast, lung adenocarcinoma, and hepatocellular carcinoma), but not the corresponding normal tissues, express high levels of myositis autoantigens. It has been also demonstrated that in affected muscles from myositis patients, regenerating myoblasts overexpress myositis specific autoantigens and notably the expression of these autoantigens by tumour cells as well as by regenerating myoblasts, indicates a possible antigenic similarity between the two cell populations (Casciola-Rosen et al., 2005).

9.4 Sjögren's syndrome

The link between Sjögren's syndrome (SS) and non-Hodgkin's lymphoma (NHL) is one of the strongest among all the known associations between systemic autoimmune diseases and malignancies. The occurrence of NHL has been reported to be as much as 44-fold greater in Sjögren's syndrome than in the general population (Kovács et al., 2010). In the majority of patients, the histopathologic type of lymphoma is mucosa-associated lymphoid tissue (MALT) type B cell lymphoma, i.e. extranodal marginal zone B cell lymphoma, and in about 30% of SS patients, other types of NHL can be observed. In SS, the predominant cellular components of the focal lymphocytic infiltration in the salivary glands are CD4+T lymphocytes. The evolution of a malignant proliferation of B-lymphocytes from this inflammatory infiltration is due to a complex process. The ultimate step in this process is the transition from benign B cell proliferation to malignant expansion. The uncontrolled expansion of B-lymphocytes is a result of various genetic alterations, typically translocations involving immunoglobulin gene loci and proto-oncogenes or other genes involved in cell-cycle regulation (Kovács et al., 2010).

10. Conclusion

The relationship between autoimmunity and cancer has been investigated, focusing on implication of immune system, apoptosis and new therapeutic agents for autoimmune diseases. Autoimmune diseases, characterized by chronic inflammatory state, with continuous antigenic stimulation, may contribute to haematological malignancies and solid tumours development. However , the role of new therapeutic agents, as biologic drugs used more frequently in autoimmune diseases treatment, is controversial and need further studies in depth, since they may be involved in cancer onset, as well. The autoimmune diseases, as rheumatoid disorders, systemic lupus erythematosus or myositis may occur before or concomitant with a tumour, as paraneoplastic syndromes, which regress after cancer removal.

Apoptosis is a critical regulator of cellular and humoral immune responses, appearing to play a critical role in the deletion of lymphocytes after an inflammatory state, as well as in the control of tumour cell survival, leading to unchecked tumour growing, if the genes of apoptosis show some mutations. Therefore, understanding normal apoptosis mechanisms is critical for developing a better know-how from which to undertake strategies for improving autoimmune diseases and cancer therapy.

In addition, it is an interesting task the different immune responses against autoantigen occurring during autoimmunity and cancer, which are involved in alterations of immunological tolerance and maintenance of immunological tolerance, respectively. Thus it is easy to understand that immunological tolerance in cancer and autoimmune disease has opposite effects in the patient: in cancer patients it stimulates the growth of the cancer, but in patients with autoimmune disease immunological tolerance may stop the attack by autoantibodies and thereby benefit the patient. In fact, cancer cells are able to employ a pseudo-autoimmune status (cancer associated autoimmune disease) and induce immunological tolerance by producing autoantibodies to tumour antigens derived from impaired clearance of apoptotic cells, resulting in an increase of regulatory T cells, thus increasing tolerance toward tumour cells.

However, further investigations are needed to better define new therapeutic strategies controlling inflammatory components, responsible of both autoimmunity and cancer progression.

11. References

Abu-Shakra, M.; Buskila, D.; Ehrenfeld, M. et al. (2001) Cancer and autoimmunity: autoimmune and rheumatic features in patients with malignancies, *Ann Rheum Dis*, Vol.60,pp.433-440

Adachi, M.; Suematsu, S.; Kondo, T. et al. (1995). Targeted mutation in the Fas gene causes hyperplasia in peripheral lymphoid organs and liver. *Nature Genet*, Vol.11, pp. 294–300

Afzali, B.; Lombardi, G.; Lechler, R.I. et al. (2007) The role of T helper 17 (Th17) and regulatory T cells   (Treg) in human organ transplantation and autoimmune disease, *Clin Exp Immunol*, Vol. 148,pp. 32–46

Amoura, Z.; Piette, J.C.; Bach, J.F. et al. (1999) The key role of nucleosomes in Lupus. *Arthritis Rheum*, Vol. 42, pp833-843

Andrai, C.; Csiki, Z.; Ponyi, A. et al. (2006) Paraneoplastic rheumatic syndromes. *Rheumatol Int*. Vol. 26, pp.376–82.

Anthoney, D.A.; McIlwrath, A.J.; Gallagher, W.M. et al. (1996). Microsatellite Instability, Apoptosis, and Loss of p53 Function in Drug-resistant Tumour Cells. *Cancer Res*, Vol.56, pp. 1374- 1381

Askling, J.; Fored, C.M.; Brandt, L. et al. (2005a) Risks of solid cancers in patients with rheumatoid arthritis and after treatment with tumour necrosis factor antagonists, *Ann Rheum Dis*, Vol. 64, pp.1421-6

Askling, J.; Fored, S.M.; Baecklund, E. et al. (2005b) Haematopoietic malignancies in rheumatoid arthritis: lymphoma risk and characteristics after exposure to tumour necrosis factor antagonists, *Ann Rheum Dis*, Vol.64, pp. 1414-20.

Attardi, L.D. & Jacks, T. (1999). The role of p53 in tumour suppression: lessons from mouse models. *Cell Mol. Life Sci.*, Vol.55, pp.48–63

Baechler, E.C.; Batliwalla, F.M.; Karypis, G. et al. (2003). Interferon-inducible gene expression signature in peripheral blood cells of patients with severe lupus. *Proc. Natl. Acad. Sci.* USA, Vol.100, pp. 2610–2615

Bardeesy, N.; Beckwith, J.B. & Pelletier, J. (1995) Clonal expansion and attenuated apoptosis in Wilms' tumours are associated with p53 gene mutations. *Cancer Res.*, Vol.55, pp.215–219

Bazzoni, F. & Beutler, B. (1996) The tumor necrosis factor ligand and receptor families. *N Engl J Med*, Vol.334, pp. 1717-1725

Becker, J.C.; Winkler, B.; Klingert, S. et al. (1994) Antiphospholipid syndrome associated with immunotherapy for patients with melanoma, *Cancer*, Vol.73, No. (6), pp.1621- 4

Bei, R.; Masuelli, L.; Palumbo, C. et al. (2009) A common repertoire of autoantibodies is shared by cancer and autoimmune disease patients: inflammation in their induction and impact on tumour growth. *Cancer Lett*, Vol. 281, pp.8–23

Bernatsky, S.; Clarke, A. & Ramsey-Goldman, R. (2002) Malignancy and systemic lupus erythematosus. *Curr Rheumatol Rep*, Vol.4, No. (4), pp.351–8

Bernatsky, S.; Ramsey-Goldman, R. & Clarke, A. (2006) Malignancy and autoimmunity, *Curr Opin Rheumatol*, Vol.18, pp.129–34

Bernatsky, S.; Lee, J.L. & Rahme, E. (2007) Non-Hodgkin's lymphoma — meta-analyses of the effects of corticosteroids and non-steroidal anti-inflammatories. *Rheumatology*; Vol. 46, pp.690–4

Biancone, L.; Orlando, A.; Kohn, A. et al. (2006) Infliximab and newly diagnosed neoplasia in Crohn's disease: a multicentre matched pair study. *Gut*, Vol.55, pp.228-33

Bickston, S.J.; Lichtenstein, G.R.; Arseneau K.O. et al. (1999) The Relationship Between Infliximab Treatment and Lymphoma in Crohn's Disease. *Gastroenterology*, Vol. 117, pp.1433–1437

Boldin, M.P.; Goncharov, T.M.; Goltsev, Y.V. et al. (1996). Involvement of MACH, a novel MORT1/FADD-interacting protease, in Fas/APO-1- and TNF receptor-induced cell death. *Cell*, Vol.85, pp. 803-815

Bolstad, A.I.; Wargelius, A.; Nakken, B. et al. (2000). Fas and Fas ligand gene polymorphisms in primary Sjögren's syndrome. *J Rheumatol*, Vol.27, pp.2397–2405

Bongartz, T.; Sutton, A.J.; Sweeting, M.J. et al. (2006) Anti-TNF antibody therapy in rheumatoid arthritis and the risk of serious infections and malignancies: systematic review and meta-analysis of rare harmful effects in randomized controlled trials, *JAMA*, Vol. 295, pp.2275-85

Briani, C.; Doria, A.; Sarzi-Puttini, P. et al. (2006) Update on idiopathic inflammatory myopathies. *Autoimmunity*, Vol. 39, pp.161–70

Brown, C.J.; Lain, S.; Verma, C.S. et al. (2009). Awakening guardian angels: drugging the p53 pathway. *Nat Rev Cancer*, Vol.9, No.12, pp. 862-873

Brown, E.R.; Charles, K.A.; Hoare, S.A. et al. (2008) A clinical study assessing the tolerability and biological effects of infliximab, a TNF-alpha inhibitor, in patients with advanced cancer, *Ann Oncol*, Vol. 19,pp.1340-6

Brown, S.L.; Greene, M.H.; Gershon, S.K. et al. (2002) Tumour necrosis factor antagonist therapy and lymphoma development, *Arthritis Rheum*, Vol.46, pp.3151-8

Brunner, T.; Mogil, R.J.; La Face, D. et al. (1995). Cell-autonomous Fas (CD95)/Fas-ligand interaction mediates activation-induced apoptosis in T-cell hybridomas. *Nature*, Vol.373, pp. 441–444.

Buchbinder, R.; Forbes, A.; Hall, S. et al. (2001) Incidence of malignant disease in biopsy-proven inflammatory myopathy. A population-based cohort study. *Ann Intern Med*, Vol. 134, pp.1087–95.

Burge, D. (2003) Etanercept and squamous cell carcinoma. *J Am Acad Dermatol*, Vol. 49,pp.358-9.

Burnet, F.M. (1988). 'The Clonal Selection Theory of Acquired Immunity', In: *Milestones in Immunology: A Historical Exploration*, Debra Jan Bibel (Ed.), 185-187, Science Tech, London

Cao, D.; Malmström, V.; Baecher-Allan, C. et al. (2003) Isolation and functional characterization of regulatory CD25bright CD4+ T cells from the target organ of patients with rheumatoid arthritis, *Eur J Immunol*; Vol. 33, No. (1), pp. 215–223.

Casciola-Rosen, L.; Nagaraju, K.; Plots, P. et al. (2005) Enhanced autoantigen expression in regenerating muscle cells in idiopathic inflammatory myopathy. *J Exp Med*, Vol.4, pp.591–601

Catrina, A.I.; Ulfgren, A.K.; Lindblad, S. et al. (2002). Low levels of apoptosis and high FLIP expression in early rheumatoid arthritis synovium. *Ann Rheum Dis*, Vol.61, pp.934-936

Cellier, C.; Delabesse, E.; Helmer, C. et al. (2000) Refractory sprue, coeliac disease, and enteropathy associated T-cell lymphoma. *Lancet*, Vol.356, pp.203–8

Cepika, A.M.; Marinic, I.; Morovic-Vergles, J. et al. (2007) Effect of steroids on the frequency of regulatory T cells and expression of FOXP3 in a patient with systemic lupus erythematosus: A two-year follow-up, *Lupus*, Vol. 16, No.(5), pp.374–377

Chakravarty, E. & Genovese, M.C. (2003) Rheumatic syndromes associated with malignancy. *Curr Opin Rheumatol*, Vol. 15, No. , pp.35–43

Chang, J.; Clark, G.M.; Allred, D.C. et al. (2003). Survival of patients with metastatic breast carcinoma: importance of prognostic markers of the primary tumour. *Cancer*, Vol.97, No.3, pp. 545-553

Chen, M.L.; Pittet, M.J.; Gorelik, L. et al. (2005) Regulatory T cells suppress tumour-specific CD8 T cell cytotoxicity through TGF-beta signals *in vivo*, *Proc Natl Acad Sci U S A*, Vol. 102, pp. 419-424

Chinnaiyan, A.M.; O'Rourke, K.; Tewari, M. et al. (1995). FADD, a novel death domain-containing protein interacts with the death domain of Fas and initiates apoptosis. *Cell*, Vol.81, pp. 505-512

Ciric, B.; El-behi, M.; Cabrera, R. et al. (2009) IL-23 drives pathogenic IL-17- producing CD8+ T cells, *J Immunol*, Vol.182, pp.5296–5305.

Conrad, K. (2000) Autoantibodies in cancer patients and in persons with a higher risk of cancer development. In: *Cancer and autoimmunity*, Shoenfeld, Y. & Gershwin, M.F. (Eds.), 159-74, Elsevier, The Netherlands.

Coussens, L.M. & Werb, Z. (2002) Inflammation and cancer, *Nature*, Vol.420, pp.860–7

Curiel,T.J.; Coukos, G.; Zou, L. et al (2004) Specific recruitment of regulatory T cells in ovarian carcinoma fosters immune privilege and predicts reduced survival, *Nat Med*, Vol. 10, pp. 942-949

Dewan, P.; Jawad, A.; Goldsmith, P. et al. (2009) Melanoma in patients with rheumatoid arthritis treated with antitumour necrosis factor: cause or coincidence? Report of two cases, *British Journal of Dermatology, Vol.* 161, pp1399–1424

Dighiero, G. (1998) Autoimmunity and B-cell malignancies *Hematol Cell Ther*, Vol.40, pp.1–9

Eisenlohr, L.C. & Rothstein, J.L. (2006) Oncogenic inflammation and autoimmune disease, *Autoimmun Rev, Vol.* 6, pp.*107–14*

Emlen, W.; Niebur, J., & Kadera, R. (1994). Accelerated in vitro apoptosis of lymphocytes from patients with systemic lupus erythematosus. *J Immunol*, Vol.152, pp. 3685-3692

Engels, E.A. (2007) Infectious agents as causes of non-Hodgkin lymphoma. *Cancer Epidemiol Biomarkers Prev*, Vol.16, pp.401–4

Erickson, S.L.; de Sauvage, F.J.; Kikly, K. et al. (1994) Decreased sensitivity to tumour-necrosis factor but normal T-cell development in TNF receptor-2–deficient mice, *Nature*, Vol.372, pp. 560–563

Eskes, R.; Desagher, S.; Antonsson, B. et al. (2000). Bid induces the oligomerization and insertion of Bax into the outer mitochondrial membrane. *Mol Cell Biol*, Vol.20, pp. 929-935

Feldmann, M.; Elliott, M.J.; Woody, J. et al. (1997) Anti-tumour necrosis factor alpha therapy of RA, *Adv Immunol*, Vol.64, pp.283–350

Fernandes, R.S.; Kirszberg, C.; Rumjanek, V.M. et al. (2006) On the molecular mechanisms for the highly procoagulant pattern of C6 glioma cells, *J Thromb Haemost*, Vol.4, pp.1546–52

Finazzi, G. (1997) The Italian registry of antiphospholipid antibodies, *Haematologica*, Vol. 82, No. (1), pp.101–5

Firestein, G.S.; Nguyen, K.; Aupperle, K.R. et al. (1996). Apoptosis in rheumatoid arthritis: p53 overexpression in rheumatoid arthritis synovium. *Am J Pathol*, Vol.149, pp. 2143-2151

Gascoyne, R.D.; Adomat, S.A.; Krajewski, S. et al. (1997). Prognostic significance of Bcl-2 protein expression and Bcl-2 gene rearrangement in diffuse aggressive non-Hodgkin's lymphoma. *Blood*, Vol.90, No.1, pp. 244-251

Goodnow, C.C. (2007) Multistep pathogenesis of autoimmune disease, *Cell*; Vol.130,pp. 25–35

Hill, C.L.; Zhang, Y.; Sigurgeirsson, B. et al. (2001) Frequency of specific cancer types in dermatomyositis and polymyositis: a population-based study. *Lancet*, Vol. 357, pp.96–100.

Holzelova, E.; Vonarbourg, C.; Stolzenberg, M.C. et al. (2004) Autoimmune lymphoproliferative syndrome with somatic Fas mutations, *N Engl J Med*, Vol.351, pp.1409-18

Hori, S.; Nomura, T. & Sakaguchi, S. (2003) Control of regulatory T cell development by the transcription factor Foxp3, *Science*, Vol.299, No.(5609), pp.1057-1061

Hsu, H.; Shu, H.B.; Pan, M.G. et al. (1996). TRADD-TRAF2 and TRADD-FADD interactions define two distinct TNF Receptor 1 signal transduction pathways. *Cell*, Vol.84, pp. 299-308

Humphreys-Beher, M.G.; Peck, A.B.; Dang, H. et al. (1999). The role of apoptosis in the initiation of the autoimmune response in Sjögren's syndrome. *Clin Exp Immunol*, Vol.116, pp.383-387

Illes, A.; Varoczy, L.; Papp, G. et al. (2009) Aspects of B-cell non- Hodgkin's lymphoma development: a transition from immune-reactivity to malignancy, *Scand J Immunol*, Vol.69, No.(5), pp.387-400

Irmler, M.; Thome, M.; Hahne, M. et al. (1997). Inhibition of death receptor signals by cellular FLIP. *Nature*, Vol.388, pp. 190-195

Itoh, N. & Nagata, S. (1993). A novel protein domain required for apoptosis: mutational analysis of human Fas antigen. *J Biol Chem.*, Vol.268, pp. 10932-10937

Janicke, R.U.; Ng, P.; Sprengart, M.L. et al. (1998). Caspase-3 is required for a-fodrin cleavage but dispensable for cleavage of other death substrates in apoptosis. *J Biol Chem*, Vol.273, pp.15540-15545

Kalden, J.R.; Winkler, T.H.; Herrmann, M. et al. (1991). Pathogenesis of SLE: Immunopathology in man. *Rheumatol Int*, Vol.11, pp. 95-100

Kawakami, A.; Nakashima, T.; Sakai, H. et al. (1999). Regulation of synovial cell apoptosis by proteasome inhibitor. *Arthritis Rheum*, Vol.42, pp. 2440-2448

Kelliher, M.A.; Grimm, S.; Ishida, Y. et al. (1998). The death domain kinase RIP mediates the TNF-induced NF-kB signal. *Immunity*, Vol.8, pp. 297-303

Kim, R.; Emi, M. & Tanabe, K. (2005). Cancer cell immune escape and tumour progression by exploitation of anti-inflammatory and pro inflammatory responses. *Cancer Biol Ther*, Vol.4, pp.924-933

Kischkel, F.C.; Hellbardt, S.; Behrmann, I. et al. (1995). Cytotoxicity-dependent APO-1 (Fas/CD95)-associated proteins form a death-inducing signaling complex (DISC) with the receptor. *EMBO J*, Vol.14, pp. 5579-5588

Kiss, E.; Kovacs, L. & Szodoray, P. (2010) Malignancies in systemic lupus erythematosus, *Autoimmun Rev*, Vol.9, pp.195-9

Kolls, J.K. & Linden, A. (2004) Interleukin-17 family members and inflammation, *Immunity*,Vol. 21, p.467-476

Kormeyer, S.J. (1995) Regulators of cell death. *Trends Genet* , Vol.11, pp.101-105

Kovács, L.; Szodoray,P. & Kiss, E. (2010) Secondary tumours in Sjögren's syndrome, *Autoimmunity Reviews*, Vol.9, pp.203-206

Kryczek, I.; Banerjee, M.; Cheng, P. et al. (2009) Phenotype, distribution, generation, functional and clinical relevance of Th17 cells in the human tumour environments, *Blood*, Vol. 114, pp.1141-9

Kuhn, A.; Beissert, S. & Krammer, P.H. (2009) CD4+ CD25+ regulatory T cells in human lupus erythematosus, *Arch Dermatol Res*, Vol.301, No.(1), pp.71-81

La Cava, A. (2008) T-regulatory cells in systemic lupus erythematosus, *Lupus*, Vol.17, No.(5), pp.421–425

Landgren, O.; Engels, E.A., Pfeiffer, R.M. et al. (2006) Autoimmunity and susceptibility to Hodgkin lymphoma: a population based case–control study in Scandinavia. *J Natl Cancer Inst*,Vol. 98, pp.1321–30

Lang, K.S.; Recher, M.; Junt, T. et al. (2005). Toll-like receptor engagement converts T-cell autoreactivity into overt autoimmune disease. *Nat Med*, Vol.1, pp.138-145

Langier, S.; Sade, K. & Kivity, S. (2010) Regulatory T cells: The suppressor arm of the immune system. *Autoimmunity Reviews*, Vol.10, pp.112-115

Lawson, C.A.; Brown, A.K., Bejarano, V. et al. (2006) Early rheumatoid arthritis is associated with a deficit in the CD4+ CD25high regulatory T cell population in peripheral blood, *Rheumatology*, Vol.45, No. (10), pp.1210–1217

Lee, J.H.; Wang, L.C.; Lin, Y.T. et al. (2006) Inverse correlation between CD4+ regulatory T-cell population and autoantibody levels in paediatric patients with systemic lupus erythematosus, *Immunology*, Vol.117, No.(2),pp. 280–286

Linden, A.; Laan, M. & Anderson, G.P. (2005) Neutrophils, interleukin-17A and lung disease, *Eur Respir J*, Vol. 25, pp.159–172

Lorenz, H.M.; Herrmann, M.; Winkler, T. et al (2000). Role of apoptosis in autoimmunity. *Apoptosis*, Vol.5, pp. 443–449

Love, L.A. (1994). New environmental agents associated with lupus-like disorders. *Lupus*, Vol.3, pp. 467–471

Lovell, D.J.; Giannini, E.H.; Reiff, A. et al.. (2000) Etanercept in children with polyarticular juvenile rheumatoid arthritis. Pediatric Rheumatology Collaborative Study Group. *N Engl J Med, Vol.* 342, pp.763-9

Lowe, S.W.; Schmitt, E.M.; Smith, S.W. et al. (1993). p53 is required for radiation-induced apoptosis in mouse thymocytes. *Nature*, Vol.362, pp. 847-849

Lu, L. & Osmond, D.G. (1997). Apoptosis during B lymphopoiesis in mouse bone marrow. *J Immunol*, Vol.158, pp. 5136–5145

Maas, K.; Chan, S.; Parker, J. et al. (2002). Cutting edge: molecular portrait of human autoimmune disease. *J Immunol*, Vol.169, pp.5-9

Malaguarnera, L.; Cristaldi, E. & Malaguarnera, M. (2010) The role of immunità in elderly cancer, *Critical Reviews in Oncology/Hematology*, Vol. 74, pp. 40–60

Martin-Orozco, N. & Dong, C. (2009a) The IL-17/IL-23 axis of inflammation in cancer: Friend or foe? *Current Opinion in Investigational Drugs*, Vol.10, No.6, pp.543-9.

Martin-Orozco, N.; Muranski, P.; Chung, Y. et al. (2009b) Th17 cells promote cytotoxic T cell activation in tumour immunity, *Immunity*, Vol. 31, No (5), pp.787–798

Mc Arthur, C.; Wang, Y.; Veno, P. et al. (2002). Intracellular trafficking and surface expression of SS-A (Ro), SS-B (La), poly(ADP-ribose) polymerase and α-fodrin autoantigens during apoptosis in human salivary gland cells induced by tumour necrosis factor-α. *Arch Oral Biol*, Vol.47, pp.443-448

Mc Cubrey, J.A.; May, W.S.; Duronio, V. et al. (2000). Serine/threonine phosphorylation in cytokine signal transduction. *Leukemia*, Vol.14, pp. 9-21

Mease, P.J.; Goffe, B.S.; Metz, J. et al. (2000) Etanercept in the treatment of psoriatic arthritis and psoriasis: a randomised trial, *Lancet*, Vol.356,pp.385-90

Medh, R.D. & Thompson, E.B. (2000). Hormonal regulation of physiological cell turnover and apoptosis. *Cell Tissue Res*, Vol.301, pp. 101-124

Meenan, J.; Hommes, D.W.; van Dulleman, H. et al. (1997) The influence of TNF mAB, cA2, on circulating lymphocyte populations (abstr). *Gastroenterology*, Vol.122:A1039

Melichar, B.; Bures⌄, J. & De⌄dic⌄, K. (2006) Anorectal Carcinoma After Infliximab Therapy in Crohn's Disease: Report of a Case, *Dis Colon Rectum*, Vol. 49,pp. 1228–1233

Mevorach, D.; Zhou, J.L.; Song, X. et al (1998). Systemic exposure to irradiated apoptotic cells induces autoantibody production. *J. Exp. Med.*, Vol.188, pp. 387-392

Miyara, M.; Amoura, Z.; Parizot, C. et al. (2005) Global natural regulatory T cell depletion in active systemic lupus erythematosus, *J Immunol*,Vol.175, No.(12), pp. 8392–8400

Morgan, M.E.; Flierman, R.; van Duivenvoorde, L.M. et al. (2005) Effective treatment of collagen-induced arthritis by adoptive transfer of CD25+ regulatory T cells. *Arthritis Rheum*, Vol. 52, No.(7), pp.2212–2221.

Moriishi, K.; Huang, D.C.; Cory, S. et al. (1999). Bcl-2 family members do not inhibit apoptosis by binding the caspase activator Apaf-1. *Proc Natl Acad Sci USA*, Vol.96, pp. 9683-9688

Mountz, J.D.; Wu, J.; Cheng, J. et al (1994). Autoimmune disease: a problem of defective apoptosis. *Arthritis Rheum*, Vol.37, pp. 1415-1420

Moutsopoulos, H.M.; Chused, T.M.; Mann, D.L. et al. (1980). SjÖgren's syndrome (sicca syndrome): current issues. *Ann Intern Med*, Vol.92, pp. 212-226

Muzio, M.; Salvesen, G.S. & Dixit, V.M. (1997). FLICE induced apoptosis in a cell free system. *J Biol Chem*, Vol.272, pp. 2952-2956

Mysler, E.; Bini, P.; Drappa, J. et al. (1994). The apoptosis-1/Fas protein in human systemic lupus erythematosus. *J Clin Invest*, Vol.93, pp. 1029–1034

Nagamine, K.; Peterson, P.; Scott, H.S. et al. (1997) Positional cloning of the APECED gene. *Nat Genet*, Vol.17, pp.393–8

Naschitz, J.E. (2001) Rheumatic syndromes: clues to occult neoplasia, *Curr Opin Rheumatol*,Vol. 13, pp.62–6

Newton, K.; Harris, A.W.; Bath, M.L. et al. (1998).Smith KGC, Strasser A. A dominant interfering mutant of Fadd/Mort1 enhances deletion of autoreactive thymocytes and inhibits proliferation of mature T lymphocytes. *EMBO J*, Vol.17, pp. 706–718

Nossal, G.; Pike, B. & Boyd, A. (1982). Clonal anergy: the universally anergic B lymphocyte. *Proc Natl Acad Sci*, USA, Vol.79, No 6, pp. 2013-2017

O'Reilly, L.A.; Harris, A.W.; Tarlinton, D.M. et al. (1997). Expression of a bcl-2 transgene reduces proliferation and slows turnover of developing B lymphocytes in vivo. *J Immunol*, Vol.159, pp.2301-2311

Ohmura, Y.; Yoshikawa, K.; Saga, S. et al. (2008) Combinations of tumour-specific CD8[+] CTLs and anti-CD25 mAb provide improved immunotherapy, *Oncol Rep*, Vol.19, pp. 1265-1270

Pap, T.; Muller-Ladner, U.; Gay, R. E. et al. (2000). Fibroblast biology: role of synovial fibroblasts in the pathogenesis of rheumatoid arthritis. *Arthritis Res.*, Vol.2, pp. 361–367

Patel, Y.I. & McHugh, N.J. (2000). Apoptosis–new clues to the pathogenesis of Sjögren's syndrome?. *Rheumatology*, Vol.39, pp. 119-121

Pérez, P.; Goicovich, E.; Alliende, C. et al. (2000). Differential expression of matrix metalloproteinases in labial salivary glands of patients with primary Sjögren's syndrome. Mechanisms of exocrine parenchyma destruction. *Arthritis Rheum*, Vol.43, pp. 2807-2817

Perlman, H.; Liu, H.; Georganas, C. et al. (2001). Differential expression pattern of the anti apoptotic proteins, Bcl-2 and FLIP, in experimental arthritis. *Arthritis Rheum,* Vol.44, pp. 2899-2908

Pope, R.M. & Perlman, H. (2000). Rheumatoid Arthritis, In: *Principles of Molecular Rheumatology,* G.C. Tsokas, (Ed.), pp. 325-361, Totowa, New Jersey

Pusterla, S.; Previstali, S.; Marziali, S. et al. (2004) Antiphospholipid antibodies in lymphoma: prevalence and clinical significance. *Hematol J,* Vol.5, No.(4), pp.341–6

Racanelli, V.; Prete, M.; Minoia, C. et al. (2008) Rheumatic disorders as paraneoplastic syndromes, *Autoimmunity Rev,* Vol.7, pp.352–8

Ramsey-Goldman, R.; Mattai, S.A.; Schilling, E. et al. (1998) Increased risk of malignancy in patients with systemic lupus erythematosus. *J Invest Med* Vol. 46, pp.217–22

Ran, S.; Downes, A. & Thorpe, P.E. (2002) Increased exposure of anionic phospholipids on the surface of tumour blood vessels. *Cancer Res,* Vol.62, pp.6132–40

Ranger, A.M.; Zha, J.; Harada, H. et al. (2003). Bad-deficient mice develop diffuse large B cell lymphoma. *Proc Natl Acad Sci,* USA, Vol.100, No.16, pp.9324-9329

Rayet, B. & Gelinas, C. (1999). Aberrant rel/nfkb genes and activity in human cancer. *Oncogene,* Vol.18, pp. 6938–6947

Reed, J. (1999). Dysregulation of Apoptosis in Cancer. *J. Clin. Oncol,* Vol.17, No. 9 (September) p. 2941

Reinstein, E. & Shoenfeld, Y. (2007) Antiphospholipid syndrome and cancer, *Clin Rev Allergy Immunol,* Vol.32, No.(2), pp.184–7

Rieux-Laucat, F.; Le Deist, F.; Hivroz, C. et al. (1995). Mutations in Fas associated with human lymphoproliferative syndrome and autoimmunity. *Science,* Vol.268, pp. 1347–1349

Rosenquist, R. (2008) Introduction: the role of inflammation, autoimmune disease and infectious agents in development of leukaemia and lymphoma. *J Intern Med,* Vol.264, pp. 512–3

Russell, J.H. & Ley, T.J. (2002). Lymphocyte-mediated cytotoxicity. *Annu Rev Immunol,* Vol.20, pp. 323-70

Sakaguchi, S. (2004) Naturally arising CD4_ regulatory T cells for immunologic self-tolerance and negative control of immune responses. *Annu Rev Immunol,* Vol. 22, pp.531–562

Sawamura, M.; Yamaguchi, S.; Murakami, H. et al. (1994) Multiple autoantibody production in a patient with splenic lymphoma, *Ann Hematol,* Vol. 68, No. (5), pp251–4

Scaffidi, C.; Schmitz, I.; Zha, J. et al. (1999). Differential modulation of apoptosis sensitivity in CD95 type I and type II cells. *J Biol Chem,* Vol.274, pp. 22532-22538

Schuetz, C.; Niehues, T.; Friedrich, W. et al. (2010) Autoimmunity, autoinflammation and lymphoma in combined immunodeficiency (CID). *Autoimmunity Reviews,* Vol.9, pp. 477–482

Schuler, M.; Bossy-Wetzel, E.; Goldstein, J.C. et al. (2000). p53 induces apoptosis by caspase activation through mitochondrial cytochrome c release. *J Biol Chem,* Vol.275, No.10, pp. 7337-7342

Scott, R.S.; McMahon, E.J.; Pop, S.M. et al. (2001). Phagocytosis and clearance of apoptotic cells is mediated by MER. *Nature,* Vol.411, pp. 207-211

Sekine, C.; Yagita, H.; Kobata, T. et al. (1996). Fas-mediated stimulation induces IL-8 sercretion by rheumatoid arthritis synoviocytes independently of CPP32-mediated apoptosis. *Biochem Biophys Res Commun*, Vol.228, pp. 14-20

Sentman, C.L.; Shutter, J.R.; Hockenbery, D. et al. (1991). bcl-2 inhibits multiple forms of apoptosis but not negative selection in thymocytes. *Cell*, Vol.67, pp. 879–88

Silink, M. (2002) Childhood diabetes: a global perspective, *Horm Res*, Vol.57, pp.1–5

Skarstein, K.; Nerland, A.H.; Eidsheim, M. et al. (1997). Lymphoid cell accumulation in salivary glands of autoimmune MRL mice can be due to impaired apoptosis. *Scand J Immunol*, Vol.46, pp.373–378

Skopouli, F.N.; Fox, P.C.; Galanopoulou, V. et al. (1991). T cell subpopulations in the labial minor salivary gland histopathologic lesion of SjÖgren's syndrome. *J Rheumatol*, Vol.18, pp.210-214

SLEGEN; Harley, J.B.; Alarcon-Riquelme, M.E.; et al. (2008). Genome-wide association scan in women with systemic lupus erythematosus identifies susceptibility variants in ITGAM, PXK, KIAA1542 and other loci. *Nat Genet*, Vol 40, pp. 204–209

Soengas, M.S.; Alarcon, R.M.; Yoshida, H. et al. (1999). apaf-1 and caspase-9 in p53-dependent apoptosis and tumour inhibition. *Science*, Vol.284, pp.156-159

Strasser, A.; Harris, A.W.; Huang, D.C.S. et al. (1995). Bcl- 2 and Fas/APO-1 regulate distinct pathways to lymphocyte apoptosis. *EMBO J*, Vol.14, pp. 6136–6147

Straus, S.E.; Sneller, M.; Lenardo, M.J.; et al. (1999) An inherited disorder of lymphocyte apoptosis: the autoimmune lymphoproliferative syndrome. Ann Intern Med, Vol. 130, No.7, pp. 591-601.

Suarez, F.; Lortholary, O.; Hermine, O. et al. (2006) Infection-associated lymphomas derived from marginal zone B cells: a model of antigen-driven lymphoproliferation. *Blood*, Vol.107, pp3034–44

Szekanecz, E.; András, C.; Sándor, Z. et al. (2006) Malignancies and soluble tumour antigens in rheumatic diseases, *Autoimmun Rev*, Vol. 6, pp.42–7

Tartaglia, L.A.; Ayres, T.M.; Wong, G.H.W. et al. (1993). A novel domain within the 55 kd TNF receptor signals cell death. *Cell*, Vol.74, pp. 845-853

Tincani, A.; Taraborelli, M. & Cattaneo, R. (2010) Antiphospholipid antibodies and malignancies. *Autoimmunity Reviews*, Vol.9, pp.200-202

Tsimberidou, A.M. & Giles, F.J. (2002) TNF-alpha targeted therapeutic approaches in patients with hematologic malignancies. *Expert Rev Anticancer Ther*, Vol.2, pp.277-86

Tsimberidou, A.M.; Giles, F.J.; Duvic, M. et al. (2004) Pilot study of etanercept in patients with relapsed cutaneous T-cell lymphomas, *J Am Acad Dermatol*, Vol.51, pp.200-4

Turbyville, J.C. & Rao, V.K. (2010) The autoimmune lymphoproliferative syndrome: a rare disorder providing clues about normal tolerance. *Autoimmun Rev*, Vol.9, pp.488–93

Ueda, H.; Howson, J.M.; Esposito, L. et al. (2003). Association of the T-cell regulatory gene CTLA4 with susceptibility to autoimmune disease. *Nature*, Vol. 423, pp. 506-511

Ulbricht, K.U.; Schmidt, R.E. & Witte T. (2003). Antibodies against alpha- fodrin in Sjögren's syndrome. *Autoimmunity Rev*, Vol.2, pp. 109-113

Utz, P.J. & Anderson, P. (1998). Posttranslational protein modifications, apoptosis and the bypass of tolerance to autoantigens. *Arthritis Rheum*, Vol.41, pp. 1152-1160

Van Parijs, L.; Peterson, D.A. & Abbas, A.K. (1998). The Fas/Fas ligand pathway and Bcl-2 regulate T cell responses to model self and foreign antigens. *Immunity*, Vol.8, pp. 265–274

Vidalino, L.; Doria, A.; Quarta, S. et al. (2009) SERPINB3, apoptosis and autoimmunity. *Autoimmunity Reviews, Vol. 9*, pp. 108–112

Vogt, E.; Ng, A.K. & Rote, N.S. (1997) Antiphosphatidylserine antibody removes annexin-V and facilitates the binding of prothrombin at the surface of a choriocarcinoma model of trophoblast differentiation, *Am J Obstet Gynecol*, Vol. 177, No.(4), pp.964–72

Von Muhlen, C.A. & Tan, E.M. (1995). Autoantibodies in the diagnosis of syotemic rheumatic diseases. *Semin Arthritis Rheum*, Vol.24, pp. 323-358

Wakata, N.; Kurihara, T.; Saito, E. et al. (2002) Polymyositis and dermatomyositis associated with malignancy: a 30-year retrospective study, *Int J Dermatol*, Vol.41, pp. 729–34

Wallach, D. (1997). Cell death induction by TNF: a matter of self control. *Trends Biochem Sci*, Vol.22, pp. 107–109

Wan, Y.Y. & Flavell, R.A. (2007) Regulatory T-cell functions are subverted and converted owing to attenuated Foxp3 expression. *Nature* , Vol. 15, No.445(7129), pp. 766-70

Ward, J.M.; Nikolov, N.P.; Tschetter, J.R. et al. (2004). Progressive glomerulonephritis and histiocytic sarcoma associated with macrophage functional defects in CYP1B1-deficient mice. *Toxicol Pathol*, Vol.32, pp.710-718

Watson, M.L.; Rao, J.K.; Gilkeson, G.S. et al. (1992). Genetic analysis of MRL-lpr mice: Relationship of the Fas apoptosis gene to disease manifestations and renal disease-modifying loci. *J Exp Med*, Vol.176, pp. 1645–1656

Weaver, C.T.; Hatton, R.D.; Mangan, P.R. et al. (2007) IL-17 family cytokines and the expanding diversity of effector T cell lineages. *Annu Rev Immunol*, Vol. 25, pp.821–852

Weiner, H.L. (2001) Induction and mechanism of action of transforming growth factor-b-secreting Th3 regulatory cells. *Immunol Rev*, Vol. 182, pp.207–214

Williams, G.M. (2008) Antitumour necrosis factor-alpha therapy and potential cancer inhibition, *Eur J Cancer Prev*, Vol.17, pp.169-77

Yamaguchi, Y.; Seta, N.; Kaburaki, J. et al. (2007) Excessive exposure to anionic surfaces maintains autoantibody response to beta(2)-glycoprotein I in patients with antiphospholipid syndrome, *Blood*, Vol. 110, pp.4312–8

Yang, X.O.; Nurieva, R.; Martinez, G.J. et al. (2008) Molecular antagonism and plasticity of regulatory and inflammatory T cell programs, *Immunity*, Vol.29, pp.44–56

Ye, P.; Garvey, P.B.; Zhang, P. et al. (2001) Interleukin-17 and lung host defence against Klebsiella pneumoniae infection, *Am J Respir Cell Mol Biol* Vol. 25, pp.335–340

Yeh, W.C.; Shahinian, A.; Speiser, D. et al. (1997). Early lethality, functional NF-kB activation, and increased sensitivity to TNF-induced cell death in TRAF2- deficient mice. *Immunity*, Vol.7, pp. 715-725

Zampieri, S.; Valente, M.; Adami, N. et al. (2010) Polymyositis, dermatomyositis and malignancy: a further intringuing link, *Autoimmun Rev*, Vol 9, pp.449–53

Zhang, J.; Cado, D.; Chen, A. et al. (1998). Fas-mediated apoptosis and activation-induced T-cell proliferation are defective in mice lacking FADD/Mort1. *Nature*, Vol.392, pp. 296–299

Zheng, S.G., Wang, J.H.; Gray, J.D. et al. (2004) Natural and induced CD4+CD25+ cells educate CD4+CD25- cells to develop suppressive activity: the role of IL-2, TGF-beta, and IL-10, *J Immunol*, Vol.172, pp. 5213-5221

Zinkel, S.S.; Hurov, K.E.; Ong, C. et al. (2005). A role for proapoptotic BID in the DNA-damage response. *Cell*, Vol.122, No.4, pp.579-591

Zintzaras, E.; Voulgarelis, M. & Moutsopoulos, H.M. (2005) The risk of lymphoma development in autoimmune diseases: a meta-analysis. *Arch Intern Med*, Vol. 165, No.(20), pp. 2337–44

Zou, W. (2005). Immunosuppressive networks in the tumour environment and their therapeutic relevance. *Nat Rev Cancer*, *Vol.* 5, pp.263–267

Zuckerman, E.; Toubi, E.; Golan, T.D. et al. (1995) Increased thromboembolic incidence in anti-cardiolipin-positive patients with malignancy. *Br J Cancer*, Vol. 72, No. (2), pp.447–51.

5

Autoimmune Disorders and Lymphomas

Dolcetti R.[1], Ponzoni M.[2,3], Mappa S.[2,4] and Ferreri A.J.M.[2]
[1]Cancer Bioimmunotherapy Unit, Dept of Oncology,
National Cancer Institute CRO-IRCCS,
[2]Unit of Lymphoid Malignancies, Dept of Onco-Hematology,
[3]Pathology Unit, [4]Internal Medicine Unit; San Raffaele Scientific Institute
Italy

1. Introduction

Patients affected by autoimmune diseases have demonstrated an increased risk of developing lymphoid malignancies. Non-Hodgkin lymphomas (NHL) have consistently been associated with several autoimmune conditions, such as, by way of example, rheumatoid arthritis (RA), Sjögren syndrome (SS) and systemic lupus erythematosus (SLE). Similarly, even if based on fewer studies, an increased risk of malignant lymphomas has also been associated with celiac disease, dermatitis herpetiformis, Hashimoto's thyroiditis, and autoimmune haemolytic anemia. An association between other autoimmune conditions, such as inflammatory bowel diseases (Crohn's disease and ulcerative colitis), psoriasis and systemic sclerosis, and a higher risk of lymphoproliferative disorders has not been consistently proven (Askling *et al*, 2005, von Roon *et al*, 2007, Boffetta *et al*, 2001, Gelfand *et al*, 2006, Chatterjee *et al*, 2005). The magnitude of these associations varies widely among different studies. Reported relative risk is about two-fold in RA, 9-18 fold in SS, 3-6 fold in SLE, celiac disease and Hashimoto thyroiditis, and 2-10 fold in dermatitis herpetiformis. Epidemiologic analysis by NHL subtype have shown that diffuse large B-cell lymphoma (DLBCL) is more frequently associated with RA and SS, while extranodal marginal zone lymphoma, in the respective target organs, is strongly associated with SS (Theander *et al*, 2004) and Hashimoto's thyroiditis. Celiac disease is associated with a 520-fold increased risk of enteropathy-associated T-cell lymphoma of the small intestine (EATL). Autoimmune conditions of the skin including psoriasis, pemphigus and discoid lupus erythematosus have an increased risk of T-cell cutaneous lymphoma (Anderson *et al*, 2009). Hodgkin lymphoma has also been associated with some autoimmune conditions, such as RA, SLE and sclerodermia. On the other hand, it is still unclear why other autoimmune conditions, such as type 1 mellitus diabetes, multiple sclerosis, and sarcoidosis do not present an increased risk of lymphoma development. The exact mechanism of lymphomagenesis in the contest of autoimmunity remains largely unexplained, but it may be related to chronic antigenic stimulation, chronic inflammatory response and deficiency in immunesurveillance, promoting a multistep process of genetic instability resulting in accumulation of genetic alterations. In addition, immunosuppressive medications (e.g., methotrexate) may concur to alter patient's immune status. In this chapter, we review the mainstream of epidemiologic studies, discuss the pathways underlying autoimmunity and lymphomas as well as mechanisms of lymphomagenesis, and summarize the characteristics of the various autoimmune diseases that may be associated with lymphoma. Therapeutic options for these clinically intriguing conditions are also discussed.

2. Epidemiologic studies

The first report of an association between autoimmunity and lymphomas was made in 1966 (Mellors, 1966). Notwithstanding the low incidence of autoimmune and lymphoproliferative disorders in the general population, large patients groups and long observation periods are needed to establish an association between these two conditions. In the past, many population-based case-control and cohort studies were carried out to confirm the consistence of an association between these two diseases. Registry-based cohort studies, which are generally based on hospital discharge diagnosis records, are able to evaluate large cohort of patients affected by different autoimmune disorders following them for the occurrence of cancer, usually using cancer registries. This method allows studying large number of patients with autoimmune diseases although lymphoma occurrence is a rare event. Despite the adequate statistical power of these studies, they may over select patients with severe disease, missing patients who are treated only as outpatients. On the other hand, case-control studies of lymphoma patients allows the evaluation of large numbers of well-characterized cancer cases, providing for a wider range of information about lymphoma subtype and covariate exposure of interest, with the disadvantage of rarity of some autoimmune disorders, the low statistical power and control selection bias. Therefore, both study designs have limitations in evaluating the consistence of this peculiar association. Another important limitation of these studies is the potential bias due to reverse causality (i.e., undiagnosed lymphoma causing paraneoplastic inflammation misclassified as rheumatic disease). Many studies have reported in fact a major risk of lymphoma development during the first year after diagnosis of autoimmune disease or have excluded from analysis this time interval. A meta-analysis of all previous available cohort studies relating SLE, RA and SS to the risk of NHL development showed that NHL is more frequent in patients affected by autoimmune diseases than in the general population, especially for SS and SLE (Zintzaras et al, 2005). Importantly, a reason for the inconsistent associations between many autoimmune conditions and NHL overall risk may lie in the molecular, morphologic and etiologic heterogeneity of the different NHL subtypes. One of the largest epidemiologic study published has performed a pooled analysis of self-reported autoimmune conditions and NHL different subtypes, including 29.423 participants in 12 case-control studies over Europe, North America and Australia (Ekstrom Smedby et al, 2008). The study concluded that an increased risk of NHL is associated only with few autoimmune disorders and that these associations are stronger for some lymphoma subtypes than others. In fact, a 6.5-fold increased risk of NHL was associated with SS, which is lower than in previous reports including only cohorts of hospitalized patients that may present a more severe form of disease. It has been observed a 250-fold increased risk of parotid gland NHL and a 1.000-fold increased risk of marginal zone B-cell lymphoma of mucosa-associated lymphoid tissue (MALT)-type of the parotid gland and an association with DLBCL. SLE has been associated with a 2.7-fold increased risk of NHL, in particular, DLBCL and MALT lymphomas. Haemolytic anaemia has been associated with DLBCL. In patients with celiac disease, an increased overall risk for NHL was not observed; only associations with entheropathy-associated T-cell lymphoma of small intestine and anaplastic large T-cell lymphoma have been detected. Regarding RA, an overall increased risk of NHL was not observed, but only a moderately increased risk in patients treated with corticosteroids or immunosuppressant. Finally, inflammatory bowel disorders, type I diabetes, sarcoidosis, pernicious anaemia, and multiple sclerosis were not associated with increased risk of NHL. Importantly, this analysis demonstrated a persistent risk of lymphoma development also after ten year of autoimmune disease duration, excluding the risk of autoimmune phenomena triggered by yet undiagnosed lymphomas. Another large population-based case-control study form the U.S. Surveillance Epidemiology and End Results-Medicare database has been conducted on 44.350 lymphoid malignancy cases (> 67 years) and 122.531 population-based controls (Anderson *et al*, 2009). Association between specific lymphoid malignancy subtypes and various autoimmune conditions has been also investigated. Although the study was limited to subjects over age 65, the strongest association by NHL subtype was observed between DLBCL and RA and SS; T-cell lymphoma and haemolytic anaemia, psoriasis, discoid lupus erythematosus, and celiac

Studies	Disease	NHL	95% CI	HL	95% CI	*p*
Zintzaras, 2005	Reumatoid arthritis	3.9 (SIR)	2.5-5.9	-	-	-
	Systemic lupus erythematosus	7.4	3.3-17	-	-	-
	Primary Sjögren syndrome	18.8	9.5-37.3	-	-	-
Engels, 2005	Reumatoid arthritis	1.3 (OR)	0.8-2.1	-	-	0.24
	Systemic lupus erythematosus	1.3	0.3-5.6	-	-	0.72
	Primary Sjögren syndrome	4.9	0.6-43	-	-	0.11
Landgren, 2006	Reumatoid arthritis	-	-	2.7 (OR)	1.9-4.0	-
	Systemic lupus erythematosus	-	-	5.8	2.2-15.1	-
	Systemic scleroderma	-	-	0.6	0.1-6.2	-
	Hashimoto thyroiditis	-	-	2.0	0.3-14	-
Ekstrom Smedby, 2008	Reumatoid arthritis	1.06 (OR)	0.87-1.29	-	-	< 0.1
	Systemic lupus erythematosus	2.69	1.68-4.3	-	-	0.39
	Primary Sjögren syndrome	4.75	1.79-12.6	-	-	0.93
	Secondary Sjögren syndrome	9.57	2.9-31.6	-	-	-
	Celiac disease	1.5	0.89-2.54	-	-	0.72
Anderson, 2009	Rheumatoid arthritis (OR)	1.2	1.1-1.3	1.5 (OR)	1.1-2.0	-
	Systemic lupus erythematosus	1.5	1.2-1.9	3.5	1.9-6.7	-
	Sjögren syndrome	1.9	1.5-2.3	1.6	0.6-4.4	-
	Systemic scleroderma	1.4	0.9-2.2	2.5	0.6-10	-
	Hashimoto thyroiditis	1.1	0.8-1.4	2.1	1.0-4.8	-
	Celiac disease	1.5	0.9-2.5	-	-	-

Table 1. Epidemiologic studies

disease; marginal zone lymphoma and SLE and haemolytic anaemia; Hodgkin lymphoma (HL) and SLE. Additional analysis excluding data for up to 5 years before the diagnosis of malignancy have been also performed to exclude reverse causality, i.e., lymphoma causing autoimmune disorder. Another population based case-control study disclosed a solid association between NHL and SS and a small increase in NHL risk associated with SLE (Engels *et al*, 2005). While most epidemiologic studies demonstrated a consistent association between autoimmunity and NHL, there are only limited data on the risk of developing HL in these settings. A population-based case-control study during a 40-year period analyzed the association between 32 autoimmune disorders and risk of developing HL (Landgren *et al*, 2006), reporting a statistically significant increased risk to develop HL in patients with personal history of RA, SLE, sarcoidosis, or ITP. In addition, personal or family history of sarcoidosis and ulcerative colitis was associated with significantly increased risk of HL.

3. Pathogenesis

The aetiology of NHL remains largely unexplained, but some well-established risk factors have been identified. Under normal conditions, B and T lymphocytes respond to antigenic stimulation in a regulated manner and proliferative responses are self-limited. Immune dysregulation, leading to a continue lymphocyte proliferation, is considered to play a major role in lymphomagenesis, as demonstrated by an increased risk of lymphoma development in states of immunosuppression (i.e. following organ transplant or hereditary and acquired immunodeficiency syndromes). In addition, the occurrence of specific subtypes of NHL in

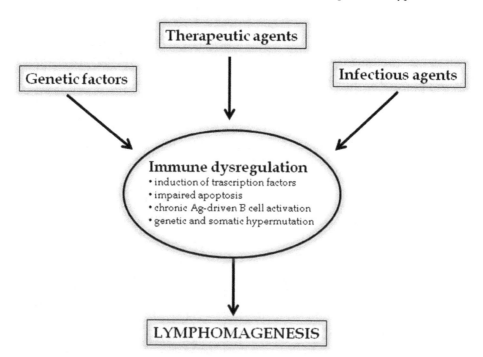

Fig. 1. Proposed pathogenetic factors of lymphomagenesis in the context of autoimmunity

the context of infectious conditions suggests a pathogenic role also for inflammation and chronic immune stimulation. Autoimmune diseases have been considered a possible predisposing factor for lymphoma development as they are characterized by impairment of immune responses leading to a loss of tolerance to self-antigens, a deregulated lymphocyte reactivity with production of autoantibodies against specific tissues and organs. It is conceivable that a sustained antigen-driven B proliferation may increase the risk of adverse genetic events that may finally result in the emergence of a neoplastic clone.

3.1 Immune dysregulation
In the development of lymphoma at primary sites, such as MALT lymphomas arising in the parotid gland during the course of SS or in the thyroid gland in the case of chronic thyroiditis, and as T-cell lymphoma in small intestine of patients with celiac disease, a critical role is played by local chronic antigen-driven stimulation leading to the genesis of organized lymphoid tissue, the so called "tertiary" lymphoid tissue, characterized by organ-specific T- or B-cell proliferation, polyclonality and, eventually, oligo-monoclonality.

3.1.1 Tertiary lymphoid tissue
Chronic inflammatory infiltrates resembling the secondary lymphoid organs have been previously described as "tertiary lymphoid organs" (Picker, 1992) and can be induced by the same mediators of lymphoid ontogenesis, such as tumor necrosis factor (TNF)-beta and other members of the TNF family (Kratz et al, 1996), through induction of transcription factors, adhesion molecules, lymphoid-tissue-homing chemokines, and other cytokines (Hjelmstrom, 2001). The transcription factor named nuclear factor kappa-B (NF-κB) is induced by TNF proteins and is involved in lymphoid tissue development through chemokines, adhesion molecules and members of the TNF family themselves. TNF proteins are also required for the normal expression of CXCL13 and CCL21, two homing chemokines crucial for lymphoid neogenesis (Ngo et al, 1999). CXCR13 is normally produced by stromal cells in lymphoid tissues and attracts naive B cells and activated and memory T cells in vitro (Legler et al, 1998). CCL21 is a ligand for the CCR7 receptor that directs the migration of naive T cells and dendritic cells. Expression of CXCL13 and CCL21 has been found in disease models of chronic inflammation characterized by lymphoid neogenesis (Hjelmstrom, 2001). Chronic autoimmune diseases are characterized by a chronic inflammatory infiltrate in the target organs, with mononuclear cells and lymphoid follicles. The thyroid gland in patients affected by Hashimoto's thyroiditis is organized in a structure that resembles a lymph node, including germinal centres, plasma cells and high endothelial venules (Knecht et al, 1981, Kabel et al, 1989). Also the thymus of patients affected by autoimmune myasthenia gravis is characterized by the presence of ectopic lymphoid follicles with germinal centres containing activated B lymphocytes and plasma cells that produce autoantibodies (Soderstrom et al, 1970, Leprince et al, 1990). SS is characterized by the presence of antigen-driven proliferation of B cells and lymphoid follicles with clonally expanded lymphocytes (Freimark et al, 1989, Stott et al, 1998). Similarly, there is an evidence for lymphoid neogenesis in the chronic synovial inflammation of patients with RA (Watson et al, 1994, Randen et al, 1995); B cell diversification, somatic hypermutation and plasma cells development occur in the synovial germinal centres (Schroder et al, 1996, Kim et al, 1999) and the homing chemokine CXCL13 seems to be present in the synovial follicles of patients with RA (Hjelmstrom, 2001).

Expansion of B self-reactive lymphocytes is normally limited by several checkpoint mechanisms able to prevent the development of both autoimmunity and lymphoma. Both such diseases may be the result of a multistep process which ends up with the elimination of such aforementioned checkpoints. This multistep process regards both inherited and somatic mutations of genes involved in these pathways. For example, germinal and somatic mutations of *Fas* are associated with both autoimmune diseases and lymphoproliferative disorders, probably by inhibition of apoptosis. Somatic mutations occur physiologically in lymphocytes, during the course of somatic hypermutation of immunoglobulin genes in the germinal centre of lymphoid follicles of lymph nodes and spleen. VDJ recombination, isotype switching and somatic hypermutation, requiring double strand break and DNA rejoining, are susceptible to error and are known to activate oncogenes and inactivate tumour suppression mechanisms. Secondly, the epidemiological evidence of overlapping pathogenesis between autoimmunity and lymphoma may be explained by an enhanced lymphocyte proliferation resulting in increased rates of somatic mutations (Goodnow, 2007). Acquisition of distinct chromosomal translocations among reactive B cells, such as the t(11;18) in the course of *Helicobacter pylori*-positive chronic gastritis, is known to promote lymphomagenesis. Conversely, a similar risk was not found in other settings characterized by chronic immune responses, such as allergic diseases (Soderberg *et al*, 2006) or inflammatory bowel disease (Smedby *et al*, 2006).

3.1.2 Triad autoimmunity-lymphoproliferation-lymphoma in Sjögren's Syndrome

Among all autoimmune diseases, SS better reflects the mechanism of the triad autoimmunity-lymphoproliferation-lymphoma. The underlying chronic inflammation, in fact, promotes the formation of organized lymphoid tissue, with a crucial role played by TNF-beta, characterized by the presence of high endothelial venules, dendritic cells and follicular dendritic cells, antigen-driven clonal proliferation of B cells, and lymphoid follicles with clonally expanded lymphocytes (Stott *et al*, 1998, Harris, 1999). The SS-associated chronic lymphoproliferation varies from benign to MALT-type lesions, MALT lymphomas, and even aggressive lymphomas (Burke, 1999). In fact, chronic antigen-driven polyclonal B-cell activation in SS seems to support selection and expansion of auto-reactive B-cell clones through the processes of class switch recombination and somatic hypermutation (Stott *et al*, 1998). Subsequent studies confirmed the selective accumulation of a B cell population characterized by a high rate of mutations in productively rearranged VL chain genes (Jacobi *et al*, 2002, Gellrich *et al*, 1999). The genetic instability associated with DNA hypermutation can favour the escape of malignant B cell clones with the consequent development of an overt B-cell lymphoma (Royer *et al*, 1997). The processes of class switch recombination and somatic hypermutation seem to critically depend on the enzyme activation-induced cytidine deaminase (AID). It has been shown (Bombardieri *et al*, 2007) that AID deaminase is expressed within follicular dendritic cell networks of the salivary gland of patients with SS, in a comparable way to that of secondary lymphoid organs, supporting the hypothesis that ectopic lymphoid tissue recapitulates the molecular setting necessary for local autoantibody production and B-cell expansion. The evolution of a non-malignant B-cell clone present in the parotid gland of a single patient with SS followed at multiple time points over a 7-year period to overt B-cell lymphoma has been documented (Gasparotto *et al*, 2003). In this case, lymphoma evolution occurred in a different site (lung) from that of the primary localization of B-cell proliferation (parotid gland), providing evidence that the pulmonary neoplastic clone derived from the salivary gland clone, possibly through the acquisition of oncogenic alterations in cell regulatory genes able to confer a more aggressive phenotype.

3.1.3 *BAFF* deregulation and apoptotic resistance

Whether local antigen-driven stimulation and chronic inflammatory processes are important for the development of distant (typically nodal) NHL such as DLBCL is not yet known. Disease severity and inflammatory load are important determinants of NHL development in SS and RA (Theander *et al*, 2006, Baecklund *et al*, 2006a), with an increased risk of occurrence of DLBCL in these autoimmune disorders (Smedby *et al*, 2008), including factors related to cytokine profile, T cell subset balance and apoptotic resistance (Theander *et al*, 2006, Eguchi, 2001). In RA and SLE, apoptotic resistance is increased and mediated by *Bcl-2* expression, activation of NF-κB by inflammatory cytokines and growth factors, and abnormalities in the expression of B-cell activating factor (*BAFF*) (Eguchi, 2001, Mackay *et al*, 2005). BAFF is a critical regulator of B-cell homeostasis, and its excessive production causes multiple autoimmune symptoms in mice models and compromises apoptosis of autoreactive B cells. Deregulated BAFF expression has been described to lead to disease progression and perpetuation of humoral autoimmunity. Patients affected by systemic autoimmune diseases, such as SS, RA and SLE, have increased levels of BAFF in serum and synovial fluid with respect to healthy people. Moreover, serum levels of BAFF in SS correlate with the level of autoantibodies, and with rheumatoid factor in patients with RA. *BAFF* has been therefore proposed to play a major role in the development of SS and to contribute in the development of B-cell malignancies. In SS patients, the overexpression of *BAFF* can cause an excessive immunoglobulin production. In salivary glands of patients with SS, the reduced level of apoptosis among BAFF-expressing cells might lead to maintain signalling for tissue-infiltrating B cells to proliferate and to become autoantibody-producing plasma cells, contributing to germinal centres formation and lymphoma development. Finally, mice carrying a BAFF transgene become highly susceptible to lymphoproliferation, autoimmunity and lymphoma development (Mackay *et al*, 1999). The possible pathogenetic role of BAFF in SS and lymphomagenesis has led to the development of agents neutralizing BAFF as a new therapeutic option for such patients (Szodoray & Jonsson, 2005). Belimumab, the fully human recombinant IgG monoclonal antibody to soluble B-lymphocyte stimulator human antibody (anti-Blys; LymphoStat-B) binds soluble BAFF and prevents interaction with its receptor (Baker *et al*, 2003). Encouraging results have been reported by two large phase III randomized controlled trials of belimumab versus placebo in seropositive SLE patients with stable disease receiving standard of care treatment. The study showed that belimumab improved several markers of disease activity (in the central nervous system, vascular, musculoskeletal, immunologic and cutaneous) and promoted reduction of average steroid dose compared to placebo. Belimumab also determined significant changes in immunologic parameters, such as reduction of IgG and IgM and autoantibodies, increase in C3 and C4 levels, reduction of circulating CD20+ B cells (Thanou-Stavraki & Sawalha, 2011). In summary, a continuous antigen-driven stimulation in a microenvironment where normal regulatory mechanisms are absent may promote both autoimmunity and lymphoma development.

3.2 Genetic factors

Several studies explored the relationship between genetic factors and development of lymphoid malignancies in the different settings of autoimmunity. It has been suggested that some inherited mutations could be involved in pathogenesis of both diseases. For example, inherited mutations of the *TNFSRF6* gene, which encodes the transmembrane protein *Fas* (CD59), a major mediator of lymphocyte apoptosis, lead to a genetic defect in apoptosis responsible of a familial syndrome called "autoimmune lymphoproliferative syndrome of childhood" (ALPS or Canale-Smith syndrome) characterized by chronic, non-malignant diffuse lymphadenopathy and hepatosplenomegaly together with hypergammaglobulinemia, autoantibodies and/or overt autoimmune diseases. These patients are at high risk of developing lymphomas, almost exclusively of the B-cell immunophenotype (HL, follicular, Burkitt and T-cell rich B-cell lymphoma) (Jackson & Puck, 1999) with an incidence of 13% (6 out 46) among cases studied at the US National Institute of Health, with intervals from the onset of ALPS of 6-48 years (Mackay & Rose, 2001). However, previous population-based case control studies have failed to demonstrate that a family history of autoimmune disease is a risk factor for lymphoma development. A multicenter US study on 759 patients observed that a family history of dermatomyositis was associated with NHL, but not family history of 14 other autoimmune diseases (Engels *et al*, 2005). A statistically significant increase in risk of HL among patients with a family history of sarcoidosis or ulcerative colitis has been reported, but no association with a family history of other autoimmune conditions has been demonstrated (Landgren *et al*, 2006). Finally, an association between the risk of lymphoma development and a family history of a wide range of autoimmune diseases has not been detected in a population-based case-control study on 24,728 NHL patients (Mellemkjaer *et al*, 2008). Likewise, an increased risk of lymphoma occurrence among the first-degree relatives of RA patients has not been proven (Ekstrom *et al*, 2003). Therefore, studies evaluating whether genetic factors play a major role in lymphoma development have failed to prove a consistent association in the context of most autoimmune diseases and available data about inherited mutations are still inconsistent.

3.3 Therapeutic agents

The role played by autoimmune disease therapy in the subsequent lymphoma development was extensively analyzed, although with inconclusive results. This seems to be due to a selection bias related to the fact that patients requiring therapy usually show a more aggressive disease. Thus, the comparison between treated and untreated patients may result in a falsely increased treatment-associated risk. Disease modifying anti-rheumatic drugs (DMARDs) such as methotrexate and azathioprine have been suggested to increase the relative risk of malignant lymphoma (Baecklund *et al*, 2006b, Bernatsky *et al*, 2008, Askling *et al*, 2009, Wolfe & Michaud, 2007). However, several large population-based studies failed to demonstrate an increased risk linked to methotrexate *per se* (Baecklund et al, 2006b, Mariette et al, 2002, Wolfe & Michaud, 2004). Corticosteroids, a mainstream of treatment of inflammatory diseases, have never been consistently associated with lymphoma development (Baecklund *et al*, 2006b). Studies about the relationship between nonsteroidal anti-inflammatory drugs (NSAID) and lymphoma are also inconsistent (Baecklund *et al*, 2006b, Sorensen *et al*, 2003). The only exception is constituted by 8 cases of hepatosplenic $\gamma\delta$ T-cell lymphoma diagnosed among young patients treated with infliximab or adalimumab for inflammatory bowel disease. All patients were receiving concomitant immunosuppressive therapy with azathioprine or prednisone and it was not possible to ascertain if anti-TNF medication had an exclusive role in the pathogenesis of these lymphomas (Mackey *et al*, 2007). Conversely, although it has not been definitively demonstrated, postponing therapy could contribute to lymphoma development; this could be due to a chronic worsening of the inflammatory microenvironment promoted by uncontrolled disease. In a population-based case-control study (Smedby et al, 2006), an increased risk of lymphoma occurrence was detected in patients with RA treated with NSAIDs, corticosteroids and other immunosuppressants but it was not confirmed in untreated patients. This may be related to the fact that the first cohort of patients had a more severe disease with higher levels of chronic inflammation that contributed to lymphoma development.

3.3.1 NSAIDs and steroids

Regular use of aspirin and NSAIDs has been hypothesized to be associated with reduced risk of development of colorectal cancer (RR= 0.5-0.8), and possibly of other cancers as stomach, breast, lung, pancreas, and ovary. Decreased cancer risk may be related to inhibition of prostaglandin synthesis, enhancement of cellular immune response or induction of apoptosis. RA patients, who frequently use long-lasting high doses of both aspirin and other NSAIDs, have a decreased risk of colorectal cancer and possibly female breast cancer (Beauparlant et al, 1999). Some prospective cohort and case-control studies analyzed the association between aspirin and non-aspirin NSAID use and risk of NHL with contradictory results. An inverse association was documented in a population-based case-control study (OR=0.72; 95% CI= 0.56-0.91) (Holly et al, 1999) and a near significant association between regular use of aspirin and moderate decrease of NHL has also been reported in another hospital-based case-control study in men (OR= 0.82; 95% CI= 0.65-1.04), while women who used acetaminophen regularly experienced a 71% elevation in the risk of B-cell NHL (OR= 1.71; 95% CI 1.18-2.50) (Baker et al, 2005). A potential protective effect of analgesic use on NHL risk in women but not in men has also been reported (Beiderbeck et al, 2003). Conversely, a positive association between use of aspirin or acetaminophen and NHL has been observed among women, but not among men (RR=1.96; 95% CI=0.56-3.08) in a population-based study (Bernstein & Ross, 1992) and a suggestive positive association has also been reported in a prospective study cohort (RR=1.40; 95% CI= 0.99-1.97). This association was lost when aspirin was evaluated alone (Cerhan et al, 2003). Finally, no association between aspirin and other analgesics and lymphoma or leukaemia was observed in two other hospital-based case-control studies (Rosenberg et al, 1995, Cartwright et al, 1988) and in a large study cohort (Sorensen et al, 2003). Although the exact reason of this gender discrepancies is unclear, a different response to pharmacologic agents could be referred to women's lower body weight and high percentage of body fat or to endocrine milieu (Meibohm et al, 2002). In fact, clearance of both aspirin and acetaminophen positively correlates with body size and is faster in man rather than women (Miners et al, 1986) and some metabolizing enzymes are induced by hormones. Treatment with corticosteroids is one of the mainstreams of the management of systemic inflammatory diseases, because of their strong and fast anti-inflammatory effects. A linkage between corticosteroids and lymphoma risk was suspected in some studies (Bernstein & Ross, 1992, Kato et al, 2002, Zhang et al, 2004), whereas this association was excluded by others (Engels et al, 2005, Smedby et al, 2006, Beiderbeck et al, 2003, Chang et al, 2005). For example, a markedly reduced risk of lymphoma associated with steroid treatment has been observed in RA patients, also after adjustment for disease severity (Baecklund et al, 2006a). Also a case-control study of 378 patients with RA-associated lymphoma demonstrated that treatment with oral steroids was associated with a 30% reduced risk of lymphoma (OR=0.69; 95%

CI=0.51-0.94); this feature remained also after adjustment for DMARDs treatment, disease activity and use of intra-articular steroids. Moreover, treatment up to 2 years showed no protective effect, while a treatment of more than 2 years was associated with a markedly reduced risk. Analysis by lymphoma subtype showed the strongest association between oral steroids and DLBCL (Hellgren *et al*, 2010b). The reduced lymphoma risk associated with steroid therapy might be explained by a reduced inflammatory activity induced by these drugs. Conversely, a meta-analysis of case-control and cohort studies reported between 1992 and 2006 failed to prove an increased risk of lymphoma development over the last decades during which there has been an increased use of immunomodulatory drugs such as corticosteroids and NSAID, disproving thus any possible link between therapy and cancer (Bernatsky *et al*, 2007).

3.3.2 Anti-TNF agents

The use of biologic drugs as antagonists of TNF has been extensively evaluated for safety profile both in randomized (Bongartz *et al*, 2006, Leombruno *et al*, 2009) and observational studies (Wolfe & Michaud, 2007, Setoguchi *et al*, 2006, Askling *et al*, 2005). TNF plays an important role in tumour growth control and host defence, and biologic therapy targeting TNF determines an important immunomodulation, raising thus the concern of a possible increased risk of malignancies in patients treated with anti-TNF antibodies. Regarding short-term cancer risk, meta-analysis of clinical trials suggested an increased risk of cancer development (Bongartz *et al*, 2006, Leombruno *et al*, 2009, Bongartz *et al*, 2009), but observational studies did not confirm these results. Randomized controlled trials provide balanced groups for analysis and a well-selected study population but, on the other hand, considering that the time interval from the onset of cancer until its clinical manifestation is counted in years and not in months, any long-term effect of therapy cannot be correctly estimated using data from clinical trials. In addition, the overall number of cancers in these trials is modest, particularly in the control arm. In a review of data from the MedWatch post-market adverse event surveillance system of FDA, 26 cases of spontaneous lymphoproliferative disorders following treatment with etanercept or infliximab have been reported, with an estimated incidence of 19.9 per 10.000 person-year for etanercept and 6.6 per 100.000 person-year for infliximab (Brown *et al*, 2002). These concerns were confirmed also by a meta-analysis of cancer risk in patients affected by RA treated with infliximab or adalimumab in randomized controlled trials, excluding patients treated with etanercept (Bongartz *et al*, 2006), which reported a pooled odds ratio for malignancy in the TNF treated vs. untreated patients of 3.3 (95% CI 1.2-9.1) in a dose-dependent manner. However, included trials were heterogeneous in terms of disease activity, disease duration and previous or concomitant DMARD treatment and usually lasted between 3 months and 1 year, a relatively short interval for estimating cancer incidence. A subsequent update of this meta-analysis with additional data reported an odds ratio of 2.02 (Costenbader *et al*, 2006). Conversely, these results were not confirmed by another meta-analysis assessing 18 randomized controlled trials for a total of 8.808 RA patients (Leombruno *et al*, 2009). Observational studies provide a major number of patients and longer follow-up, but they have also some limitations. The first one is the non-random assignment to treatment, patients with more severe arthritis being more likely treated, and so that outcome could be related to severity of disease rather than treatment. Other limitations may be due to less selected study subjects and introduced bias such as age, sex, smoking history, disease activity and baseline use of corticosteroids. Another bias could be introduced by physician's decision not to prescribe anti-TNF treatment to a patient with a history of malignancies. Finally, last reason for the divergence between data from trials and from observational studies is the control chosen in the latter. In fact, patients newly starting therapy with anti-TNF should be compared with patients newly starting therapy with other agents for the same disease (Ray, 2003). In Sweden, patients treated with anti-TNF drugs were included in a regional register since the introduction of etanercept and infliximab in 1999 (Geborek *et al*, 2002). A study comparing 757 patients treated with etanercept or infliximab from 1999 to 2002 with 800 patients who received conventional therapy showed no increased risk in solid tumors in anti-TNF treated patients, but, interestingly, five cases of lymphoma were identified among these patients (1.603 person-year), and, compared with conventional-therapy cohort, the relative risk of lymphoma in patients treated with anti-TNF agents was 4.9 (95% CI 0.9-26.2) (Geborek *et al*, 2005). Lymphoma incidence from follow–up of 18.572 American RA patients compared with general population allowed to detect 29 cases of lymphoma, with an overall relative risk for lymphoma of 1.9 in patients with RA not treated with TNF antagonists and tripled (2.9) in patients receiving treatment with TNF antagonists; 2.6 in those receiving infliximab with or without etanercept; and 3.8 in those receiving etanercept with or without infliximab (Wolfe & Michaud, 2004). The increased risk in the TNF antagonist treated group might be due to the fact that patients with the highest risk of lymphoma received TNF antagonists. Consequently, the authors were unable to conclude whether the increased standardized rate ratios were related to RA or truly associated with the drugs. Additionally, this study was not adjusted for patient characteristics other than age and sex. Analysis of cancer risk in TNF antagonists users using a Swedish registry of anti-TNF treated patients and community-based RA patients detected five cases of lymphoma per 1.603 person-year in the treated group and two cases per 3.948 person-year in the comparison group (Franklin *et al*, 2005). The adjusted hazard ratio for lymphoma was 4.9 in anti-TNF treated group, suggesting a large increase in risk. Again, RA severity in patients never treated with anti-TNF agents may be minor. The comparison between a cohort of 4.160 RA patients treated with anti-TNF agents with 53.067 patients with untreated RA, showed that patients with RA are at increased risk of lymphomas in line with previous estimations, and using these expected RA rates as reference, that patients treated with TNF antagonists were not at any additional increased lymphoma risk compared with untreated patients (Askling *et al*, 2005). A cohort study using patients with RA treated with methotrexate (MTX) as a control group did not show any significant increase in the risk of cancer in biologic DMARDS users. This particular control group has been chosen because of similar disease severity between patients treated with these two strategies, and investigators have concluded that it is unlikely that RA patients who have received biologic agents have a greater risk of lymphoproliferative disorders compared with those treated with MTX (Setoguchi *et al*, 2006). A single observational study has reported relative risk for cancer occurrence per single anti-TNF agent (infliximab, etanercept, adalimumab), finding a positive association between biologic therapy and skin cancers, but not with other malignancies, with a median time of exposure of 3.0 years, for any of the three agents separately. However, patients were not followed-up from the start of anti-TNF therapy and so any assessment of risk per time since treatment start was not carried out (Wolfe & Michaud, 2007). Finally, the largest population-based study with the longest observation period investigating cancer risks associated with anti-TNF therapy in RA patients has failed to prove an overall increase of risk during the first 6 years after treatment start and during follow-up time. In fact patients treated with anti-TNF drugs had the same cancer risk of naïve patients and of those starting MTX or DMARDs combination therapy. Incidence or relative risk of cancer does not increase with time nor with duration of active therapy (Askling *et al*, 2009).

Studies	Overall	95% CI	Infliximab	95% CI	Etanercept	95% CI	Adalimumab	95% CI
Wolfe, 2004	1.9 (SIR)	1.3-2.7	2.6	1.4-4.5	3.8	1.9-7.5	-	-
Geborek, 2005	11.5 (SIR)	3.7-26.9	-	-	-	-	-	-
Askling, 2005	1.9 (SIR)	1.7-2.1	-	-	-	-	-	-
Setoguchi, 2006	1.11 (HR)	0.51-2.37	-	-	-	-	-	-
Wolfe, 2007	1.7 (SIR)	1.3-2.2	0.9	0.4-2.1	1.3	0.6-2.8	1.3	0.2-10
Leombruno, 2008	1.26 (OR)	0.52-3.06	-	-	-	-	-	-

Table 2. Lymphoma risk and anti-TNF agents

3.3.3 Methotrexate

Methotrexate (MTX) is a widely used DMARD in the context of autoimmune diseases. RA patients treated with MTX may develop a lymphoproliferative disorder (LPD) resembling lymphomas occurring in immunosuppressed patients (Ellman *et al*, 1991, Kingsmore *et al*, 1992, Liote *et al*, 1995). LPD develops in RA patients at a frequency 2.0-5-fold higher than in general population. MTX-LPD is classified along with other iatrogenic immunodeficiency-related LPDs by WHO classification (Swerdlow *et al*, 2008) and, among these, DLBCL accounts for about 50% of cases, with frequent extranodal involvement and HL for 10-20% of cases. MTX-LPD and non-MTX-LPD seem to share similar clinical findings in RA patients, such as sex, age, primary site, stage and outcome (5-year OS: 59% vs. 53%) (Hoshida *et al*, 2007). Conversely, other papers did not confirm increased incidence of lymphoma in MTX-treated RA patients, even after long-term follow-up (Moder *et al*, 1995, Bologna *et al*, 1997, Kremer, 1997, Weinblatt *et al*, 1998). In a prospective series of 18.572 RA patients, treatment with MTX alone has not been associated with an increased standardized incidence ratio for lymphoma with respect to untreated patients (1.7 vs 1.0) (Wolfe & Michaud, 2004). These results confirmed those reported in a 3-year national prospective study on French RA patients treated with MTX. Investigators have found no increase in lymphoma risk among treated patients compared with French general population. However, in the latter study, authors did not even find an increased lymphoma risk in RA patients overall compared to general population (Mariette *et al*, 2002). There are some case reports of lymphoma regression after MTX discontinuation in patients treated for autoimmune diseases (Liote *et al*, 1995, Kamel *et al*, 1993, Salloum *et al*, 1996). Complete remission occurred generally within 4 weeks after discontinuation of MTX and appeared to persist over a median follow-up of 15 months (4-60). On the other hand, partial remission occurred in a time interval longer than four weeks, often about 2-3 months later (Rizzi *et al*, 2009). Regression of LPD after MTX discontinuation can be considered an evidence of the carcinogenic potential of MTX. This drug in fact is capable to directly induce reactivation of Epstein-Barr virus (EBV) infection with release of virions (Feng *et al*, 2004). An immunodeficient state provides the conditions for the development of lymphoma possibly through the activation of the oncogenic EBV. The EBV positive rate among patients affected by autoimmune disease and lymphoma is about 30% (Hoshida *et al*, 2007, Kamel *et al*, 1993). Moreover, patients affected by RA have an elevated number of EBV-infected circulating B lymphocytes and a major T-cell defect in EBV-specific suppression (Tosato *et al*, 1984). Taken together, the oncogenic role of EBV, the impaired immune response of RA patients to EBV and the additional immunosuppressive effect of MTX may account for EBV-positive lymphoma development in a small number of RA patients treated with MTX (Baecklund *et al*, 1998). The monoclonal antibody rituximab is currently used for the treatment of LPD after allogeneic transplantation. There are still few reports about its use for MTX-LPDs and more studies are warranted to elucidate its potential therapeutic role in this context.

4. Autoimmune entities

	Most frequent subtype	Risk factors
Rheumatoid arthritis	Diffuse large B- cell lymphoma	High inflammatory activity Male gender
Sjögren syndrome	MALT lymphoma	Low serum immunoglobulins levels High serum $\beta2$ microglobulin level Disappearance of a positive rheumatoid factor Hypocomplementemia Low CD4 levels Palpable purpura, parotid gland enlargement
Systemic lupus erythematosus	Diffuse large B- cell lymphoma	Autoimmune haemolytic anaemia Leukopenia Chronic thrombocytopenia Salivary gland swellings Pulmonary infiltrates and/or recurrent pneumonia
Hashimoto's thyroiditis	MALT lymphoma and diffuse large B-cell lymphoma	-
Systemic sclerosis	B-cell lymphomas	-
Celiac disease	Entheropathy-type T-cell lymphoma	Inadequate gluten-free diet
Dermatitis herpetiformis	Entheropathy-type T-cell lymphoma	Inadequate gluten-free diet

Table 3. Most frequent histologic subtypes associated with singular autoimmune entities and known risk factors

4.1 Rheumatoid arthritis

RA is a multisystem chronic autoimmune disorder affecting joint and almost any organ system, with inflammatory nodules formation, interstitial lung disease and leukocytoclastic vasculitis (Turesson & Matteson, 2004). Several studies have demonstrated that patients with RA have a 2-fold increased risk of developing lymphoma (Ekstrom et al, 2003, Franklin et al, 2006) and a link between disease severity and lymphoma risk exist (Smedby et al, 2006, Baecklund et al, 2006a). A nested case-control study performed to determine factors predisposing to lymphoma development in RA patients demonstrated that a high inflammatory activity is the greater risk factor with a an odds ratio of 25.8 compared with low inflammatory activity (Baecklund et al, 1998). Furthermore, a study on Felty syndrome, a complication of severe RA, reported a 13-fold relative risk for lymphoma compared with that of general population (Gridley et al, 1994). Men affected by RA display a higher standardized incidence ratio for the development of NHL and HL than female (Gridley et al, 1993). Finally, a personal history of lymphoma in the years preceding diagnosis of autoimmune disease is not more common in patients affected by RA than expected in general population, while the increased risk of lymphoma development occurs in the first 10 years from RA diagnosis. This proves that shared susceptibility or common risk factors are not the major explanation for this increased risk, but it indicates a critical link between the RA disease or its therapy and the subsequent lymphoma development (Hellgren et al, 2010a). Interestingly, the reported relative risk rates remained relatively constant over time despite therapeutic changes occurred in RA.

4.1.1 Pathogenesis

The increased risk of lymphoma development in RA patients may arise from the interaction of multiple factors: activation of autoimmune B lymphocytes, chronic inflammation, poor EBV control and immunosuppressive therapy (Balandraud et al, 2005). It has been hypothesized that a constant immune stimulation of B cells by auto-antigens may result in both synovitis and lymphocyte activation, finally leading to malignant transformation (Symmons, 1985). Evidence of a B-cell activation is derived from the finding of increased levels of B cell activating factors in RA patients, such as BLy and APRIL, which are produced in the synovial lesions and can drive B cell expansion (Mackay et al, 2005, Seyler et al, 2005). Moreover, several studies have also reported oligoclonal B cell expansion both in the synovium and in the peripheral blood of RA patients (Berek & Kim, 1997). Whether the increased risk is entirely a consequence of the disease and/or of its treatment is not yet fully ascertained. Patients with RA may lack immunocompetence, being more susceptible to lymphoma development, or immunosuppressive treatment may concur to weaken the patient's immune response. Therefore, lymphoma in RA could be due to a too strong or insufficient immunosuppressive therapy (Weyand et al, 2006). A matched case-control study on 378 consecutive Swedish RA patients in whom lymphoma occurred between 1964 and 1995 and 378 healthy controls showed that 48% of lymphoma cases were DLBCLs, and, within those, EBV infection was detected in 12% of lymphomas. Approximately half of the patients had received corticosteroids; 44% had received intra-articular injection of steroids; over 70% of patients had been treated with DMARDs, most frequently antimalarial agents; a few patients had received azathioprine (6%) or MTX (6%) and none had received anti-TNF therapy. An increased lymphoma risk was found only in the azathioprine-treated group, while oral steroids proved to reduce this risk (OR 0.6), especially the intra-articular steroid treatment (OR 0.2). Patients affected both by RA and lymphoma had received similar treatment than those without lymphoma (Baecklund et al, 2006a). In a Japanese cohort of RA patients not treated with immunosuppressive drugs, DLBCL was again the most frequently detected histotype and EBV was present in 30% of cases. Four cases were HL, all of them EBV positive (Hoshida et al, 2004). The increased risk of NHL development could be referred to the impaired capacity of RA patients to control infection of EBV (Balandraud et al, 2005). EBV is an oncogenic herpes virus involved in the pathogenesis of several lymphomas in the context of states of immunodeficiency (Young & Rickinson, 2004, Ambinder, 2003). EBV is not usually found in DLBCL of immunocompetent patients (Ambinder, 2003). EBV-related lymphomagenesis is characteristic in the setting of organ or bone marrow transplantation and congenital or acquired immunodeficiency disorders (Loren et al, 2003). Patients affected by RA have an impaired immune response to EBV. High serum titre of anti-EBV specific antibodies have been detected in some RA patients (Alspaugh et al, 1981), EBV-specific CD8+ T cells have been found in synovial fluid (Tan et al, 2000) and EBV DNA was isolated from the joints of RA patients (Edinger et al, 1999). An impaired control of the outgrowth of EBV infected cells in vitro was also observed (Tosato et al, 1981). This hypothesis is also supported by studies of EBV load in RA patients. In fact an increase in shedding of EBV in saliva and in the proportion of EBV-infected circulating B cells in RA patients has been shown (Tosato et al, 1984, Yao et al, 1986). The mean EBV load in peripheral blood of RA patients is more than 8-fold greater than in normal healthy control, similarly to what occurs in transplant recipients (Balandraud et al, 2003). Nonetheless, the overall incidence of EBV positivity in NHL reported in previous cohorts is 24% (Baecklund et al, 2006a, Mariette et al, 2002), too low to entirely justify the increased incidence of lymphomas among these patients.

4.1.2 Lymphoma subtypes

DLBCL is the most common lymphoma subtype in RA patients, with a prevalence of 48%-67% among all NHL (Mariette et al, 2002, Baecklund et al, 2003), a slightly higher incidence with respect to the general population of western countries, where DLCBL represents the 30-40% of all NHL. DLBCLs can be further subdivided into germinal centre-like (GC) and activated B cell-like subtypes by gene expression profiling, characterized by a different cellular origin and a different prognosis. The majority of RA patients develops a DLBCL of non GC subtype, particular those with a severe and longstanding disease. These lymphomas are characterized by advanced stage at diagnosis, rapid progression and a worse prognosis (5-year OS: 16% vs. 33% for the GC subtypes). In those patients presenting a severe disease and a continuous immune stimulation, the proliferative drive might determine an increased risk of genetic aberrations, particularly in the peripheral activated B cells, the expansion of an uncontrolled peripheral B cell clone and therefore the development of a non-GC DLBCL. Otherwise, alternative pathways are also probably involved in lymphomagenesis, since only a minor proportion of DLBCL are of GC subtype (30%) and other lymphoma subtypes have also been reported in RA patients (Baecklund et al, 2006a). The human germinal-centre associated lymphoma protein (HGAL) is a marker of GC B cell derivation, expressed in the cytoplasm of GC lymphocytes and in lymphomas of GC derivation (Lossos et al, 2003, Natkunam et al, 2005), which inhibits cell migration in normal GC cells and lymphoma cells (Lu et al, 2007). HGAL immunoreactivity has been found in 38 (34%) of 111 RA-DLBCLs (Baecklund et al, 2006b), a lower proportion than that reported in DLBCL in general (68%)

(Natkunam *et al*, 2005), but not surprising giving the fact that the majority of RA-DLBCLs are of the non-GC type. HGAL expression has been associated with a limited-stage disease and better survival. The expression of HGAL as a GC marker may thus been associated with a better clinical course in RA-DLBCLs.

4.2 Sjögren Syndrome

SS is a chronic systemic autoimmune disease clinically characterized by dry mouth (xerostomia) and dry eyes (keratoconjunctive sicca) (Kassan & Moutsopoulos, 2004). It is distinguished by a lymphoproliferative sialadenitis (LESA) with lymphocyte infiltration of salivary ducts, ductal epithelial cell proliferation and apoptosis (Daniels, 1984). This disorder can occur either alone, known as primary SS, or in the context of other systemic autoimmune disorders, such as RA, systemic sclerosis, SLE, which is known as secondary SS. Compared with the general population, an increased risk of developing NHL during the course of such disease was reported (Kassan *et al*, 1978, Ioannidis *et al*, 2002). Patients affected by SS, in fact, have an increased relative risk of 28 fold to develop extranodal MALT lymphoma (MZL) of the salivary gland and a 11-fold increased risk of developing a DLBCL arising *de novo* or by transformation of a previous indolent lymphoma (Smedby *et al*, 2006). Relative risk to develop a lymphoma is 8.7 for patients with primary SS form and 4.5 for patients with a secondary SS (Kauppi *et al*, 1997). NHL is the major complication during the course of the disease, with a prevalence of 4.3% (Voulgarelis *et al*, 1999). The high risk of lymphoma development suggests that it originates locally as a consequence of chronic lymphocyte activation due to the autoimmune setting.

4.2.1 Pathogenesis

Lymphocytes have a central role in the pathogenesis of both SS and lymphoma, but whether T or B lymphocytes play the leading role is controversial. From one side, biopsies of salivary and lachrymal glands are characterized by a mixed infiltrate of predominant CD4 and CD8 T cells, showing restriction of TCR usage (Adamson *et al*, 1983). On the other side, primary SS is characterized by increased monoclonal Ig and by the development of lymphomas of B-cell type. A B-cell mediated autoimmune response occurs in the salivary glands. A wide variety of nuclear auto-antigens are immune targets in SS patients. Anti-nuclear antibody as anti-SSA/Ro and anti-SSB/La are detectable in 70-85% of patients (Jonsson *et al*, 2003). The cause of B-cell hyperactivity in primary SS is not known. Exocrine glands of SS patients show an accumulation of B cells clustering in benign polyclonal aggregates (Brandtzaeg & Johansen, 2005), harbouring mutated IgVH genes and therefore being GC, marginal zone or memory B cells. Successively, an evolution from benign to malignant B lymphoproliferation has been described in the course of primary SS, but not of secondary (Anderson & Talal, 1972). Initial benign polyclonal clusters of B-cells enlarge to organize lymphoid follicle-like structures with germinal centres (GCs), in which plasma cells differentiate. The role of local antigens is crucial for the development of these extralymphoid GCs (Youinou *et al*, 2010). The evolution from a benign B-cell aggregate to a malignant lymphoma may be therefore the consequence of the autoimmune response through the selection and expansion of a monoclonal B-cell clone (Friedman *et al*, 1991). Mutations of *p53* are also involved in lymphoma development in these patients (Tapinos *et al*, 1999). Approximately 20% of SS patients exhibits monoclonal Igs in the serum and urine and mixed monoclonal cryoglobulinemia (MMC) with an IgMk monoclonal rheumatoid factor (RF) component (Youinou *et al*, 1988, Tzioufas *et al*, 1986). Monoclonality therefore correlates with the transition from the autoimmune state to NHL. Various studies on clonality have demonstrated that SS patients with the same and persistent monoclonal B-cell expansion in follow-up biopsies are at higher risk of lymphoma developing. MALT lymphoma cells are found only in glands for years and a subsequent spread outside the salivary may involve the lymph nodes and other extranodal organs (Royer *et al*, 1997).

4.2.2 Clinical characteristics

The development of a malignant lymphoproliferation occurs only in a subset of SS patients and is characterized by the emergence of clinical and serologic parameters in the initial phases of disease, the monitoring of which is important for early detection of malignancy and timely therapeutic intervention (Tzioufas *et al*, 1986, Moutsopoulos *et al*, 1983). Usually, median age at lymphoma diagnosis is 58 years, and the median time from SS diagnosis is 7.5 years (Voulgarelis *et al*, 1999). MZL is the most common histologic subtype, but also follicular lymphoma, lymphoplasmacytoid lymphoma and DLBCL have been reported (Kassan *et al*, 1978, Valesini *et al*, 1997, Mariette, 1999). MZL in SS patients is generally localized at diagnosis (stage I and II) and is characterized by a small tumour burden, good performance status and normal lactate dehydrogenase serum levels. The salivary glands are the most commonly involved organs, with parotid gland enlargement being the main presenting symptom, but near 20% of these lymphomas involve other extra-nodal sites, such as stomach, nasopharynx, skin, liver, kidney, and lung, justifying indeed the importance of a complete staging at diagnosis. Bone marrow involvement is rare (10% of cases) and B symptoms are uncommon. Other clinical manifestations are skin vasculitis, peripheral nerve and renal involvement, anemia, lymphopenia, monoclonal immunoglobulins and mixed monoclonal cryoglobulinemia (MMC) (Voulgarelis *et al*, 1999). Indolent lymphomas arisen in SS patients experience high-grade transformation, mostly in DLBCLs, in about 10% of cases. This evolution is characterized by nodal and extra-nodal dissemination and a unfavourable prognosis, with a median overall survival shorter than two years (Voulgarelis *et al*, 1999). It has been proven by immunohistochemical and genotypic studies that such DLBCLs arise from the same clone as indolent lymphomas, as a consequence of genetic alterations such as p53 allelic loss or mutation, hypermethylation of p15 and p16 genes, deletion of p16 gene (Du *et al*, 1996, Neumeister *et al*, 1997).

4.2.3 Risk factors

Some risk factors for lymphoma development have been identified in SS patients. Lymphoma risk seems to increase with disease severity, expressed by decreased levels of serum immunoglobulins, high serum β2-microglobulin levels and disappearance of a previous positive rheumatoid factor (FR) (Anderson & Talal, 1972, Anaya *et al*, 1996); parotid gland enlargement, splenomegaly, lymphadenopathy (Kassan *et al*, 1978); low C4 levels and palpable purpura (Ioannidis *et al*, 2002, Skopouli *et al*, 2000); MMC (Tzioufas *et al*, 1996). A higher relative risk of developing lymphoproliferative disorders in patients with an early onset of disease has been suggested, with a significant and independent association between lymphoma development and low C4 levels (Ramos-Casals *et al*, 2005). An adverse prognostic value of low levels of C3 (Theander *et al*, 2004), vasculitis, severe involvement in parotid scintigraphy, hypocomplementaemia and/or cryoglobulins at diagnosis (Brito-

Zeron *et al*, 2007) have been proposed in patients with primary SS. Patients with such risk factors should be closely monitored.

4.2.4 Lymphoma treatment

Many patients with localized MALT lymphoma may be managed with a "wait and watch" policy, with a median overall survival of 6.4 years (Voulgarelis *et al*, 1999). In a retrospective study (Ambrosetti *et al*, 2004), no difference in outcome between patients treated with surgery, radiotherapy or chemotherapy and those who were not treated has been reported. Single-agent chemotherapy is indicated (alkylating agents; purine analogues; monoclonal antibody rituximab) for multiple extra-nodal disease. The purine analogue cladribine has been associated with a 75% complete remission rate in patients with SS-associated MALT lymphoma (Voulgarelis *et al*, 2002); while the efficacy of the anti-CD20 monoclonal antibody rituximab is controversial (Pijpe *et al*, 2005, Quartuccio *et al*, 2009). Combined chemotherapy (CHOP-like regimens) should be reserved to patients with high tumour burden or aggressive lymphoma. R-CHOP regimen has been associated with complete remission (duration 10-23 months) in four patients with SS-aggressive NHL. Importantly, certain signs and symptoms of MC type II (purpura, peripheral neuropathy and arthralgias) significantly improved with treatment, the levels of circulating cryoglobulins and RF decreased, and C4 levels returned to normal (Voulgarelis *et al*, 2006).

4.3 Systemic Lupus Erythematosus

SLE is a systemic autoimmune disease characterized by variable severity and a multisystem involvement, including cardiovascular, musculoskeletal, excretory, respiratory, and neurological involvement. Prognosis of SLE patients has considerably improved during the last decades, with an increase in 5-year survival from <50% before 1955 to >90% nowadays (Moss *et al*, 2002), due to the use of novel therapeutic options. Nevertheless, the incidence of late complications seems to be increased and mortality due to malignancies remains higher than that of general population (Nossent *et al*, 2007). This could be referred to the common pathogenic pathways in lupus and cancer. Lupus and various malignancies share some risk factors, such as genetic predisposition, viral infections (EBV), hormones (insulin-like growth factor, prolactin, oestrogen, and growth hormone) (Bernatsky *et al*, 2002, Poole *et al*, 2009). Another shared characteristic is represented by antiphospholipid antibodies, frequently present in both diseases and recently associated with cancer development (Tincani *et al*, 2010). SLE has been associated with a 2.7 - 4.1 fold increased risk of NHL development (Ekstrom Smedby *et al*, 2008, Abu-Shakra *et al*, 1993, Ekstrom *et al*, 2003), and some studies have also suggested a link between SLE and HL (Landgren *et al*, 2006, Bernatsky *et al*, 2007). A multi-site international cohort study calculated a standardized incidence ratio (SIR) for all hematologic malignancies of 2.75 and for NHL of 3.64 (Bernatsky *et al*, 2005b). As far as HL, same authors observed a SIR of 2.4 in another large multi-site international cohort (Bernatsky *et al*, 2007). The pooled analysis combining these data with those of other large cohort studies provided a SIR estimate for HL in SLE of 3.16. Generally, aggressive lymphomas, such as DLBCL are more common in SLE patients (Smedby *et al*, 2006, Simon *et al*, 2007, Bernatsky *et al*, 2005a, Lofstrom *et al*, 2007). In general population, DLBCL accounts for 30% of all lymphomas, but in SLE patients this percentage is between 38% and 64% (Smedby *et al*, 2006, Bernatsky *et al*, 2005a, King & Costenbader, 2007). No subtyping into germinal-centre like or activated B-cell like subtype has been reported.

4.3.1 Pathogenesis

Concerning genetic predisposition, a possible reason for the increased risk of NHL in SLE is that distinct major histocompatibility complex (MHC)-haplotypes may predispose to both disorders (Okada *et al*, 1991). The role of immunosuppressive therapy is controversial; it may impair immune defence resulting in an increased risk of lymphomagenesis. However, SLE patients who have never been treated with immunosuppressive agents have the highest rate of NHL incidence during the first year from diagnosis, suggesting that the increased risk is not related to cumulative doses of therapy (Kiss *et al*, 2010). A nested case-cohort study performed to assess the HR for cancer within a multi-site international SLE cohort after exposure to immunosuppressive drugs (anti-malarial drugs, systemic glucocorticoids, NSAIDs, aspirin) showed an adjusted HR for overall cancer risk of 0.82. This risk seems to be higher when only haematological malignancies are considered (Bernatsky *et al*, 2008). In addition to extrinsic risk factors, there are also defects in the immune system contributing to the development of both SLE and lymphomas, as the abnormal B-cell activation due to the chronic and persistent antigen-stimulation, cell-cycle deregulation and impaired apoptosis, which leads to uncontrolled cell proliferation, an exaggerated humoral autoimmune response and the increased risk of oncogene translocation (Illes *et al*, 2009). The impaired immune response in SLE is thus characterized by the accumulation of activated self-reactive B and T cells (Xu & Wiernik, 2001). Many studies have underlined the role of impaired apoptosis in this process. For example, the MRL/lpr mouse, a murine SLE model, has defects in the *Fas* gene, leading to defects in apoptosis and subsequent development of SLE (Watanabe-Fukunaga *et al*, 1992). Mice with mutations of *PTEN*, a tumor suppressor gene, which impairs the *Fas*-mediated elimination of activated lymphocytes, develop SLE characterized by ANA antibodies, glomerulonephritis and lymphadenopathies (Di Cristofano *et al*, 1999). Also *bcl-2*, a proto-oncogene involved in the majority of B NHL, is highly expressed in SLE (Aringer *et al*, 1994), causing prolonged survival of auto-reactive B cells and thus favouring malignant transformation (Xu & Wiernik, 2001). The persistent clonal expansion of benign hyperactive B and T cells retained in lymph node of SLE patients in response to self-antigens exposes these cells to DNA damage, ultimately leading to neoplastic transformation (Xu & Wiernik, 2001). Increased serum levels of type-I Interferons (IFNs a/b) is also associated with active SLE disease (Theofilopoulos *et al*, 2005). The IFNs are cytokines that inhibit cell proliferation and modulate cell survival (Banchereau & Pascual, 2006), and also inhibit apoptosis induced by signalling through B-cell receptor (Su & David, 1999). The p202a murine protein is a member of the interferon-inducible p200-protein family (Choubey & Kotzin, 2002). Increased levels of the p202 protein in splenic B cells of B6.Nba2 SLE susceptible mice determine defects of apoptosis and accumulation of B cells in the spleen (Xin *et al*, 2006) probably by inhibiting p53-mediated transcriptional activation of genes that encode pro-apoptotic proteins as well as transcriptional repression of genes that encode anti-apoptotic proteins. It is therefore possible that increased levels of p202 in B cells also contribute to enhance the risk of developing B-cell malignancies (Veeranki & Choubey, 2010). The murine p202 protein does not have any human homologue, but the human IFI16 protein, a member of the p200-protein family, is functionally similar. An increased expression of IFI16 protein in normal human cells determines cellular growth arrest and up to 29% of SLE patients present high auto-antibodies titres to the IFI16 protein (Choubey *et al*, 2008). IFI16 protein binds p53, so basal and IFN-induced increased levels of IFI16 in SLE patients may inhibit the p53 mediated transcription of target genes (Choubey *et al*, 2008). Finally, SLE patients have high plasma levels of BAFF (Do & Chen-Kiang, 2002), which activates NF-kB (Laabi & Strasser, 2000). Mice overexpressing BAFF develop a SLE-like disease and exhibit B-cell activation (Mackay *et al*, 1999). Also the increased level of IFI16 protein in B cells is capable to activate the NF-kB transcription factor, which persistent activation has been related to the development of B cell malignancies (Vallabhapurapu & Karin, 2009). In addition, NF-kB induces IL-6 expression (Choubey & Panchanathan, 2008). Overall, these results suggest that the triad IFI16/NF-kB/IL-6 could be involved in the development of B-cell malignancies in SLE patients. Recently, it was also shown that antiribosomal-P-protein (anti-P) antibodies, present in nearly 15-20% of patients with SLE active disease, cross react with phospholipids (Caponi *et al*, 2007), enhancing the production of TNF-alfa and IL-6 by monocytes (Toubi & Shoenfeld, 2007), which increases proliferation of normal and clonal B cells. The role of EBV in the pathogenesis of lymphoma in SLE patients has not been fully investigated. An increased prevalence of EBV infection in young patients with SLE has been reported (James *et al*, 1997) and there are some observations that, in some cases, EBV may be a trigger of lymphomagenesis in SLE (Verdolini *et al*, 2002). In contrast, in a retrospective study analyzing lymphoma development in a large cohort of SLE patients, EBV positivity was found only in 17% of cases (King & Costenbader, 2007). Whether EBV infection causes SLE and/or lymphoma independently has not yet been ascertained.

4.3.2 Clinical characteristics

The emerge of NHL in a SLE patient is clinically difficult to recognize in the current practice, due to the fact that many lymphoma characteristics are already part of the autoimmune disease (lymphadenopathy, fever, weight loss, hepato-splenomegaly, cytopenias, autoantibodies), raising the possibility that SLE might be a paraneoplastic syndrome appearing in the context of the lymphoid malignancy. Some clinical SLE characteristics as haematological manifestations (autoimmune haemolytic anaemia, leukopenia, hyperglobulinemia, chronic thrombocytopenia) (King & Costenbader, 2007), sicca symptoms/salivary gland swellings, pulmonary infiltrates, and/or recurrent pneumonia (Lofstrom *et al*, 2007) have been associated with increased risk of developing lymphoma. The common involvement of mucosal membranes, salivary glands and lung parenchyma in patients developing a lymphoma could be due to the fact that, in an immune-deficient patient, an impaired barrier for exogenous agents, as viruses, favour recurrent infections, which may be involved in lymphomagenesis. Median age at lymphoma diagnosis is 50 years, with a median time interval from SLE diagnosis of 17.8 years (King & Costenbader, 2007). Diffuse large B cell lymphoma is the most common subtype (King & Costenbader, 2007). After diagnosis of NHL a 5-year survival probability of 47%-50% has been estimated (Bernatsky *et al*, 2005b, Lofstrom *et al*, 2007), and mortality in patients with both diseases is usually due to progressive B-cell malignancy (Xu & Wiernik, 2001).

4.4 Hashimoto's thyroiditis

Hashimoto's thyroiditis (HT) is an autoimmune chronic inflammatory disease of the thyroid, histologically characterized by a severe and progressive lymphocytic infiltration causing destruction of the glandular parenchyma and consequent goitre development and hypothyroidism. It commonly affects middle-aged women (Aozasa, 1990). The activation of CD4+ T lymphocytes specific for thyroid antigens is considered the trigger of the autoimmune process in HT (Weetman & McGregor, 1994, Dayan & Daniels, 1996). Autoantibodies produced in HT are specific for thyreoglobulin, thyroperoxidase and the thyroid stimulating hormone receptor (TSH-R). The first two antibodies are not detected in all patients. Antibodies against TSH-R block the activation of this receptor, causing the functional impairment of the thyroid. On the other side, activated CD4+ T cells recruit cytotoxic CD8+ T cells and B cells into the thyroid causing the direct killing of thyroid cells. Patients affected by HT are at increased risk of developing primary thyroid lymphoma (PTL) with a relative risk of 67 fold for marginal zone B-cell lymphoma of MALT-type (Holm et al, 1985). Lymphoma typically occurs 20-30 years after the diagnosis of thyroiditis (Pedersen & Pedersen, 1996). HT is not only associated with thyroidal MALT lymphoma, but also with other extranodal lymphomas. In a retrospective study on 80 patients affected by MALT lymphoma, 13 (16%) had a concomitant diagnosis of HT; four of these patients had thyroidal lymphoma and nine had extra-thyroidal lymphomas (gastric, orbital, small intestinal, and salivary gland lymphomas) (Troch et al, 2008). PTL represents 5% of all thyroid malignancies (Staunton & Greening, 1973) and MALT lymphoma represent 25% of all PTLs (Thieblemont et al, 2002, Derringer et al, 2000). About 50% of patients diagnosed with PTL have a clinical history of HT (Niitsu et al, 2007, Rossi, 2009), even if only 0.5% of patients with HT develop PTL.

4.4.1 Pathogenesis

It has been hypothesized that the chronic antigenic stimulation caused by the autoimmune and inflammatory process in HT leads to the proliferation of newly formed lymphoid tissue and ultimately to malignant transformation. The thyroid gland does not contain native lymphoid tissue (Holm et al, 1985, Isaacson, 1997). The lymphoid tissue present in HT thyroid gland share many features with MALT (Hyjek & Isaacson, 1988). The presence of clonal B-cell populations has been demonstrated in HT thyroid specimens also in patients without evidence of lymphoma development (Saxena et al, 2004). The clonal IgH gene rearrangements carried by thyroid lymphomas may already be evident in the oligoclonal rearrangements characterizing HT, and a fraction of thyroid lymphomas use the same IgH utilized by anti-thyroid auto-antibodies (Rossi, 2009, Moshynska & Saxena, 2008). IGVH genes are extensively targeted by aberrant somatic hypermutation in thyroid DLBCL, MALT and follicular lymphoma, and also in 2 of 14 (14.3%) patients affected by HT, suggesting that these genetic alterations represent an early step in the process of B-cell lymphomagenesis. This aberrant activity of somatic hypermutation may introduce activating mutations and may cause genetic instability, favouring chromosomal translocation (Takakuwa et al, 2009).

4.4.2 Clinical characteristics

Patients developing a PTL clinically present a rapid growth of a thyroid mass, associated with hoarseness, stridor or, less commonly, with dysphagia or dyspnoea. The presence of B symptoms is uncommon in indolent subtypes (Ansell et al, 1999). Up to 90% of patients usually presents with early stage I or II lymphoma (Graff-Baker et al, 2010). The most common histologic subtypes are B cell-type, in particular MALT lymphomas and DLBCL. The other histological subtypes are exceptional (Thieblemont et al, 2002). MALT lymphoma is an indolent lymphoma, with a 5-year disease-free survival of over 95% (Graff-Baker et al, 2010) and the disease tends to remain localized for a long time. Conversely, aggressive DLBCL usually arise from a pre-existing MALT lymphoma and a component of residual MALT lymphoma can be still found (Niitsu et al, 2007). DLBCL has a dismal prognosis despite polychemotherapic regimens, with a 5 year probability of survival of 44% (Thieblemont *et al*, 2002). Only rare cases of HL of the thyroid have been reported in the literature, but any association with underlying thyroiditis cannot be ascertained because of the small number of cases (Wang *et al*, 2005). Older age at diagnosis is associated with decreased disease-free survival (Graff-Baker *et al*, 2010). Tissue biopsies should be considered the gold standard for histological diagnosis (Thieblemont *et al*, 2002).

4.4.3 Therapy

Local treatment, such as surgical excision and radiotherapy, could represent a valid treatment strategy for patients with stage I or II MALT lymphoma of the thyroid gland (Tsang *et al*, 2003). Complete surgical resection improves prognosis over incomplete resection, with a 5-year OS of 100% (Thieblemont *et al*, 2002), although most authors currently believe that total thyroidectomy is unnecessary, exposing patients to the risks of surgery (recurrent laryngeal nerve damage and hypoparathyroidism) without conferring any survival advantage (Tupchong *et al*, 1986, Ruggiero *et al*, 2005, Klyachkin *et al*, 1998). Involved field radiotherapy is associated with a 5-year OS of 90% (Laing *et al*, 1994). Nonetheless, patients with thyroid malignant lymphoma treated with radiotherapy seem to have a higher incidence of hypothyroidism than those treated with chemotherapy (Tamura *et al*, 1981). Localized treatment plays a minor role in DLBCL, which requires aggressive anthracycline-based chemotherapy regimens (CHOP or CHOP-like), associated with rituximab, a monoclonal antibody directed against B-cell specific antigen CD20, and followed by involved-field radiotherapy. Chemotherapy alone may be considered in selected patients younger than 60 years and with no adverse prognostic factors (Reyes *et al*, 2005). Rituximab is effective for autoimmune thyroid diseases such as Grave's disease (El Fassi *et al*, 2007a, El Fassi *et al*, 2007b). The use of rituximab monotherapy in three cases of HT-related thyroid MALT lymphoma has also been reported. Rituximab monotherapy determined a significant decrease of anti-thyroid autoantibody levels, but it is still unknown whether thyroid dysfunction can be restored, and its use remains still controversial in HT (Kahara *et al*, 2011).

4.5 Systemic sclerosis

Systemic sclerosis (SSc) is a multisystem inflammatory disease with autoimmune features. It is characterized by vascular abnormalities and fibrosis of the skin and internal organs. Some retrospective studies have reported an increased risk of malignancies in SSc patients (Abu-Shakra *et al*, 1993, Rosenthal *et al*, 1993, Derk *et al*, 2006), but data on the link between SSc and lymphoproliferative disorders are still controversial. This association was first proposed in 1953 (ZATUCHNI *et al*, 1953) and successively several epidemiological studies have been performed to explore this risk (Chatterjee *et al*, 2005, Hill *et al*, 2003, Duncan & Winkelmann, 1979). A number of sporadic case reports have underlined the association between SSc and NHL, particularly with aggressive B-cell subtypes (Arnaud *et al*, 2006, Derk *et al*, 2004, Haviv *et al*, 1997) and some authors observed an increased risk of NHL among SSc patients, primarily within the first year after the onset of disease, but not beyond 4 years of follow up (Landgren *et al*, 2006, Mellemkjaer *et al*, 2008, Rosenthal *et al*, 1993). Conversely, other studies failed to demonstrate a consistent association between SSc and lymphomas (Chatterjee *et al*, 2005, Rosenthal *et al*, 1995, Roumm & Medsger, 1985). In some cases, systemic sclerosis could even represent a paraneoplastic syndrome (Vettori *et al*, 2010). In a population-based cohort study from south-west England to determine if patients with scleroderma have an increased risk of malignancy compared with general population, the highest risk among patients affected by scleroderma was found for haematological malignancies, especially for NHL (RR=25.8) (Siau *et al*, 2010). Another retrospective analysis of 218 Hungarian patients with SSc followed during a period of 12 years showed lymphoma development in three of them (1.38%), all of B cell phenotype, within 2 years after the onset of SSc. The incidence of lymphoma in this cohort was 38.3 cases per 100.000 patients per year (Szekanecz *et al*, 2008). Considering 24 studies analyzed in a review, characteristics associated to NHL development are old age, female sex, diffuse cutaneous subset and early disease. B-cell lymphoma represents the most frequent histotype and the interval between diagnosis of SSc and lymphoma onset is usually short (Vettori *et al*, 2010). Some sporadic cases have also reported an association with HL (Rosenthal *et al*, 1993, Duggal *et al*, 2002, Kedar *et al*, 1979, Hall *et al*, 1978).

4.5.1 Pathogenesis

The pathophysiological relationship between scleroderma and malignancy remains poorly understood. There might be multiple pathways leading to cancer in general, and lymphoproliferative disorders in particular. B cells have many pathogenic roles in SSc (Sato *et al*, 2004). SSc patients are indeed characterized by alterations of the B-cell homeostasis, such as expansion of naïve cells, decreased number of circulating but activated memory cells and defective natural killer cells activity (Sato *et al*, 2004, Horikawa *et al*, 2005). Therefore, altered B cell functions may be responsible of the higher incidence of B NHL. Also TGF-β, a cytokine involved in the regulation of connective tissue proteins, which is highly expressed in SSc tissues, might play an important role since dysregulated signalling of the TGF-β is capable to induce tumorigenesis (Grady, 2005). Moreover, the malignant transformation might be a consequence of chronic tissue damage. Finally, EBV-encoded small RNAs have been detected in the majority of DLBCLs associated with systemic rheumatic diseases, including SSc (Kojima *et al*, 2006). In conclusion, a clear relationship between SSc and NHL has not yet been ascertained and further studies with higher number of patients are required to clarify the coexistence of these two entities.

4.6 Celiac disease

Celiac disease (CD) is a chronic autoimmune enteropathy affecting small-intestine, triggered by gluten proteins from wheat, barley and rye. The small-intestinal mucosal injury caused by the autoimmune response determines malabsorption which results in gastrointestinal symptoms (diarrhoea, weight loss, abdominal pain, anorexia, lactose intolerance, abdominal distension and irritability) and/or non-gastrointestinal features (iron-deficiency anaemia, dermatitis herpetiformis, chronic fatigue, joint pain/inflammation, migraines, depression, attention-deficit disorder, epilepsy, osteoporosis/osteopenia, infertility and/or recurrent fetal loss, vitamin deficiencies, short stature, failure to thrive, delayed puberty, dental defects and autoimmune disorders). The diagnosis of CD is based on histologic characteristics of small-bowel biopsy and on clinical and histological remission after a strict gluten-free diet. The presence of circulating CD-associated antibodies, such as IgA against the endomysium of connective tissue and against tissue transglutaminase, at time of diagnosis and their normalization after a gluten-free diet support the diagnosis of CD. Most CD patients display specific pairs of allelic variants in two HLA genes, HLA-DQA1 and

HLA-DQB1. Adhering to a strict gluten-free diet usually results in healing of the damaged small-intestinal mucosa and improvement of intestinal absorption. A gluten-free diet is sufficient to treat the majority of patients. Two–5% of patients with adult-onset CD, especially those diagnosed above the age of 50, does not respond to a gluten-free diet (Tack et al, 2010a). Refractory celiac disease (RCD) is defined when clinical and histological symptoms recur after a good response to a gluten-free diet or persist after more than 12 months of strict diet. Patients affected by CD are at increased risk of lymphoma development, not only primary gastrointestinal, but at any site. The occurrence of an EATL is the main cause of death in RCD patient. About 50-60% of patients with RCD type II develop an EATL within 5 years (Al-Toma et al, 2007, Di Sabatino & Corazza, 2009, Daum et al, 2003). Despite the strong association between CD and EATL, the majority of lymphomas associated with CD are of different histologies, such as DLBCL and peripheral T cell lymphomas (Catassi et al, 2002, Mearin et al, 2006, Smedby et al, 2005, Halfdanarson et al, 2010).

4.6.1 Epidemiology

Earlier estimates of risk of NHL in CD amply varies, from no increased risk (Collin et al, 1994) to a 42-fold (Holmes et al, 1989) or a 69-fold increased risk of NHL (Corrao et al, 2001). A significant increased risk of NHL among CD patients has been reported, with a SIR of 2.2 (95% CI 1.3-3.6) for B-cell NHL and 3.6 (95% CI 2.3-5.2) for lymphomas of non-intestinal origin (Smedby et al, 2005), most common subtype being DLBCL. The RR for T cell NHL was 50-fold increased. Patients with B-cell lymphomas have been demonstrated to have a better prognosis that those with T cell NHL (Halfdanarson et al, 2010). To investigate the frequency of CD among patients with NHL a prospective, multi-centre case-control study was conducted in 10 European countries between 1998 and 2002, showing that patients with CD have a significantly increased risk of developing NHL (OR=2.6 95%CI=1.4-4.9) in comparison with the general population. Importantly, the increased frequency of CD in NHL occurred in those celiac patients diagnosed clinically before screening and not in undiagnosed CD (Mearin et al, 2006). Another large nationwide population-based study assessed and compared risk of developing a lymphoproliferative disease among three different classes of subjects: patients affected by CD, patients with small bowel intestinal inflammation and patients with latent CD. It was showed an increased risk of lymphoproliferative malignancy (HR=2.82 95% CI 2.36-3.37) associated with the presence of a biopsy-proven CD, even after 5 years of follow up, but not with latent CD. The increased risk regarded NHL of the T cell and the B cell type as well as HL (Elfstrom et al, 2011). The risk of developing a lymphoma in CD patients is related to the age of diagnosis of CD. As a matter of fact, mean age at diagnosis of patients who develops a cancer is higher than that of patients who did not (Silano et al, 2007). This could be due to the diagnostic delay causing a prolonged period of dietary exposure to gluten (Holmes et al, 1989, Corrao et al, 2001). The risk of developing a malignancy in patients with CD who adhere to a gluten-free diet for five consecutive years or more is not increased compared with that of general population (Holmes et al, 1989, Lewis et al, 1996, Silano et al, 2008).

4.6.2 EATL

EATL is an intestinal tumour of intraepithelial T lymphocytes, usually presenting as a neoplasm composed of large lymphoid cells and often associated with necrosis and an inflammatory background, including large number of histiocytes and eosinophils. The adjacent intestinal mucosa frequently shows enteropathy with villous atrophy, crypt hyperplasia, increased *lamina propria* lymphocytes and plasma cells and intraepithelial lymphocytosis (Chott *et al*, 1998). In 10-20% of cases, lymphoma is composed of monomorphic medium-sized cells with no inflammatory background and rare necrosis (type II EATL) and may occur sporadically, not associated with CD. EATL more often occurs in the jejunum or ileum as one or more ulcerating mucosal lesions that invade the wall of intestine and frequently cause perforation. The time interval between diagnosis of CD and development of lymphoma varies from 2 months to more than 5 years (Ilyas *et al*, 1995). HLA genotyping shows that patients with EATL have the CD-associated DQA1*0501, DQB1*0201 phenotype, and additional HLA-DR/DQ alleles may increase the risk of lymphoma (Wright, 1995).

4.6.2.1 Pathogenesis

RCD patients can be classified as RCD type I and type II. Type-II RCD patients have >20% phenotypically aberrant intraepithelial lymphocytes (IEL), expressing cytoplasmatic CD3, but lacking surface expression of CD3, CD4 and CD8, while type-I RCD patients have normal IEL (Cellier *et al*, 2000, Patey-Mariaud De Serre *et al*, 2000). IEL with aberrant phenotype also show monoclonal T-cell receptor (TCR)-gamma rearrangement (Bagdi *et al*, 1999), suggesting that these cells constitute a neoplastic population. Moreover, in those patients with type II RCD who subsequently develop EATL, the IEL share the same monoclonal TCR-gamma as the subsequent T-cell lymphoma (Cellier *et al*, 2000, Cellier *et al*, 1998, Daum *et al*, 2005, Ashton-Key *et al*, 1997) and carry gain of chromosome 1q in common with 16% of EATL (Verkarre *et al*, 2003). Therefore, type II RCD may be considered an example of cryptic intraepithelial T-cell lymphoma (Daum *et al*, 2001). CD30+ IEL in RCD II seem to indicate a worse prognosis, including risk of developing lymphoma (Farstad *et al*, 2002). Also interleukin 15 (IL15) might play a role in lymphomagenesis. Uncontrolled overexpression of IL15 by enterocytes in patients with type-II RCD promotes and maintain activation of IEL, favouring the emergence of T-cell clonal proliferations and the subsequent transformation into EATL (Mention *et al*, 2003).

4.6.2.2 Clinical characteristics and prognosis

EATL often present at older age (mean > 60 years) and in patients with a reduced performance status. In most cases disease is disseminated at diagnosis. Patients generally present with abdominal pain, often associated with jejunal perforation, weight loss, diarrhoea or bowel obstruction. Since obstruction and perforation are frequent, many cases are diagnosed at laparotomy. EATL is characterized by multifocal presentation in 10-25% of cases. Neurologic symptoms are reported in approximately 6% of adults with CD, of which cerebellar ataxia is the most frequent one. EATL is an aggressive malignancy that, if untreated, leads to death due to multifocal intestinal perforation caused by refractory malignant ulcers. The prognosis of EATL is very poor compared with that of intestinal B cell lymphomas (Domizio *et al*, 1993). It shows low chemosensitivity, rapid tumour growth and a tendency to dissemination with about 80% of patients experiencing relapse, even after 5 years of follow up, and a 1- and 5-year survival rates of 31-39% and 8-20% respectively (Al-Toma *et al*, 2007, Daum *et al*, 2003). Overall, the dismal prognosis of these patients reflects in part late diagnosis and in part the poor performance status due to the compromised immunological and nutritional status (Gale *et al*, 2000). Stage is the main prognostic factor, with a 5-year cause-specific survival higher than 60% for patients with limited disease and 25% for those with advanced stage (d'Amore et al, 1994, Chott et al, 1992).

4.6.2.3 Therapy

A standard treatment for patients with EATL has not been established, and reported results are overall unsatisfactory. Most patients with EATL are managed with a surgical approach as the primary strategy. Even if surgery is not a curative approach, debulking and resection of masses at high risk of perforation following chemotherapy or occlusion are frequently indicated in these patients. Involved-field radiotherapy 35 Gy was indicated in some patients with bulky disease or incomplete resection (Novakovic et al, 2006), but it is used almost exclusively with palliative purposes. Combined treatment modality with debulking surgery followed by systemic anthracycline-containing polichemotherapy, with or without consolidation radiotherapy, showed an ORR of 58%, a 5-year FFS of 3% and a 5-year OS of 20-25% (Domizio et al, 1993, Gale et al, 2000, d'Amore et al, 1994, Morton et al, 1993). Many patients are unable to complete the chemotherapy program and do not receive radiotherapy due to rapid disease progression, poor nutritional and performance status, associated with local and systemic complications (Daum et al, 2003, Gale et al, 2000). Given the dismal prognosis of patients treated with conventional chemotherapy, some authors assessed feasibility and activity of high-dose chemotherapy supported by autologous stem cell transplantation as upfront treatment of EATL, with conflicting results. Most of these studies are based on small retrospective series of patients with disomogeneous characteristics, and utilizing different conditioning regimens (Al-Toma et al, 2007, Bishton & Haynes, 2007). High-dose chemotherapy with IVE/MTX (ifosfamide, vincristine, etoposide, methotrexate) followed by ASCT has been associated with significantly better outcome in comparison with historical controls treated with conventional anthracycline-based chemotherapy. In fact, patients treated with IVE/MTX-ASCT had an improved remission rate (69% vs. 42%); lower death rates and higher 5-year PFS and OS (52% vs. 22% and 60% vs. 22%, respectively) (Sieniawski et al, 2010). Interestingly, chemotherapy supported by ASCT may also prevent EATL development in patients with RCD (Meijer et al, 2004). In fact, in a retrospective series of 18 patients with RCD type II, 13 patients successfully underwent conditioning with fludarabine and melphalan supported by ASCT, with a significant reduction of the aberrant T-cells in duodenal biopsies associated with improvement in clinical well-being and normalization of hematologic and biochemical markers. After a follow up > 2 years EATL developed only in one transplanted patients, with a 4-year survival rate of 66% (Tack et al, 2010b). Alemtuzumab, a humanized anti-CD52 monoclonal antibody has been rarely used in EATL. The combination of gemcitabine and alemtuzumab has been successfully used in an elderly patients with poor performance status and extra-intestinal dissemination of EATL both at diagnosis and relapse (Soldini et al, 2008). Another patient with EATL was treated with alemtuzumab-CHOP combination at diagnosis in a prospective phase II trial on T-cell lymphomas achieving a short-lasting complete remission (Gallamini et al, 2007). Moreover, alemtuzumab was successfully used in the treatment of a patient with RCD at high risk of developing EATL, obtaining a total recovery of duodenal biopsy (Vivas et al, 2006). Patients with refractory or relapsed EATL and without formal contraindications should be therefore managed with high-dose chemotherapy supported by ASCT. Two patients in CR were treated with allogeneic SCT with reduced intensity conditioning regimen, with a HLA identical sibling donor. Both patients relapsed within few months after transplantation (van de Water et al, 2010).

4.7 Dermatitis herpetiformis

Dermatitis herpetiformis (DH) is a gluten-sensitive skin disease characterized by an itchy, blistering rash which diagnosis is based on the presence of granular IgA deposits in the epidermal-dermal junction observed by direct immunofluorescence. About 75-80% of patients have an associated gluten-sensitive enteropathy with villous atrophy identical to that found in CD, even if gastrointestinal symptoms are rare, and the remaining show increased amount of γδ receptor bearing T lymphocytes in the jejunal mucosa (Savilahti et al, 1992, Reunala, 1998). Both enteropathy and cutaneous rash recover with a gluten-free diet and relapse when diet is withdrawn (Fry et al, 1973, Reunala et al, 1977), suggesting that DH might be a cutaneous manifestation of CD. Moreover, almost all patients affected by DH carry the HLA alleles DQA1*0501 and DQB1*0201 typical of CD (Fronek et al, 1991). Since 1970, it is thought that patients with DH but without clinical sign of CD have an increased risk of developing cancer (Gjone & Nordoy, 1970), and some cases of patients with DH and lymphoma were reported (Jenkins et al, 1983, Reunala et al, 1982). The first large population-based cohort study assessing lymphoma risk in DH included 976 patients affected by DH without concomitant CD diagnosed from 1964 to 1983 in Sweden (Sigurgeirsson et al, 1994). The RR of developing cancer resulted 1.4 (95% CI= 1.1-1.7) in male patients and 1.2 (95% CI= 0.8-1.7) in female patients. This increased risk lost significance if lymphomas were excluded from analysis. In fact, analyzing cancer by subtype, it was found only a significant association with NHL (RR 5.4 95% CI= 2.2-11.1 in male patients and 4.5 95% CI=0.9-13.2 in female patients). The median time between the first admission to hospital and diagnosis of lymphoma was 4 years and the median age at diagnosis was 64 years. Most lymphomas were localized outside the gastrointestinal tract and were of the B cell phenotype. Only one case was classified as EATL. DH indeed is not only associated with EATL, but also with B-cell lymphomas, which may occur both within and outside the gastrointestinal tract as nodal or extranodal disease (Hervonen et al, 2005, Viljamaa et al, 2006). One possible reason for this discrepancy may be the less severe small bowel damage in DH with respect to that in CD. Occurrence of malignancy was assessed in another DH-patient cohort mainly treated with dapsone and gluten-free diet compared with patients affected by CD and general population (Collin et al, 1996). This study cohort included 305 consecutive Finnish patients diagnosed with DH from 1970 to 1992 and 383 patients diagnosed with CD. The only significantly increased SIR was that for NHL among patients with DH (10.3; 95% CI 2.8-26.3), while the overall incidence of other malignancies was not increased. Of four patients who developed NHL, three were adhering to a gluten-free diet, but two for less than five years, which is probably a too short period to exhibit a protective effect against malignancy (Holmes et al, 1989). Extension of the follow up period for a further 12 years confirmed that patients who have adhered to a strict gluten-free diet for more than 5 years have no increased risk of developing lymphoma compared to the general population (Lewis et al, 1996), supporting the protective role of a gluten-free diet against lymphoma development in DH (Hervonen et al, 2005). Moreover, three patients had abnormal small bowel villous architecture, while one patient had normal mucosa, implying that a normal small bowel mucosa in DH does not protect from lymphoma. Another retrospective cohort study has reported a 2-fold increased risk for malignant lymphoma (SIR=1.9; 95% CI 0.8-3.9) (Askling et al, 2002). Importantly, NHL occurrence seems to be reduced in DH patients whose diagnosis was made over the recent years (Viljamaa et al, 2006) maybe due to a less adherence of patients to a gluten-free diet in the past, not considered as essential as nowadays in DH. First-degree relatives of patients with DH or CD have an higher risk of developing a gluten-sensitive enteropathy (Hervonen *et al*, 2002). This is not true for lymphoma risk, as demonstrated in a large series of patients with DH and their first-degree relatives, where three lymphoma cases (0.2%) were diagnosed among 1.825 first-degree relatives, compared with the prevalence in the general population of 0.1%. The aetiopathology of lymphoma development in patients with DH is unknown, but several mechanisms may be involved, such as the polyclonal stimulation of B or T lymphocytes by gluten in the gastrointestinal tract, leading to the transformation in a malignant clone.

5. Conclusions

The relationship existing between autoimmunity and cancer continues to fascinate clinicians and physicians. Many pathogenic and therapeutic overlaps have been demonstrated so far in these two intriguing and closely interrelated fields but several challenges remain open to future development. The exact pathogenic mechanism connecting both diseases remain still poorly understood and additional studies will explore genetic, biologic and inflammatory mechanisms underlying lymphoma development. Further epidemiologic studies are needed to ascertain which host factors may predispose in the setting of an autoimmune disease to develop a malignancy in general, and a lymphoproliferative disorder in particular, in order to define more accurately the pre-treatment risk. Finally, more surveillance studies will clarify if novel immunomodulatory treatments increase or decrease lymphoma risk. A more clear elucidation of these critical issues will lead to the development of novel therapeutic options able to improve the prevention and/or treatment of lymphomas in the setting of autoimmunity.

6. References

Abu-Shakra, M., Guillemin, F. & Lee, P. (1993) Cancer in systemic sclerosis. *Arthritis and Rheumatism*, 36, 460-464.

Adamson, T.C.,3rd, Fox, R.I., Frisman, D.M. & Howell, F.V. (1983) Immunohistologic analysis of lymphoid infiltrates in primary sjogren's syndrome using monoclonal antibodies. *Journal of Immunology (Baltimore, Md.: 1950)*, 130, 203-208.

Alspaugh, M.A., Henle, G., Lennette, E.T. & Henle, W. (1981) Elevated levels of antibodies to epstein-barr virus antigens in sera and synovial fluids of patients with rheumatoid arthritis. *The Journal of Clinical Investigation*, 67, 1134-1140.

Al-Toma, A., Verbeek, W.H., Hadithi, M., von Blomberg, B.M. & Mulder, C.J. (2007) Survival in refractory coeliac disease and enteropathy-associated T-cell lymphoma: Retrospective evaluation of single-centre experience. *Gut*, 56, 1373-1378.

Ambinder, R.F. (2003) Epstein-barr virus-associated lymphoproliferative disorders. *Reviews in Clinical and Experimental Hematology*, 7, 362-374.

Ambrosetti, A., Zanotti, R., Pattaro, C., Lenzi, L., Chilosi, M., Caramaschi, P., Arcaini, L., Pasini, F., Biasi, D., Orlandi, E., D'Adda, M., Lucioni, M. & Pizzolo, G. (2004) Most cases of primary salivary mucosa-associated lymphoid tissue lymphoma are associated either with sjoegren syndrome or hepatitis C virus infection. *British Journal of Haematology*, 126, 43-49.

Anaya, J.M., McGuff, H.S., Banks, P.M. & Talal, N. (1996) Clinicopathological factors relating malignant lymphoma with sjogren's syndrome. *Seminars in Arthritis and Rheumatism*, 25, 337-346.

Anderson, L.A., Gadalla, S., Morton, L.M., Landgren, O., Pfeiffer, R., Warren, J.L., Berndt, S.I., Ricker, W., Parsons, R. & Engels, E.A. (2009) Population-based study of autoimmune conditions and the risk of specific lymphoid malignancies. *International Journal of Cancer.Journal International Du Cancer*, 125, 398-405.

Anderson, L.G. & Talal, N. (1972) The spectrum of benign to malignant lymphoproliferation in sjogren's syndrome. *Clinical and Experimental Immunology*, 10, 199-221.

Ansell, S.M., Grant, C.S. & Habermann, T.M. (1999) Primary thyroid lymphoma. *Seminars in Oncology*, 26, 316-323.

Aozasa, K. (1990) Hashimoto's thyroiditis as a risk factor of thyroid lymphoma. *Acta Pathologica Japonica*, 40, 459-468.

Aringer, M., Wintersberger, W., Steiner, C.W., Kiener, H., Presterl, E., Jaeger, U., Smolen, J.S. & Graninger, W.B. (1994) High levels of bcl-2 protein in circulating T lymphocytes, but not B lymphocytes, of patients with systemic lupus erythematosus. *Arthritis and Rheumatism*, 37, 1423-1430.

Arnaud, L., Chryssostalis, A., Terris, B., Pavy, S., Chaussade, S., Kahan, A. & Allanore, Y. (2006) Systemic sclerosis and gastric MALT lymphoma. *Joint, Bone, Spine : Revue Du Rhumatisme*, 73, 105-108.

Ashton-Key, M., Diss, T.C., Pan, L., Du, M.Q. & Isaacson, P.G. (1997) Molecular analysis of T-cell clonality in ulcerative jejunitis and enteropathy-associated T-cell lymphoma. *The American Journal of Pathology*, 151, 493-498.

Askling, J., Linet, M., Gridley, G., Halstensen, T.S., Ekstrom, K. & Ekbom, A. (2002) Cancer incidence in a population-based cohort of individuals hospitalized with celiac disease or dermatitis herpetiformis. *Gastroenterology*, 123, 1428-1435.

Askling, J., Brandt, L., Lapidus, A., Karlen, P., Bjorkholm, M., Lofberg, R. & Ekbom, A. (2005) Risk of haematopoietic cancer in patients with inflammatory bowel disease. *Gut*, 54, 617-622.

Askling, J., van Vollenhoven, R.F., Granath, F., Raaschou, P., Fored, C.M., Baecklund, E., Dackhammar, C., Feltelius, N., Coster, L., Geborek, P., Jacobsson, L.T., Lindblad, S., Rantapaa-Dahlqvist, S., Saxne, T. & Klareskog, L. (2009) Cancer risk in patients with rheumatoid arthritis treated with anti-tumor necrosis factor alpha therapies: Does the risk change with the time since start of treatment? *Arthritis and Rheumatism*, 60, 3180-3189.

Askling, J., Fored, C.M., Baecklund, E., Brandt, L., Backlin, C., Ekbom, A., Sundstrom, C., Bertilsson, L., Coster, L., Geborek, P., Jacobsson, L.T., Lindblad, S., Lysholm, J., Rantapaa-Dahlqvist, S., Saxne, T., Klareskog, L. & Feltelius, N. (2005) Haematopoietic malignancies in rheumatoid arthritis: Lymphoma risk and characteristics after exposure to tumour necrosis factor antagonists. *Annals of the Rheumatic Diseases*, 64, 1414-1420.

Baecklund, E., Ekbom, A., Sparen, P., Feltelius, N. & Klareskog, L. (1998) Disease activity and risk of lymphoma in patients with rheumatoid arthritis: Nested case-control study. *BMJ (Clinical Research Ed.)*, 317, 180-181.

Baecklund, E., Sundstrom, C., Ekbom, A., Catrina, A.I., Biberfeld, P., Feltelius, N. & Klareskog, L. (2003) Lymphoma subtypes in patients with rheumatoid arthritis: Increased proportion of diffuse large B cell lymphoma. *Arthritis and Rheumatism*, 48, 1543-1550.

Baecklund, E., Iliadou, A., Askling, J., Ekbom, A., Backlin, C., Granath, F., Catrina, A.I., Rosenquist, R., Feltelius, N., Sundstrom, C. & Klareskog, L. (2006a) Association of chronic inflammation, not its treatment, with increased lymphoma risk in rheumatoid arthritis. *Arthritis and Rheumatism*, 54, 692-701.

Baecklund, E., Backlin, C., Iliadou, A., Granath, F., Ekbom, A., Amini, R.M., Feltelius, N., Enblad, G., Sundstrom, C., Klareskog, L., Askling, J. & Rosenquist, R. (2006b) Characteristics of diffuse large B cell lymphomas in rheumatoid arthritis. *Arthritis and Rheumatism*, 54, 3774-3781.

Bagdi, E., Diss, T.C., Munson, P. & Isaacson, P.G. (1999) Mucosal intra-epithelial lymphocytes in enteropathy-associated T-cell lymphoma, ulcerative jejunitis, and refractory celiac disease constitute a neoplastic population. *Blood*, 94, 260-264.

Baker, J.A., Weiss, J.R., Czuczman, M.S., Menezes, R.J., Ambrosone, C.B. & Moysich, K.B. (2005) Regular use of aspirin or acetaminophen and risk of non-hodgkin lymphoma. *Cancer Causes & Control : CCC*, 16, 301-308.

Baker, K.P., Edwards, B.M., Main, S.H., Choi, G.H., Wager, R.E., Halpern, W.G., Lappin, P.B., Riccobene, T., Abramian, D., Sekut, L., Sturm, B., Poortman, C., Minter, R.R., Dobson, C.L., Williams, E., Carmen, S., Smith, R., Roschke, V., Hilbert, D.M., Vaughan, T.J. & Albert, V.R. (2003) Generation and characterization of LymphoStat-B, a human monoclonal antibody that antagonizes the bioactivities of B lymphocyte stimulator. *Arthritis and Rheumatism*, 48, 3253-3265.

Balandraud, N., Roudier, J. & Roudier, C. (2005) What are the links between epstein-barr virus, lymphoma, and tumor necrosis factor antagonism in rheumatoid arthritis? *Seminars in Arthritis and Rheumatism*, 34, 31-33.

Balandraud, N., Meynard, J.B., Auger, I., Sovran, H., Mugnier, B., Reviron, D., Roudier, J. & Roudier, C. (2003) Epstein-barr virus load in the peripheral blood of patients with rheumatoid arthritis: Accurate quantification using real-time polymerase chain reaction. *Arthritis and Rheumatism*, 48, 1223-1228.

Banchereau, J. & Pascual, V. (2006) Type I interferon in systemic lupus erythematosus and other autoimmune diseases. *Immunity*, 25, 383-392.

Beauparlant, P., Papp, K. & Haraoui, B. (1999) The incidence of cancer associated with the treatment of rheumatoid arthritis. *Seminars in Arthritis and Rheumatism*, 29, 148-158.

Beiderbeck, A.B., Holly, E.A., Sturkenboom, M.C., Coebergh, J.W., Stricker, B.H. & Leufkens, H.G. (2003) No increased risk of non-hodgkin's lymphoma with steroids, estrogens and psychotropics (netherlands). *Cancer Causes & Control : CCC*, 14, 639-644.

Berek, C. & Kim, H.J. (1997) B-cell activation and development within chronically inflamed synovium in rheumatoid and reactive arthritis. *Seminars in Immunology*, 9, 261-268.

Bernatsky, S., Lee, J.L. & Rahme, E. (2007) Non-hodgkin's lymphoma--meta-analyses of the effects of corticosteroids and non-steroidal anti-inflammatories. *Rheumatology (Oxford, England)*, 46, 690-694.

Bernatsky, S., Clarke, A. & Ramsey-Goldman, R. (2002) Malignancy and systemic lupus erythematosus. *Current Rheumatology Reports*, 4, 351-358.

Bernatsky, S., Ramsey-Goldman, R., Isenberg, D., Rahman, A., Dooley, M.A., Sibley, J., Boivin, J.F., Joseph, L., Armitage, J., Zoma, A. & Clarke, A. (2007) Hodgkin's lymphoma in systemic lupus erythematosus. *Rheumatology (Oxford, England)*, 46, 830-832.

Bernatsky, S., Joseph, L., Boivin, J.F., Gordon, C., Urowitz, M., Gladman, D., Fortin, P.R., Ginzler, E., Bae, S.C., Barr, S., Edworthy, S., Isenberg, D., Rahman, A., Petri, M., Alarcon, G.S., Aranow, C., Dooley, M.A., Rajan, R., Senecal, J.L., Zummer, M., Manzi, S., Ramsey-Goldman, R. & Clarke, A.E. (2008) The relationship between cancer and medication exposures in systemic lupus erythaematosus: A case-cohort study. *Annals of the Rheumatic Diseases*, 67, 74-79.

Bernatsky, S., Ramsey-Goldman, R., Rajan, R., Boivin, J.F., Joseph, L., Lachance, S., Cournoyer, D., Zoma, A., Manzi, S., Ginzler, E., Urowitz, M., Gladman, D., Fortin, P.R., Edworthy, S., Barr, S., Gordon, C., Bae, S.C., Sibley, J., Steinsson, K., Nived, O., Sturfelt, G., St Pierre, Y. & Clarke, A. (2005a) Non-hodgkin's lymphoma in systemic lupus erythematosus. *Annals of the Rheumatic Diseases*, 64, 1507-1509.

Bernatsky, S., Boivin, J.F., Joseph, L., Rajan, R., Zoma, A., Manzi, S., Ginzler, E., Urowitz, M., Gladman, D., Fortin, P.R., Petri, M., Edworthy, S., Barr, S., Gordon, C., Bae, S.C., Sibley, J., Isenberg, D., Rahman, A., Aranow, C., Dooley, M.A., Steinsson, K., Nived, O., Sturfelt, G., Alarcon, G., Senecal, J.L., Zummer, M., Hanly, J., Ensworth, S., Pope, J., El-Gabalawy, H., McCarthy, T., St Pierre, Y., Ramsey-Goldman, R. & Clarke, A. (2005b) An international cohort study of cancer in systemic lupus erythematosus. *Arthritis and Rheumatism*, 52, 1481-1490.

Bernstein, L. & Ross, R.K. (1992) Prior medication use and health history as risk factors for non-hodgkin's lymphoma: Preliminary results from a case-control study in los angeles county. *Cancer Research*, 52, 5510s-5515s.

Bishton, M.J. & Haynes, A.P. (2007) Combination chemotherapy followed by autologous stem cell transplant for enteropathy-associated T cell lymphoma. *British Journal of Haematology*, 136, 111-113.

Boffetta, P., Gridley, G. & Lindelof, B. (2001) Cancer risk in a population-based cohort of patients hospitalized for psoriasis in sweden. *The Journal of Investigative Dermatology*, 117, 1531-1537.

Bologna, C., Picot, M.C., Jorgensen, C., Viu, P., Verdier, R. & Sany, J. (1997) Study of eight cases of cancer in 426 rheumatoid arthritis patients treated with methotrexate. *Annals of the Rheumatic Diseases*, 56, 97-102.

Bombardieri, M., Barone, F., Humby, F., Kelly, S., McGurk, M., Morgan, P., Challacombe, S., De Vita, S., Valesini, G., Spencer, J. & Pitzalis, C. (2007) Activation-induced cytidine deaminase expression in follicular dendritic cell networks and interfollicular large B cells supports functionality of ectopic lymphoid neogenesis in autoimmune sialoadenitis and MALT lymphoma in sjogren's syndrome. *Journal of Immunology (Baltimore, Md.: 1950)*, 179, 4929-4938.

Bongartz, T., Warren, F.C., Mines, D., Matteson, E.L., Abrams, K.R. & Sutton, A.J. (2009) Etanercept therapy in rheumatoid arthritis and the risk of malignancies: A systematic review and individual patient data meta-analysis of randomised controlled trials. *Annals of the Rheumatic Diseases*, 68, 1177-1183.

Bongartz, T., Sutton, A.J., Sweeting, M.J., Buchan, I., Matteson, E.L. & Montori, V. (2006) Anti-TNF antibody therapy in rheumatoid arthritis and the risk of serious infections and malignancies: Systematic review and meta-analysis of rare harmful effects in randomized controlled trials. *JAMA : The Journal of the American Medical Association*, 295, 2275-2285.

Brandtzaeg, P. & Johansen, F.E. (2005) Mucosal B cells: Phenotypic characteristics, transcriptional regulation, and homing properties. *Immunological Reviews,* 206, 32-63.

Brito-Zeron, P., Ramos-Casals, M., Bove, A., Sentis, J. & Font, J. (2007) Predicting adverse outcomes in primary sjogren's syndrome: Identification of prognostic factors. *Rheumatology (Oxford, England),* 46, 1359-1362.

Brown, S.L., Greene, M.H., Gershon, S.K., Edwards, E.T. & Braun, M.M. (2002) Tumor necrosis factor antagonist therapy and lymphoma development: Twenty-six cases reported to the food and drug administration. *Arthritis and Rheumatism,* 46, 3151-3158.

Burke, J.S. (1999) Are there site-specific differences among the MALT lymphomas--morphologic, clinical? *American Journal of Clinical Pathology,* 111, S133-43.

Caponi, L., Anzilotti, C., Longombardo, G. & Migliorini, P. (2007) Antibodies directed against ribosomal P proteins cross-react with phospholipids. *Clinical and Experimental Immunology,* 150, 140-143.

Cartwright, R.A., McKinney, P.A., O'Brien, C., Richards, I.D., Roberts, B., Lauder, I., Darwin, C.M., Bernard, S.M. & Bird, C.C. (1988) Non-hodgkin's lymphoma: Case control epidemiological study in yorkshire. *Leukemia Research,* 12, 81-88.

Catassi, C., Fabiani, E., Corrao, G., Barbato, M., De Renzo, A., Carella, A.M., Gabrielli, A., Leoni, P., Carroccio, A., Baldassarre, M., Bertolani, P., Caramaschi, P., Sozzi, M., Guariso, G., Volta, U., Corazza, G.R. & Italian Working Group on Coeliac Disease and Non-Hodgkin's-Lymphoma. (2002) Risk of non-hodgkin lymphoma in celiac disease. *JAMA : The Journal of the American Medical Association,* 287, 1413-1419.

Cellier, C., Delabesse, E., Helmer, C., Patey, N., Matuchansky, C., Jabri, B., Macintyre, E., Cerf-Bensussan, N. & Brousse, N. (2000) Refractory sprue, coeliac disease, and enteropathy-associated T-cell lymphoma. french coeliac disease study group. *Lancet,* 356, 203-208.

Cellier, C., Patey, N., Mauvieux, L., Jabri, B., Delabesse, E., Cervoni, J.P., Burtin, M.L., Guy-Grand, D., Bouhnik, Y., Modigliani, R., Barbier, J.P., Macintyre, E., Brousse, N. & Cerf-Bensussan, N. (1998) Abnormal intestinal intraepithelial lymphocytes in refractory sprue. *Gastroenterology,* 114, 471-481.

Cerhan, J.R., Anderson, K.E., Janney, C.A., Vachon, C.M., Witzig, T.E. & Habermann, T.M. (2003) Association of aspirin and other non-steroidal anti-inflammatory drug use with incidence of non-hodgkin lymphoma. *International Journal of Cancer.Journal International Du Cancer,* 106, 784-788.

Chang, E.T., Smedby, K.E., Hjalgrim, H., Schollkopf, C., Porwit-MacDonald, A., Sundstrom, C., Tani, E., d'Amore, F., Melbye, M., Adami, H.O. & Glimelius, B. (2005) Medication use and risk of non-hodgkin's lymphoma. *American Journal of Epidemiology,* 162, 965-974.

Chatterjee, S., Dombi, G.W., Severson, R.K. & Mayes, M.D. (2005) Risk of malignancy in scleroderma: A population-based cohort study. *Arthritis and Rheumatism,* 52, 2415-2424.

Chott, A., Dragosics, B. & Radaszkiewicz, T. (1992) Peripheral T-cell lymphomas of the intestine. *The American Journal of Pathology,* 141, 1361-1371.

Chott, A., Haedicke, W., Mosberger, I., Fodinger, M., Winkler, K., Mannhalter, C. & Muller-Hermelink, H.K. (1998) Most CD56+ intestinal lymphomas are CD8+CD5-T-cell lymphomas of monomorphic small to medium size histology. *The American Journal of Pathology*, 153, 1483-1490.

Choubey, D. & Panchanathan, R. (2008) Interferon-inducible Ifi200-family genes in systemic lupus erythematosus. *Immunology Letters*, 119, 32-41.

Choubey, D. & Kotzin, B.L. (2002) Interferon-inducible p202 in the susceptibility to systemic lupus. *Frontiers in Bioscience : A Journal and Virtual Library*, 7, e252-62.

Choubey, D., Deka, R. & Ho, S.M. (2008) Interferon-inducible IFI16 protein in human cancers and autoimmune diseases. *Frontiers in Bioscience : A Journal and Virtual Library*, 13, 598-608.

Collin, P., Pukkala, E. & Reunala, T. (1996) Malignancy and survival in dermatitis herpetiformis: A comparison with coeliac disease. *Gut*, 38, 528-530.

Collin, P., Reunala, T., Pukkala, E., Laippala, P., Keyrilainen, O. & Pasternack, A. (1994) Coeliac disease--associated disorders and survival. *Gut*, 35, 1215-1218.

Corrao, G., Corazza, G.R., Bagnardi, V., Brusco, G., Ciacci, C., Cottone, M., Sategna Guidetti, C., Usai, P., Cesari, P., Pelli, M.A., Loperfido, S., Volta, U., Calabro, A., Certo, M. & Club del Tenue Study Group. (2001) Mortality in patients with coeliac disease and their relatives: A cohort study. *Lancet*, 358, 356-361.

Costenbader, K.H., Glass, R., Cui, J. & Shadick, N. (2006) Risk of serious infections and malignancies with anti-TNF antibody therapy in rheumatoid arthritis. *JAMA : The Journal of the American Medical Association*, 296, 2201; author reply 2203-4.

d'Amore, F., Brincker, H., Gronbaek, K., Thorling, K., Pedersen, M., Jensen, M.K., Andersen, E., Pedersen, N.T. & Mortensen, L.S. (1994) Non-hodgkin's lymphoma of the gastrointestinal tract: A population-based analysis of incidence, geographic distribution, clinicopathologic presentation features, and prognosis. danish lymphoma study group. *Journal of Clinical Oncology : Official Journal of the American Society of Clinical Oncology*, 12, 1673-1684.

Daniels, T.E. (1984) Labial salivary gland biopsy in sjogren's syndrome. assessment as a diagnostic criterion in 362 suspected cases. *Arthritis and Rheumatism*, 27, 147-156.

Daum, S., Cellier, C. & Mulder, C.J. (2005) Refractory coeliac disease. *Best Practice & Research.Clinical Gastroenterology*, 19, 413-424.

Daum, S., Ullrich, R., Heise, W., Dederke, B., Foss, H.D., Stein, H., Thiel, E., Zeitz, M. & Riecken, E.O. (2003) Intestinal non-hodgkin's lymphoma: A multicenter prospective clinical study from the german study group on intestinal non-hodgkin's lymphoma. *Journal of Clinical Oncology : Official Journal of the American Society of Clinical Oncology*, 21, 2740-2746.

Daum, S., Weiss, D., Hummel, M., Ullrich, R., Heise, W., Stein, H., Riecken, E.O., Foss, H.D. & Intestinal Lymphoma Study Group. (2001) Frequency of clonal intraepithelial T lymphocyte proliferations in enteropathy-type intestinal T cell lymphoma, coeliac disease, and refractory sprue. *Gut*, 49, 804-812.

Dayan, C.M. & Daniels, G.H. (1996) Chronic autoimmune thyroiditis. *The New England Journal of Medicine*, 335, 99-107.

Derk, C.T., Conway, R.T. & Jimenez, S.A. (2004) Primary B-cell lymphoma of the tongue in a patient with systemic sclerosis. *Oral Oncology*, 40, 103-106.

Derk, C.T., Rasheed, M., Artlett, C.M. & Jimenez, S.A. (2006) A cohort study of cancer incidence in systemic sclerosis. *The Journal of Rheumatology*, 33, 1113-1116.

Derringer, G.A., Thompson, L.D., Frommelt, R.A., Bijwaard, K.E., Heffess, C.S. & Abbondanzo, S.L. (2000) Malignant lymphoma of the thyroid gland: A clinicopathologic study of 108 cases. *The American Journal of Surgical Pathology*, 24, 623-639.

Di Cristofano, A., Kotsi, P., Peng, Y.F., Cordon-Cardo, C., Elkon, K.B. & Pandolfi, P.P. (1999) Impaired fas response and autoimmunity in pten+/- mice. *Science (New York, N.Y.)*, 285, 2122-2125.

Di Sabatino, A. & Corazza, G.R. (2009) Coeliac disease. *Lancet*, 373, 1480-1493.

Do, R.K. & Chen-Kiang, S. (2002) Mechanism of BLyS action in B cell immunity. *Cytokine & Growth Factor Reviews*, 13, 19-25.

Domizio, P., Owen, R.A., Shepherd, N.A., Talbot, I.C. & Norton, A.J. (1993) Primary lymphoma of the small intestine. A clinicopathological study of 119 cases. *The American Journal of Surgical Pathology*, 17, 429-442.

Du, M.Q., Xu, C.F., Diss, T.C., Peng, H.Z., Wotherspoon, A.C., Isaacson, P.G. & Pan, L.X. (1996) Intestinal dissemination of gastric mucosa-associated lymphoid tissue lymphoma. *Blood*, 88, 4445-4451.

Duggal, L., Gupta, S., Aggarwal, P.K., Sachar, V.P. & Bhalla, S. (2002) Hodgkin's disease and scleroderma. *The Journal of the Association of Physicians of India*, 50, 1186-1188.

Duncan, S.C. & Winkelmann, R.K. (1979) Cancer and scleroderma. *Archives of Dermatology*, 115, 950-955.

Edinger, J.W., Bonneville, M., Scotet, E., Houssaint, E., Schumacher, H.R. & Posnett, D.N. (1999) EBV gene expression not altered in rheumatoid synovia despite the presence of EBV antigen-specific T cell clones. *Journal of Immunology (Baltimore, Md.: 1950)*, 162, 3694-3701.

Eguchi, K. (2001) Apoptosis in autoimmune diseases. *Internal Medicine (Tokyo, Japan)*, 40, 275-284.

Ekstrom Smedby, K., Vajdic, C.M., Falster, M., Engels, E.A., Martinez-Maza, O., Turner, J., Hjalgrim, H., Vineis, P., Seniori Costantini, A., Bracci, P.M., Holly, E.A., Willett, E., Spinelli, J.J., La Vecchia, C., Zheng, T., Becker, N., De Sanjose, S., Chiu, B.C., Dal Maso, L., Cocco, P., Maynadie, M., Foretova, L., Staines, A., Brennan, P., Davis, S., Severson, R., Cerhan, J.R., Breen, E.C., Birmann, B., Grulich, A.E. & Cozen, W. (2008) Autoimmune disorders and risk of non-hodgkin lymphoma subtypes: A pooled analysis within the InterLymph consortium. *Blood*, 111, 4029-4038.

Ekstrom, K., Hjalgrim, H., Brandt, L., Baecklund, E., Klareskog, L., Ekbom, A. & Askling, J. (2003) Risk of malignant lymphomas in patients with rheumatoid arthritis and in their first-degree relatives. *Arthritis and Rheumatism*, 48, 963-970.

El Fassi, D., Clemmensen, O., Nielsen, C.H., Silkiss, R.Z. & Hegedus, L. (2007a) Evidence of intrathyroidal B-lymphocyte depletion after rituximab therapy in a patient with graves' disease. *The Journal of Clinical Endocrinology and Metabolism*, 92, 3762-3763.

El Fassi, D., Nielsen, C.H., Bonnema, S.J., Hasselbalch, H.C. & Hegedus, L. (2007b) B lymphocyte depletion with the monoclonal antibody rituximab in graves' disease: A controlled pilot study. *The Journal of Clinical Endocrinology and Metabolism*, 92, 1769-1772.

Elfstrom, P., Granath, F., Ekstrom Smedby, K., Montgomery, S.M., Askling, J., Ekbom, A. & Ludvigsson, J.F. (2011) Risk of lymphoproliferative malignancy in relation to small intestinal histopathology among patients with celiac disease. *Journal of the National Cancer Institute*, 103, 436-444.

Ellman, M.H., Hurwitz, H., Thomas, C. & Kozloff, M. (1991) Lymphoma developing in a patient with rheumatoid arthritis taking low dose weekly methotrexate. *The Journal of Rheumatology*, 18, 1741-1743.

Engels, E.A., Cerhan, J.R., Linet, M.S., Cozen, W., Colt, J.S., Davis, S., Gridley, G., Severson, R.K. & Hartge, P. (2005) Immune-related conditions and immune-modulating medications as risk factors for non-hodgkin's lymphoma: A case-control study. *American Journal of Epidemiology*, 162, 1153-1161.

Farstad, I.N., Johansen, F.E., Vlatkovic, L., Jahnsen, J., Scott, H., Fausa, O., Bjorneklett, A., Brandtzaeg, P. & Halstensen, T.S. (2002) Heterogeneity of intraepithelial lymphocytes in refractory sprue: Potential implications of CD30 expression. *Gut*, 51, 372-378.

Feng, W.H., Cohen, J.I., Fischer, S., Li, L., Sneller, M., Goldbach-Mansky, R., Raab-Traub, N., Delecluse, H.J. & Kenney, S.C. (2004) Reactivation of latent epstein-barr virus by methotrexate: A potential contributor to methotrexate-associated lymphomas. *Journal of the National Cancer Institute*, 96, 1691-1702.

Franklin, J., Lunt, M., Bunn, D., Symmons, D. & Silman, A. (2006) Incidence of lymphoma in a large primary care derived cohort of cases of inflammatory polyarthritis. *Annals of the Rheumatic Diseases*, 65, 617-622.

Franklin, J.P., Symmons, D.P. & Silman, A.J. (2005) Risk of lymphoma in patients with RA treated with anti-TNFalpha agents. *Annals of the Rheumatic Diseases*, 64, 657-658.

Freimark, B., Fantozzi, R., Bone, R., Bordin, G. & Fox, R. (1989) Detection of clonally expanded salivary gland lymphocytes in sjogren's syndrome. *Arthritis and Rheumatism*, 32, 859-869.

Friedman, D.F., Cho, E.A., Goldman, J., Carmack, C.E., Besa, E.C., Hardy, R.R. & Silberstein, L.E. (1991) The role of clonal selection in the pathogenesis of an autoreactive human B cell lymphoma. *The Journal of Experimental Medicine*, 174, 525-537.

Fronek, Z., Cheung, M.M., Hanbury, A.M. & Kagnoff, M.F. (1991) Molecular analysis of HLA DP and DQ genes associated with dermatitis herpetiformis. *The Journal of Investigative Dermatology*, 97, 799-802.

Fry, L., Seah, P.P., Riches, D.J. & Hoffbrand, A.V. (1973) Clearance of skin lesions in dermatitis herpetiformis after gluten withdrawal. *Lancet*, 1, 288-291.

Gale, J., Simmonds, P.D., Mead, G.M., Sweetenham, J.W. & Wright, D.H. (2000) Enteropathy-type intestinal T-cell lymphoma: Clinical features and treatment of 31 patients in a single center. *Journal of Clinical Oncology : Official Journal of the American Society of Clinical Oncology*, 18, 795-803.

Gallamini, A., Zaja, F., Patti, C., Billio, A., Specchia, M.R., Tucci, A., Levis, A., Manna, A., Secondo, V., Rigacci, L., Pinto, A., Iannitto, E., Zoli, V., Torchio, P., Pileri, S. & Tarella, C. (2007) Alemtuzumab (campath-1H) and CHOP chemotherapy as first-line treatment of peripheral T-cell lymphoma: Results of a GITIL (gruppo italiano terapie innovative nei linfomi) prospective multicenter trial. *Blood*, 110, 2316-2323.

Gasparotto, D., De Vita, S., De Re, V., Marzotto, A., De Marchi, G., Scott, C.A., Gloghini, A., Ferraccioli, G. & Boiocchi, M. (2003) Extrasalivary lymphoma development in sjogren's syndrome: Clonal evolution from parotid gland lymphoproliferation and role of local triggering. *Arthritis and Rheumatism*, 48, 3181-3186.

Geborek, P., Crnkic, M., Petersson, I.F., Saxne, T. & South Swedish Arthritis Treatment Group. (2002) Etanercept, infliximab, and leflunomide in established rheumatoid arthritis: Clinical experience using a structured follow up programme in southern sweden. *Annals of the Rheumatic Diseases,* 61, 793-798.

Geborek, P., Bladstrom, A., Turesson, C., Gulfe, A., Petersson, I.F., Saxne, T., Olsson, H. & Jacobsson, L.T. (2005) Tumour necrosis factor blockers do not increase overall tumour risk in patients with rheumatoid arthritis, but may be associated with an increased risk of lymphomas. *Annals of the Rheumatic Diseases,* 64, 699-703.

Gelfand, J.M., Shin, D.B., Neimann, A.L., Wang, X., Margolis, D.J. & Troxel, A.B. (2006) The risk of lymphoma in patients with psoriasis. *The Journal of Investigative Dermatology,* 126, 2194-2201.

Gellrich, S., Rutz, S., Borkowski, A., Golembowski, S., Gromnica-Ihle, E., Sterry, W. & Jahn, S. (1999) Analysis of V(H)-D-J(H) gene transcripts in B cells infiltrating the salivary glands and lymph node tissues of patients with sjogren's syndrome. *Arthritis and Rheumatism,* 42, 240-247.

Gjone, E. & Nordoy, A. (1970) Dermatitis herpetiformis, steatorrhoea, and malignancy. *British Medical Journal,* 1, 610.

Goodnow, C.C. (2007) Multistep pathogenesis of autoimmune disease. *Cell,* 130, 25-35.

Grady, W.M. (2005) Transforming growth factor-beta, smads, and cancer. *Clinical Cancer Research: An Official Journal of the American Association for Cancer Research,* 11, 3151-3154.

Graff-Baker, A., Sosa, J.A. & Roman, S.A. (2010) Primary thyroid lymphoma: A review of recent developments in diagnosis and histology-driven treatment. *Current Opinion in Oncology,* 22, 17-22.

Gridley, G., Klippel, J.H., Hoover, R.N. & Fraumeni, J.F.,Jr. (1994) Incidence of cancer among men with the felty syndrome. *Annals of Internal Medicine,* 120, 35-39.

Gridley, G., McLaughlin, J.K., Ekbom, A., Klareskog, L., Adami, H.O., Hacker, D.G., Hoover, R. & Fraumeni, J.F.,Jr. (1993) Incidence of cancer among patients with rheumatoid arthritis. *Journal of the National Cancer Institute,* 85, 307-311.

Halfdanarson, T.R., Rubio-Tapia, A., Ristow, K.M., Habermann, T.M., Murray, J.A. & Inwards, D.J. (2010) Patients with celiac disease and B-cell lymphoma have a better prognosis than those with T-cell lymphoma. *Clinical Gastroenterology and Hepatology: The Official Clinical Practice Journal of the American Gastroenterological Association,* 8, 1042-1047.

Hall, S.W., Gillespie, J.J. & Tenczynski, T.F. (1978) Generalized lipodystrophy, scleroderma, and hodgkin's disease. *Archives of Internal Medicine,* 138, 1303-1304.

Harris, N.L. (1999) Lymphoid proliferations of the salivary glands. *American Journal of Clinical Pathology,* 111, S94-103.

Haviv, Y.S., Ben-Yehuda, A., Polliack, A. & Safadi, R. (1997) Lymphoma and systemic sclerosis--an uncommon association or possible coincidence of two disorders with a fatal outcome. *European Journal of Haematology,* 59, 194-196.

Hellgren, K., Smedby, K.E., Feltelius, N., Baecklund, E. & Askling, J. (2010a) Do rheumatoid arthritis and lymphoma share risk factors?: A comparison of lymphoma and cancer risks before and after diagnosis of rheumatoid arthritis. *Arthritis and Rheumatism,* 62, 1252-1258.

Hellgren, K., Iliadou, A., Rosenquist, R., Feltelius, N., Backlin, C., Enblad, G., Askling, J. & Baecklund, E. (2010b) Rheumatoid arthritis, treatment with corticosteroids and risk of malignant lymphomas: Results from a case-control study. *Annals of the Rheumatic Diseases,* 69, 654-659.

Hervonen, K., Vornanen, M., Kautiainen, H., Collin, P. & Reunala, T. (2005) Lymphoma in patients with dermatitis herpetiformis and their first-degree relatives. *The British Journal of Dermatology*, 152, 82-86.

Hervonen, K., Hakanen, M., Kaukinen, K., Collin, P. & Reunala, T. (2002) First-degree relatives are frequently affected in coeliac disease and dermatitis herpetiformis. *Scandinavian Journal of Gastroenterology*, 37, 51-55.

Hill, C.L., Nguyen, A.M., Roder, D. & Roberts-Thomson, P. (2003) Risk of cancer in patients with scleroderma: A population based cohort study. *Annals of the Rheumatic Diseases*, 62, 728-731.

Hjelmstrom, P. (2001) Lymphoid neogenesis: De novo formation of lymphoid tissue in chronic inflammation through expression of homing chemokines. *Journal of Leukocyte Biology*, 69, 331-339.

Holly, E.A., Lele, C., Bracci, P.M. & McGrath, M.S. (1999) Case-control study of non-hodgkin's lymphoma among women and heterosexual men in the san francisco bay area, california. *American Journal of Epidemiology*, 150, 375-389.

Holm, L.E., Blomgren, H. & Lowhagen, T. (1985) Cancer risks in patients with chronic lymphocytic thyroiditis. *The New England Journal of Medicine*, 312, 601-604.

Holmes, G.K., Prior, P., Lane, M.R., Pope, D. & Allan, R.N. (1989) Malignancy in coeliac disease--effect of a gluten free diet. *Gut*, 30, 333-338.

Horikawa, M., Hasegawa, M., Komura, K., Hayakawa, I., Yanaba, K., Matsushita, T., Takehara, K. & Sato, S. (2005) Abnormal natural killer cell function in systemic sclerosis: Altered cytokine production and defective killing activity. *The Journal of Investigative Dermatology*, 125, 731-737.

Hoshida, Y., Tomita, Y., Zhiming, D., Yamauchi, A., Nakatsuka, S., Kurasono, Y., Arima, Y., Tsudo, M., Shintaku, M. & Aozasa, K. (2004) Lymphoproliferative disorders in autoimmune diseases in japan: Analysis of clinicopathological features and epstein-barr virus infection. *International Journal of Cancer.Journal International Du Cancer*, 108, 443-449.

Hoshida, Y., Xu, J.X., Fujita, S., Nakamichi, I., Ikeda, J., Tomita, Y., Nakatsuka, S., Tamaru, J., Iizuka, A., Takeuchi, T. & Aozasa, K. (2007) Lymphoproliferative disorders in rheumatoid arthritis: Clinicopathological analysis of 76 cases in relation to methotrexate medication. *The Journal of Rheumatology*, 34, 322-331.

Hyjek, E. & Isaacson, P.G. (1988) Primary B cell lymphoma of the thyroid and its relationship to hashimoto's thyroiditis. *Human Pathology*, 19, 1315-1326.

Illes, A., Varoczy, L., Papp, G., Wilson, P.C., Alex, P., Jonsson, R., Kovacs, T., Konttinen, Y.T., Zeher, M., Nakken, B. & Szodoray, P. (2009) Aspects of B-cell non-hodgkin's lymphoma development: A transition from immune-reactivity to malignancy. *Scandinavian Journal of Immunology*, 69, 387-400.

Ilyas, M., Niedobitek, G., Agathanggelou, A., Barry, R.E., Read, A.E., Tierney, R., Young, L.S. & Rooney, N. (1995) Non-hodgkin's lymphoma, coeliac disease, and epstein-barr virus: A study of 13 cases of enteropathy-associated T- and B-cell lymphoma. *The Journal of Pathology*, 177, 115-122.

Ioannidis, J.P., Vassiliou, V.A. & Moutsopoulos, H.M. (2002) Long-term risk of mortality and lymphoproliferative disease and predictive classification of primary sjogren's syndrome. *Arthritis and Rheumatism*, 46, 741-747.

Isaacson, P.G. (1997) Lymphoma of the thyroid gland. *Current Topics in Pathology.Ergebnisse Der Pathologie*, 91, 1-14.

Jackson, C.E. & Puck, J.M. (1999) Autoimmune lymphoproliferative syndrome, a disorder of apoptosis. *Current Opinion in Pediatrics*, 11, 521-527.

Jacobi, A.M., Hansen, A., Kaufmann, O., Pruss, A., Burmester, G.R., Lipsky, P.E. & Dorner, T. (2002) Analysis of immunoglobulin light chain rearrangements in the salivary gland and blood of a patient with sjogren's syndrome. *Arthritis Research*, 4, R4.

James, J.A., Kaufman, K.M., Farris, A.D., Taylor-Albert, E., Lehman, T.J. & Harley, J.B. (1997) An increased prevalence of epstein-barr virus infection in young patients suggests a possible etiology for systemic lupus erythematosus. *The Journal of Clinical Investigation*, 100, 3019-3026.

Jenkins, D., Lynde, C.W. & Stewart, W.D. (1983) Histiocytic lymphoma occurring in a patient with dermatitis herpetiformis. *Journal of the American Academy of Dermatology*, 9, 252-256.

Jonsson, R., Gordon, T.P. & Konttinen, Y.T. (2003) Recent advances in understanding molecular mechanisms in the pathogenesis and antibody profile of sjogren's syndrome. *Current Rheumatology Reports*, 5, 311-316.

Kabel, P.J., Voorbij, H.A., de Haan-Meulman, M., Pals, S.T. & Drexhage, H.A. (1989) High endothelial venules present in lymphoid cell accumulations in thyroids affected by autoimmune disease: A study in men and BB rats of functional activity and development. *The Journal of Clinical Endocrinology and Metabolism*, 68, 744-751.

Kahara, T., Iwaki, N., Kaya, H., Kurokawa, T., Yoshida, T., Ishikura, K. & Usuda, R. (2011) Transition of thyroid autoantibodies by rituximab treatment for thyroid MALT lymphoma. *Endocrine Journal*, 58, 7-12.

Kamel, O.W., van de Rijn, M., Weiss, L.M., Del Zoppo, G.J., Hench, P.K., Robbins, B.A., Montgomery, P.G., Warnke, R.A. & Dorfman, R.F. (1993) Brief report: Reversible lymphomas associated with epstein-barr virus occurring during methotrexate therapy for rheumatoid arthritis and dermatomyositis. *The New England Journal of Medicine*, 328, 1317-1321.

Kassan, S.S. & Moutsopoulos, H.M. (2004) Clinical manifestations and early diagnosis of sjogren syndrome. *Archives of Internal Medicine*, 164, 1275-1284.

Kassan, S.S., Thomas, T.L., Moutsopoulos, H.M., Hoover, R., Kimberly, R.P., Budman, D.R., Costa, J., Decker, J.L. & Chused, T.M. (1978) Increased risk of lymphoma in sicca syndrome. *Annals of Internal Medicine*, 89, 888-892.

Kato, I., Koenig, K.L., Shore, R.E., Baptiste, M.S., Lillquist, P.P., Frizzera, G., Burke, J.S. & Watanabe, H. (2002) Use of anti-inflammatory and non-narcotic analgesic drugs and risk of non-hodgkin's lymphoma (NHL) (united states). *Cancer Causes & Control : CCC*, 13, 965-974.

Kauppi, M., Pukkala, E. & Isomaki, H. (1997) Elevated incidence of hematologic malignancies in patients with sjogren's syndrome compared with patients with rheumatoid arthritis (finland). *Cancer Causes & Control : CCC*, 8, 201-204.

Kedar, A., Khan, A.B., Mattern, J.Q., Fisher, J., Thomas, P.R. & Freeman, A.I. (1979) Autoimmune disorders complicating adolescent hodgkin's disease. *Cancer*, 44, 112-116.

Kim, H.J., Krenn, V., Steinhauser, G. & Berek, C. (1999) Plasma cell development in synovial germinal centers in patients with rheumatoid and reactive arthritis. *Journal of Immunology (Baltimore, Md.: 1950)*, 162, 3053-3062.

King, J.K. & Costenbader, K.H. (2007) Characteristics of patients with systemic lupus erythematosus (SLE) and non-hodgkin's lymphoma (NHL). *Clinical Rheumatology,* 26, 1491-1494.

Kingsmore, S.F., Hall, B.D., Allen, N.B., Rice, J.R. & Caldwell, D.S. (1992) Association of methotrexate, rheumatoid arthritis and lymphoma: Report of 2 cases and literature review. *The Journal of Rheumatology,* 19, 1462-1465.

Kiss, E., Kovacs, L. & Szodoray, P. (2010) Malignancies in systemic lupus erythematosus. *Autoimmunity Reviews,* 9, 195-199.

Klyachkin, M.L., Schwartz, R.W., Cibull, M., Munn, R.K., Regine, W.F., Kenady, D.E., McGrath, P.C. & Sloan, D.A. (1998) Thyroid lymphoma: Is there a role for surgery? *The American Surgeon,* 64, 234-238.

Knecht, H., Saremaslani, P. & Hedinger, C. (1981) Immunohistological findings in hashimoto's thyroiditis, focal lymphocytic thyroiditis and thyroiditis de quervain. comparative study. *Virchows Archiv.A, Pathological Anatomy and Histology,* 393, 215-231.

Kojima, M., Itoh, H., Shimizu, K., Saruki, N., Murayama, K., Higuchi, K., Tamaki, Y., Matsumoto, M., Hirabayashi, K., Igarishi, S., Masawa, N. & Nakamura, S. (2006) Malignant lymphoma in patients with systemic rheumatic disease (rheumatoid arthritis, systemic lupus erythematosus, systemic sclerosis, and dermatomyositis): A clinicopathologic study of 24 japanese cases. *International Journal of Surgical Pathology,* 14, 43-48.

Kratz, A., Campos-Neto, A., Hanson, M.S. & Ruddle, N.H. (1996) Chronic inflammation caused by lymphotoxin is lymphoid neogenesis. *The Journal of Experimental Medicine,* 183, 1461-1472.

Kremer, J.M. (1997) Is methotrexate oncogenic in patients with rheumatoid arthritis? *Seminars in Arthritis and Rheumatism,* 26, 785-787.

Laabi, Y. & Strasser, A. (2000) Immunology. lymphocyte survival--ignorance is BLys. *Science (New York, N.Y.),* 289, 883-884.

Laing, R.W., Hoskin, P., Hudson, B.V., Hudson, G.V., Harmer, C., Bennett, M.H. & MacLennan, K.A. (1994) The significance of MALT histology in thyroid lymphoma: A review of patients from the BNLI and royal marsden hospital. *Clinical Oncology (Royal College of Radiologists (Great Britain)),* 6, 300-304.

Landgren, O., Engels, E.A., Pfeiffer, R.M., Gridley, G., Mellemkjaer, L., Olsen, J.H., Kerstann, K.F., Wheeler, W., Hemminki, K., Linet, M.S. & Goldin, L.R. (2006) Autoimmunity and susceptibility to hodgkin lymphoma: A population-based case-control study in scandinavia. *Journal of the National Cancer Institute,* 98, 1321-1330.

Legler, D.F., Loetscher, M., Roos, R.S., Clark-Lewis, I., Baggiolini, M. & Moser, B. (1998) B cell-attracting chemokine 1, a human CXC chemokine expressed in lymphoid tissues, selectively attracts B lymphocytes via BLR1/CXCR5. *The Journal of Experimental Medicine,* 187, 655-660.

Leombruno, J.P., Einarson, T.R. & Keystone, E.C. (2009) The safety of anti-tumour necrosis factor treatments in rheumatoid arthritis: Meta and exposure-adjusted pooled analyses of serious adverse events. *Annals of the Rheumatic Diseases,* 68, 1136-1145.

Leprince, C., Cohen-Kaminsky, S., Berrih-Aknin, S., Vernet-Der Garabedian, B., Treton, D., Galanaud, P. & Richard, Y. (1990) Thymic B cells from myasthenia gravis patients are activated B cells. phenotypic and functional analysis. *Journal of Immunology (Baltimore, Md.: 1950),* 145, 2115-2122.

Lewis, H.M., Renaula, T.L., Garioch, J.J., Leonard, J.N., Fry, J.S., Collin, P., Evans, D. & Fry, L. (1996) Protective effect of gluten-free diet against development of lymphoma in dermatitis herpetiformis. *The British Journal of Dermatology,* 135, 363-367.

Liote, F., Pertuiset, E., Cochand-Priollet, B., D'Agay, M.F., Dombret, H., Numeric, P., D'Anglejan, G. & Kuntz, D. (1995) Methotrexate related B lymphoproliferative disease in a patient with rheumatoid arthritis. role of epstein-barr virus infection. *The Journal of Rheumatology,* 22, 1174-1178.

Lofstrom, B., Backlin, C., Sundstrom, C., Ekbom, A. & Lundberg, I.E. (2007) A closer look at non-hodgkin's lymphoma cases in a national swedish systemic lupus erythematosus cohort: A nested case-control study. *Annals of the Rheumatic Diseases,* 66, 1627-1632.

Loren, A.W., Porter, D.L., Stadtmauer, E.A. & Tsai, D.E. (2003) Post-transplant lymphoproliferative disorder: A review. *Bone Marrow Transplantation,* 31, 145-155.

Lossos, I.S., Alizadeh, A.A., Rajapaksa, R., Tibshirani, R. & Levy, R. (2003) HGAL is a novel interleukin-4-inducible gene that strongly predicts survival in diffuse large B-cell lymphoma. *Blood,* 101, 433-440.

Lu, X., Chen, J., Malumbres, R., Cubedo Gil, E., Helfman, D.M. & Lossos, I.S. (2007) HGAL, a lymphoma prognostic biomarker, interacts with the cytoskeleton and mediates the effects of IL-6 on cell migration. *Blood,* 110, 4268-4277.

Mackay, F., Sierro, F., Grey, S.T. & Gordon, T.P. (2005) The BAFF/APRIL system: An important player in systemic rheumatic diseases. *Current Directions in Autoimmunity,* 8, 243-265.

Mackay, F., Woodcock, S.A., Lawton, P., Ambrose, C., Baetscher, M., Schneider, P., Tschopp, J. & Browning, J.L. (1999) Mice transgenic for BAFF develop lymphocytic disorders along with autoimmune manifestations. *The Journal of Experimental Medicine,* 190, 1697-1710.

Mackay, I.R. & Rose, N.R. (2001) Autoimmunity and lymphoma: Tribulations of B cells. *Nature Immunology,* 2, 793-795.

Mackey, A.C., Green, L., Liang, L.C., Dinndorf, P. & Avigan, M. (2007) Hepatosplenic T cell lymphoma associated with infliximab use in young patients treated for inflammatory bowel disease. *Journal of Pediatric Gastroenterology and Nutrition,* 44, 265-267.

Mariette, X. (1999) Lymphomas in patients with sjogren's syndrome: Review of the literature and physiopathologic hypothesis. *Leukemia & Lymphoma,* 33, 93-99.

Mariette, X., Cazals-Hatem, D., Warszawki, J., Liote, F., Balandraud, N., Sibilia, J. & Investigators of the Club Rhumatismes et Inflammation. (2002) Lymphomas in rheumatoid arthritis patients treated with methotrexate: A 3-year prospective study in france. *Blood,* 99, 3909-3915.

Mearin, M.L., Catassi, C., Brousse, N., Brand, R., Collin, P., Fabiani, E., Schweizer, J.J., Abuzakouk, M., Szajewska, H., Hallert, C., Farre Masip, C., Holmes, G.K. & Biomed Study Group on Coeliac Disease and Non-Hodgkin Lymphoma. (2006) European multi-centre study on coeliac disease and non-hodgkin lymphoma. *European Journal of Gastroenterology & Hepatology,* 18, 187-194.

Meibohm, B., Beierle, I. & Derendorf, H. (2002) How important are gender differences in pharmacokinetics? *Clinical Pharmacokinetics,* 41, 329-342.

Meijer, J.W., Mulder, C.J., Goerres, M.G., Boot, H. & Schweizer, J.J. (2004) Coeliac disease and (extra)intestinal T-cell lymphomas: Definition, diagnosis and treatment. *Scandinavian Journal of Gastroenterology.Supplement,* (241), 78-84.

Mellemkjaer, L., Pfeiffer, R.M., Engels, E.A., Gridley, G., Wheeler, W., Hemminki, K., Olsen, J.H., Dreyer, L., Linet, M.S., Goldin, L.R. & Landgren, O. (2008) Autoimmune disease in individuals and close family members and susceptibility to non-hodgkin's lymphoma. *Arthritis and Rheumatism*, 58, 657-666.

Mellors, R.C. (1966) Autoimmune disease in NZB-bl mice. II. autoimmunity and malignant lymphoma. *Blood*, 27, 435-448.

Mention, J.J., Ben Ahmed, M., Begue, B., Barbe, U., Verkarre, V., Asnafi, V., Colombel, J.F., Cugnenc, P.H., Ruemmele, F.M., McIntyre, E., Brousse, N., Cellier, C. & Cerf-Bensussan, N. (2003) Interleukin 15: A key to disrupted intraepithelial lymphocyte homeostasis and lymphomagenesis in celiac disease. *Gastroenterology*, 125, 730-745.

Miners, J.O., Grgurinovich, N., Whitehead, A.G., Robson, R.A. & Birkett, D.J. (1986) Influence of gender and oral contraceptive steroids on the metabolism of salicylic acid and acetylsalicylic acid. *British Journal of Clinical Pharmacology*, 22, 135-142.

Moder, K.G., Tefferi, A., Cohen, M.D., Menke, D.M. & Luthra, H.S. (1995) Hematologic malignancies and the use of methotrexate in rheumatoid arthritis: A retrospective study. *The American Journal of Medicine*, 99, 276-281.

Morton, J.E., Leyland, M.J., Vaughan Hudson, G., Vaughan Hudson, B., Anderson, L., Bennett, M.H. & MacLennan, K.A. (1993) Primary gastrointestinal non-hodgkin's lymphoma: A review of 175 british national lymphoma investigation cases. *British Journal of Cancer*, 67, 776-782.

Moshynska, O.V. & Saxena, A. (2008) Clonal relationship between hashimoto thyroiditis and thyroid lymphoma. *Journal of Clinical Pathology*, 61, 438-444.

Moss, K.E., Ioannou, Y., Sultan, S.M., Haq, I. & Isenberg, D.A. (2002) Outcome of a cohort of 300 patients with systemic lupus erythematosus attending a dedicated clinic for over two decades. *Annals of the Rheumatic Diseases*, 61, 409-413.

Moutsopoulos, H.M., Steinberg, A.D., Fauci, A.S., Lane, H.C. & Papadopoulos, N.M. (1983) High incidence of free monoclonal lambda light chains in the sera of patients with sjogren's syndrome. *Journal of Immunology (Baltimore, Md.: 1950)*, 130, 2663-2665.

Natkunam, Y., Lossos, I.S., Taidi, B., Zhao, S., Lu, X., Ding, F., Hammer, A.S., Marafioti, T., Byrne, G.E.,Jr, Levy, S., Warnke, R.A. & Levy, R. (2005) Expression of the human germinal center-associated lymphoma (HGAL) protein, a new marker of germinal center B-cell derivation. *Blood*, 105, 3979-3986.

Neumeister, P., Hoefler, G., Beham-Schmid, C., Schmidt, H., Apfelbeck, U., Schaider, H., Linkesch, W. & Sill, H. (1997) Deletion analysis of the p16 tumor suppressor gene in gastrointestinal mucosa-associated lymphoid tissue lymphomas. *Gastroenterology*, 112, 1871-1875.

Ngo, V.N., Korner, H., Gunn, M.D., Schmidt, K.N., Riminton, D.S., Cooper, M.D., Browning, J.L., Sedgwick, J.D. & Cyster, J.G. (1999) Lymphotoxin alpha/beta and tumor necrosis factor are required for stromal cell expression of homing chemokines in B and T cell areas of the spleen. *The Journal of Experimental Medicine*, 189, 403-412.

Niitsu, N., Okamoto, M., Nakamura, N., Nakamine, H., Bessho, M. & Hirano, M. (2007) Clinicopathologic correlations of stage IE/IIE primary thyroid diffuse large B-cell lymphoma. *Annals of Oncology : Official Journal of the European Society for Medical Oncology / ESMO*, 18, 1203-1208.

Nossent, J., Cikes, N., Kiss, E., Marchesoni, A., Nassonova, V., Mosca, M., Olesinska, M., Pokorny, G., Rozman, B., Schneider, M., Vlachoyiannopoulos, P.G. & Swaak, A.

(2007) Current causes of death in systemic lupus erythematosus in europe, 2000--2004: Relation to disease activity and damage accrual. *Lupus*, 16, 309-317.

Novakovic, B.J., Novakovic, S. & Frkovic-Grazio, S. (2006) A single-center report on clinical features and treatment response in patients with intestinal T cell non-hodgkin's lymphomas. *Oncology Reports*, 16, 191-195.

Okada, T., Takiura, F., Tokushige, K., Nozawa, S., Kiyosawa, T., Nakauchi, H., Hirose, S. & Shirai, T. (1991) Major histocompatibility complex controls clonal proliferation of CD5+ B cells in H-2-congenic new zealand mice: A model for B cell chronic lymphocytic leukemia and autoimmune disease. *European Journal of Immunology*, 21, 2743-2748.

Patey-Mariaud De Serre, N., Cellier, C., Jabri, B., Delabesse, E., Verkarre, V., Roche, B., Lavergne, A., Briere, J., Mauvieux, L., Leborgne, M., Barbier, J.P., Modigliani, R., Matuchansky, C., MacIntyre, E., Cerf-Bensussan, N. & Brousse, N. (2000) Distinction between coeliac disease and refractory sprue: A simple immunohistochemical method. *Histopathology*, 37, 70-77.

Pedersen, R.K. & Pedersen, N.T. (1996) Primary non-hodgkin's lymphoma of the thyroid gland: A population based study. *Histopathology*, 28, 25-32.

Picker, L.J. (1992) Mechanisms of lymphocyte homing. *Current Opinion in Immunology*, 4, 277-286.

Pijpe, J., van Imhoff, G.W., Spijkervet, F.K., Roodenburg, J.L., Wolbink, G.J., Mansour, K., Vissink, A., Kallenberg, C.G. & Bootsma, H. (2005) Rituximab treatment in patients with primary sjogren's syndrome: An open-label phase II study. *Arthritis and Rheumatism*, 52, 2740-2750.

Poole, B.D., Templeton, A.K., Guthridge, J.M., Brown, E.J., Harley, J.B. & James, J.A. (2009) Aberrant epstein-barr viral infection in systemic lupus erythematosus. *Autoimmunity Reviews*, 8, 337-342.

Quartuccio, L., Fabris, M., Salvin, S., Maset, M., De Marchi, G. & De Vita, S. (2009) Controversies on rituximab therapy in sjogren syndrome-associated lymphoproliferation. *International Journal of Rheumatology*, 2009, 424935.

Ramos-Casals, M., Brito-Zeron, P., Yague, J., Akasbi, M., Bautista, R., Ruano, M., Claver, G., Gil, V. & Font, J. (2005) Hypocomplementaemia as an immunological marker of morbidity and mortality in patients with primary sjogren's syndrome. *Rheumatology (Oxford, England)*, 44, 89-94.

Randen, I., Mellbye, O.J., Forre, O. & Natvig, J.B. (1995) The identification of germinal centres and follicular dendritic cell networks in rheumatoid synovial tissue. *Scandinavian Journal of Immunology*, 41, 481-486.

Ray, W.A. (2003) Population-based studies of adverse drug effects. *The New England Journal of Medicine*, 349, 1592-1594.

Reunala, T. (1998) Dermatitis herpetiformis: Coeliac disease of the skin. *Annals of Medicine*, 30, 416-418.

Reunala, T., Helin, H., Kuokkanen, K. & Hakala, T. (1982) Lymphoma in dermatitis herpetiformis: Report on four cases. *Acta Dermato-Venereologica*, 62, 343-346.

Reunala, T., Blomqvist, K., Tarpila, S., Halme, H. & Kangas, K. (1977) Gluten-free diet in dermatitis herpetiformis. I. clinical response of skin lesions in 81 patients. *The British Journal of Dermatology*, 97, 473-480.

Reyes, F., Lepage, E., Ganem, G., Molina, T.J., Brice, P., Coiffier, B., Morel, P., Ferme, C., Bosly, A., Lederlin, P., Laurent, G., Tilly, H. & Groupe d'Etude des Lymphomes de l'Adulte (GELA). (2005) ACVBP versus CHOP plus radiotherapy for localized aggressive lymphoma. *The New England Journal of Medicine*, 352, 1197-1205.

Rizzi, R., Curci, P., Delia, M., Rinaldi, E., Chiefa, A., Specchia, G. & Liso, V. (2009) Spontaneous remission of "methotrexate-associated lymphoproliferative disorders" after discontinuation of immunosuppressive treatment for autoimmune disease. review of the literature. *Medical Oncology (Northwood, London, England)*, 26, 1-9.

Rosenberg, L., Palmer, J.R., Zauber, A.G., Warshauer, M.E., Strom, B.L., Harlap, S. & Shapiro, S. (1995) Relation of benzodiazepine use to the risk of selected cancers: Breast, large bowel, malignant melanoma, lung, endometrium, ovary, non-hodgkin's lymphoma, testis, hodgkin's disease, thyroid, and liver. *American Journal of Epidemiology*, 141, 1153-1160.

Rosenthal, A.K., McLaughlin, J.K., Gridley, G. & Nyren, O. (1995) Incidence of cancer among patients with systemic sclerosis. *Cancer*, 76, 910-914.

Rosenthal, A.K., McLaughlin, J.K., Linet, M.S. & Persson, I. (1993) Scleroderma and malignancy: An epidemiological study. *Annals of the Rheumatic Diseases*, 52, 531-533.

Rossi, D. (2009) Thyroid lymphoma: Beyond antigen stimulation. *Leukemia Research*, 33, 607-609.

Roumm, A.D. & Medsger, T.A.,Jr. (1985) Cancer and systemic sclerosis. an epidemiologic study. *Arthritis and Rheumatism*, 28, 1336-1340.

Royer, B., Cazals-Hatem, D., Sibilia, J., Agbalika, F., Cayuela, J.M., Soussi, T., Maloisel, F., Clauvel, J.P., Brouet, J.C. & Mariette, X. (1997) Lymphomas in patients with sjogren's syndrome are marginal zone B-cell neoplasms, arise in diverse extranodal and nodal sites, and are not associated with viruses. *Blood*, 90, 766-775.

Ruggiero, F.P., Frauenhoffer, E. & Stack, B.C.,Jr. (2005) Thyroid lymphoma: A single institution's experience. *Otolaryngology--Head and Neck Surgery : Official Journal of American Academy of Otolaryngology-Head and Neck Surgery*, 133, 888-896.

Salloum, E., Cooper, D.L., Howe, G., Lacy, J., Tallini, G., Crouch, J., Schultz, M. & Murren, J. (1996) Spontaneous regression of lymphoproliferative disorders in patients treated with methotrexate for rheumatoid arthritis and other rheumatic diseases. *Journal of Clinical Oncology : Official Journal of the American Society of Clinical Oncology*, 14, 1943-1949.

Sato, S., Fujimoto, M., Hasegawa, M. & Takehara, K. (2004) Altered blood B lymphocyte homeostasis in systemic sclerosis: Expanded naive B cells and diminished but activated memory B cells. *Arthritis and Rheumatism*, 50, 1918-1927.

Savilahti, E., Reunala, T. & Maki, M. (1992) Increase of lymphocytes bearing the gamma/delta T cell receptor in the jejunum of patients with dermatitis herpetiformis. *Gut*, 33, 206-211.

Saxena, A., Alport, E.C., Moshynska, O., Kanthan, R. & Boctor, M.A. (2004) Clonal B cell populations in a minority of patients with hashimoto's thyroiditis. *Journal of Clinical Pathology*, 57, 1258-1263.

Schroder, A.E., Greiner, A., Seyfert, C. & Berek, C. (1996) Differentiation of B cells in the nonlymphoid tissue of the synovial membrane of patients with rheumatoid arthritis. *Proceedings of the National Academy of Sciences of the United States of America*, 93, 221-225.

Setoguchi, S., Solomon, D.H., Weinblatt, M.E., Katz, J.N., Avorn, J., Glynn, R.J., Cook, E.F., Carney, G. & Schneeweiss, S. (2006) Tumor necrosis factor alpha antagonist use and cancer in patients with rheumatoid arthritis. *Arthritis and Rheumatism*, 54, 2757-2764.

Seyler, T.M., Park, Y.W., Takemura, S., Bram, R.J., Kurtin, P.J., Goronzy, J.J. & Weyand, C.M. (2005) BLyS and APRIL in rheumatoid arthritis. *The Journal of Clinical Investigation*, 115, 3083-3092.

Siau, K., Laversuch, C.J., Creamer, P. & O'Rourke, K.P. (2010) Malignancy in scleroderma patients from south west england: A population-based cohort study. *Rheumatology International*.

Sieniawski, M., Angamuthu, N., Boyd, K., Chasty, R., Davies, J., Forsyth, P., Jack, F., Lyons, S., Mounter, P., Revell, P., Proctor, S.J. & Lennard, A.L. (2010) Evaluation of enteropathy-associated T-cell lymphoma comparing standard therapies with a novel regimen including autologous stem cell transplantation. *Blood*, 115, 3664-3670.

Sigurgeirsson, B., Agnarsson, B.A. & Lindelof, B. (1994) Risk of lymphoma in patients with dermatitis herpetiformis. *BMJ (Clinical Research Ed.)*, 308, 13-15.

Silano, M., Volta, U., Vincenzi, A.D., Dessi, M., Vincenzi, M.D. & Collaborating Centers of the Italian Registry of the Complications of Coeliac Disease. (2008) Effect of a gluten-free diet on the risk of enteropathy-associated T-cell lymphoma in celiac disease. *Digestive Diseases and Sciences*, 53, 972-976.

Silano, M., Volta, U., Mecchia, A.M., Dessi, M., Di Benedetto, R., De Vincenzi, M. & Collaborating centers of the Italian registry of the complications of coeliac disease. (2007) Delayed diagnosis of coeliac disease increases cancer risk. *BMC Gastroenterology*, 7, 8.

Simon, Z., Tarr, T., Ress, Z., Gergely, L., Kiss, E. & Illes, A. (2007) Successful rituximab-CHOP treatment of systemic lupus erythematosus associated with diffuse large B-cell non-hodgkin lymphoma. *Rheumatology International*, 28, 179-183.

Skopouli, F.N., Dafni, U., Ioannidis, J.P. & Moutsopoulos, H.M. (2000) Clinical evolution, and morbidity and mortality of primary sjogren's syndrome. *Seminars in Arthritis and Rheumatism*, 29, 296-304.

Smedby, K.E., Baecklund, E. & Askling, J. (2006) Malignant lymphomas in autoimmunity and inflammation: A review of risks, risk factors, and lymphoma characteristics. *Cancer Epidemiology, Biomarkers & Prevention : A Publication of the American Association for Cancer Research, Cosponsored by the American Society of Preventive Oncology*, 15, 2069-2077.

Smedby, K.E., Askling, J., Mariette, X. & Baecklund, E. (2008) Autoimmune and inflammatory disorders and risk of malignant lymphomas--an update. *Journal of Internal Medicine*, 264, 514-527.

Smedby, K.E., Akerman, M., Hildebrand, H., Glimelius, B., Ekbom, A. & Askling, J. (2005) Malignant lymphomas in coeliac disease: Evidence of increased risks for lymphoma types other than enteropathy-type T cell lymphoma. *Gut*, 54, 54-59.

Smedby, K.E., Hjalgrim, H., Askling, J., Chang, E.T., Gregersen, H., Porwit-MacDonald, A., Sundstrom, C., Akerman, M., Melbye, M., Glimelius, B. & Adami, H.O. (2006) Autoimmune and chronic inflammatory disorders and risk of non-hodgkin lymphoma by subtype. *Journal of the National Cancer Institute*, 98, 51-60.

Soderberg, K.C., Jonsson, F., Winqvist, O., Hagmar, L. & Feychting, M. (2006) Autoimmune diseases, asthma and risk of haematological malignancies: A nationwide case-control study in sweden. *European Journal of Cancer (Oxford, England : 1990)*, 42, 3028-3033.

Soderstrom, N., Axelsson, J.A. & Hagelqvist, E. (1970) Postcapillary venules of the lymph node type in the thymus in myasthenia. *Laboratory Investigation; a Journal of Technical Methods and Pathology*, 23, 451-458.

Soldini, D., Mora, O., Cavalli, F., Zucca, E. & Mazzucchelli, L. (2008) Efficacy of alemtuzumab and gemcitabine in a patient with enteropathy-type T-cell lymphoma. *British Journal of Haematology*, 142, 484-486.

Sorensen, H.T., Friis, S., Norgard, B., Mellemkjaer, L., Blot, W.J., McLaughlin, J.K., Ekbom, A. & Baron, J.A. (2003) Risk of cancer in a large cohort of nonaspirin NSAID users: A population-based study. *British Journal of Cancer*, 88, 1687-1692.

Staunton, M.D. & Greening, W.P. (1973) Clinical diagnosis of thyroid cancer. *British Medical Journal*, 4, 532-535.

Stott, D.I., Hiepe, F., Hummel, M., Steinhauser, G. & Berek, C. (1998) Antigen-driven clonal proliferation of B cells within the target tissue of an autoimmune disease. the salivary glands of patients with sjogren's syndrome. *The Journal of Clinical Investigation*, 102, 938-946.

Su, L. & David, M. (1999) Inhibition of B cell receptor-mediated apoptosis by IFN. *Journal of Immunology (Baltimore, Md.: 1950)*, 162, 6317-6321.

Swerdlow, S.H., Campo, E., Harris, N.L., Jaffe, E.S., Pileri, S., Stein, H., Thiele, J. & Vardiman J.W. (2008) WHO classification of tumours of haematopoietic and lymphoid tissues.

Symmons, D.P. (1985) Neoplasms of the immune system in rheumatoid arthritis. *The American Journal of Medicine*, 78, 22-28.

Szekanecz, E., Szamosi, S., Gergely, L., Keszthelyi, P., Szekanecz, Z. & Szucs, G. (2008) Incidence of lymphoma in systemic sclerosis: A retrospective analysis of 218 hungarian patients with systemic sclerosis. *Clinical Rheumatology*, 27, 1163-1166.

Szodoray, P. & Jonsson, R. (2005) The BAFF/APRIL system in systemic autoimmune diseases with a special emphasis on sjogren's syndrome. *Scandinavian Journal of Immunology*, 62, 421-428.

Tack, G.J., Verbeek, W.H., Schreurs, M.W. & Mulder, C.J. (2010a) The spectrum of celiac disease: Epidemiology, clinical aspects and treatment. *Nature Reviews. Gastroenterology & Hepatology*, 7, 204-213.

Tack, G.J., Wondergem, M.J., Al-Toma, A., Verbeek, W.H., Schmittel, A., Machado, M.V., Perri, F., Ossenkoppele, G.J., Huijgens, P.C., Schreurs, M.W., Mulder, C.J. & Visser, O.J. (2010b) Auto-SCT in refractory celiac disease type II patients unresponsive to cladribine therapy. *Bone Marrow Transplantation*, .

Takakuwa, T., Miyauchi, A. & Aozasa, K. (2009) Aberrant somatic hypermutations in thyroid lymphomas. *Leukemia Research*, 33, 649-654.

Tamura, K., Shimaoka, K. & Friedman, M. (1981) Thyroid abnormalities associated with treatment of malignant lymphoma. *Cancer*, 47, 2704-2711.

Tan, L.C., Mowat, A.G., Fazou, C., Rostron, T., Roskell, H., Dunbar, P.R., Tournay, C., Romagne, F., Peyrat, M.A., Houssaint, E., Bonneville, M., Rickinson, A.B., McMichael, A.J. & Callan, M.F. (2000) Specificity of T cells in synovial fluid: High frequencies of CD8(+) T cells that are specific for certain viral epitopes. *Arthritis Research*, 2, 154-164.

Tapinos, N.I., Polihronis, M. & Moutsopoulos, H.M. (1999) Lymphoma development in sjogren's syndrome: Novel p53 mutations. *Arthritis and Rheumatism*, 42, 1466-1472.

Thanou-Stavraki, A. & Sawalha, A.H. (2011) An update on belimumab for the treatment of lupus. *Biologics : Targets & Therapy*, 5, 33-43.

Theander, E., Manthorpe, R. & Jacobsson, L.T. (2004) Mortality and causes of death in primary sjogren's syndrome: A prospective cohort study. *Arthritis and Rheumatism*, 50, 1262-1269.

Theander, E., Henriksson, G., Ljungberg, O., Mandl, T., Manthorpe, R. & Jacobsson, L.T. (2006) Lymphoma and other malignancies in primary sjogren's syndrome: A cohort study on cancer incidence and lymphoma predictors. *Annals of the Rheumatic Diseases*, 65, 796-803.

Theofilopoulos, A.N., Baccala, R., Beutler, B. & Kono, D.H. (2005) Type I interferons (alpha/beta) in immunity and autoimmunity. *Annual Review of Immunology*, 23, 307-336.

Thieblemont, C., Mayer, A., Dumontet, C., Barbier, Y., Callet-Bauchu, E., Felman, P., Berger, F., Ducottet, X., Martin, C., Salles, G., Orgiazzi, J. & Coiffier, B. (2002) Primary thyroid lymphoma is a heterogeneous disease. *The Journal of Clinical Endocrinology and Metabolism*, 87, 105-111.

Tincani, A., Taraborelli, M. & Cattaneo, R. (2010) Antiphospholipid antibodies and malignancies. *Autoimmunity Reviews*, 9, 200-202.

Tosato, G., Steinberg, A.D. & Blaese, R.M. (1981) Defective EBV-specific suppressor T-cell function in rheumatoid arthritis. *The New England Journal of Medicine*, 305, 1238-1243.

Tosato, G., Steinberg, A.D., Yarchoan, R., Heilman, C.A., Pike, S.E., De Seau, V. & Blaese, R.M. (1984) Abnormally elevated frequency of epstein-barr virus-infected B cells in the blood of patients with rheumatoid arthritis. *The Journal of Clinical Investigation*, 73, 1789-1795.

Toubi, E. & Shoenfeld, Y. (2007) Clinical and biological aspects of anti-P-ribosomal protein autoantibodies. *Autoimmunity Reviews*, 6, 119-125.

Troch, M., Woehrer, S., Streubel, B., Weissel, M., Hoffmann, M., Mullauer, L., Chott, A. & Raderer, M. (2008) Chronic autoimmune thyroiditis (hashimoto's thyroiditis) in patients with MALT lymphoma. *Annals of Oncology : Official Journal of the European Society for Medical Oncology / ESMO*, 19, 1336-1339.

Tsang, R.W., Gospodarowicz, M.K., Pintilie, M., Wells, W., Hodgson, D.C., Sun, A., Crump, M. & Patterson, B.J. (2003) Localized mucosa-associated lymphoid tissue lymphoma treated with radiation therapy has excellent clinical outcome. *Journal of Clinical Oncology : Official Journal of the American Society of Clinical Oncology*, 21, 4157-4164.

Tupchong, L., Hughes, F. & Harmer, C.L. (1986) Primary lymphoma of the thyroid: Clinical features, prognostic factors, and results of treatment. *International Journal of Radiation Oncology, Biology, Physics*, 12, 1813-1821.

Turesson, C. & Matteson, E.L. (2004) Management of extra-articular disease manifestations in rheumatoid arthritis. *Current Opinion in Rheumatology*, 16, 206-211.

Tzioufas, A.G., Boumba, D.S., Skopouli, F.N. & Moutsopoulos, H.M. (1996) Mixed monoclonal cryoglobulinemia and monoclonal rheumatoid factor cross-reactive idiotypes as predictive factors for the development of lymphoma in primary sjogren's syndrome. *Arthritis and Rheumatism*, 39, 767-772.

Tzioufas, A.G., Manoussakis, M.N., Costello, R., Silis, M., Papadopoulos, N.M. & Moutsopoulos, H.M. (1986) Cryoglobulinemia in autoimmune rheumatic diseases. evidence of circulating monoclonal cryoglobulins in patients with primary sjogren's syndrome. *Arthritis and Rheumatism*, 29, 1098-1104.

Valesini, G., Priori, R., Bavoillot, D., Osborn, J., Danieli, M.G., Del Papa, N., Gerli, R., Pietrogrande, M., Sabbadini, M.G., Silvestris, F. & Valsecchi, L. (1997) Differential risk of non-hodgkin's lymphoma in italian patients with primary sjogren's syndrome. *The Journal of Rheumatology*, 24, 2376-2380.

Vallabhapurapu, S. & Karin, M. (2009) Regulation and function of NF-kappaB transcription factors in the immune system. *Annual Review of Immunology*, 27, 693-733.

van de Water, J.M., Cillessen, S.A., Visser, O.J., Verbeek, W.H., Meijer, C.J. & Mulder, C.J. (2010) Enteropathy associated T-cell lymphoma and its precursor lesions. *Best Practice & Research.Clinical Gastroenterology*, 24, 43-56.

Veeranki, S. & Choubey, D. (2010) Systemic lupus erythematosus and increased risk to develop B cell malignancies: Role of the p200-family proteins. *Immunology Letters*, 133, 1-5.

Verdolini, R., Bugatti, L., Giangiacomi, M., Nicolini, M., Filosa, G. & Cerio, R. (2002) Systemic lupus erythematosus induced by epstein-barr virus infection. *The British Journal of Dermatology*, 146, 877-881.

Verkarre, V., Romana, S.P., Cellier, C., Asnafi, V., Mention, J.J., Barbe, U., Nusbaum, S., Hermine, O., Macintyre, E., Brousse, N., Cerf-Bensussan, N. & Radford-Weiss, I. (2003) Recurrent partial trisomy 1q22-q44 in clonal intraepithelial lymphocytes in refractory celiac sprue. *Gastroenterology*, 125, 40-46.

Vettori, S., Staibano, S., Mascolo, M., Ilardi, G. & Valentini, G. (2010) Non-hodgkin's lymphoma in systemic sclerosis: Case and literature review. *Clinical Rheumatology*, 29, 1-6.

Viljamaa, M., Kaukinen, K., Pukkala, E., Hervonen, K., Reunala, T. & Collin, P. (2006) Malignancies and mortality in patients with coeliac disease and dermatitis herpetiformis: 30-year population-based study. *Digestive and Liver Disease : Official Journal of the Italian Society of Gastroenterology and the Italian Association for the Study of the Liver*, 38, 374-380.

Vivas, S., Ruiz de Morales, J.M., Ramos, F. & Suarez-Vilela, D. (2006) Alemtuzumab for refractory celiac disease in a patient at risk for enteropathy-associated T-cell lymphoma. *The New England Journal of Medicine*, 354, 2514-2515.

von Roon, A.C., Reese, G., Teare, J., Constantinides, V., Darzi, A.W. & Tekkis, P.P. (2007) The risk of cancer in patients with crohn's disease. *Diseases of the Colon and Rectum*, 50, 839-855.

Voulgarelis, M., Giannouli, S., Tzioufas, A.G. & Moutsopoulos, H.M. (2006) Long term remission of sjogren's syndrome associated aggressive B cell non-hodgkin's lymphomas following combined B cell depletion therapy and CHOP (cyclophosphamide, doxorubicin, vincristine, prednisone). *Annals of the Rheumatic Diseases*, 65, 1033-1037.

Voulgarelis, M., Petroutsos, G., Moutsopoulos, H.M. & Skopouli, F.N. (2002) 2-chloro-2'-deoxyadenosine in the treatment of sjogren's syndrome-associated B cell lymphoproliferation. *Arthritis and Rheumatism*, 46, 2248-2249.

Voulgarelis, M., Dafni, U.G., Isenberg, D.A. & Moutsopoulos, H.M. (1999) Malignant lymphoma in primary sjogren's syndrome: A multicenter, retrospective, clinical study by the european concerted action on sjogren's syndrome. *Arthritis and Rheumatism*, 42, 1765-1772.

Wang, S.A., Rahemtullah, A., Faquin, W.C., Roepke, J., Harris, N.L. & Hasserjian, R.P. (2005) Hodgkin's lymphoma of the thyroid: A clinicopathologic study of five cases and review of the literature. *Modern Pathology : An Official Journal of the United States and Canadian Academy of Pathology, Inc*, 18, 1577-1584.

Watanabe-Fukunaga, R., Brannan, C.I., Copeland, N.G., Jenkins, N.A. & Nagata, S. (1992) Lymphoproliferation disorder in mice explained by defects in fas antigen that mediates apoptosis. *Nature*, 356, 314-317.

Watson, W.C., Tooms, R.E., Carnesale, P.G. & Dutkowsky, J.P. (1994) A case of germinal center formation by CD45RO T and CD20 B lymphocytes in rheumatoid arthritic subchondral bone: Proposal for a two-compartment model of immune-mediated disease with implications for immunotherapeutic strategies. *Clinical Immunology and Immunopathology*, 73, 27-37.

Weetman, A.P. & McGregor, A.M. (1994) Autoimmune thyroid disease: Further developments in our understanding. *Endocrine Reviews*, 15, 788-830.

Weinblatt, M.E., Maier, A.L., Fraser, P.A. & Coblyn, J.S. (1998) Longterm prospective study of methotrexate in rheumatoid arthritis: Conclusion after 132 months of therapy. *The Journal of Rheumatology*, 25, 238-242.

Weyand, C.M., Goronzy, J.J. & Kurtin, P.J. (2006) Lymphoma in rheumatoid arthritis: An immune system set up for failure. *Arthritis and Rheumatism*, 54, 685-689.

Wolfe, F. & Michaud, K. (2007) The effect of methotrexate and anti-tumor necrosis factor therapy on the risk of lymphoma in rheumatoid arthritis in 19,562 patients during 89,710 person-years of observation. *Arthritis and Rheumatism*, 56, 1433-1439.

Wolfe, F. & Michaud, K. (2004) Lymphoma in rheumatoid arthritis: The effect of methotrexate and anti-tumor necrosis factor therapy in 18,572 patients. *Arthritis and Rheumatism*, 50, 1740-1751.

Wright, D.H. (1995) The major complications of coeliac disease. *Bailliere's Clinical Gastroenterology*, 9, 351-369.

Xin, H., D'Souza, S., Jorgensen, T.N., Vaughan, A.T., Lengyel, P., Kotzin, B.L. & Choubey, D. (2006) Increased expression of Ifi202, an IFN-activatable gene, in B6.Nba2 lupus susceptible mice inhibits p53-mediated apoptosis. *Journal of Immunology (Baltimore, Md.: 1950)*, 176, 5863-5870.

Xu, Y. & Wiernik, P.H. (2001) Systemic lupus erythematosus and B-cell hematologic neoplasm. *Lupus*, 10, 841-850.

Yao, Q.Y., Rickinson, A.B., Gaston, J.S. & Epstein, M.A. (1986) Disturbance of the epstein-barr virus-host balance in rheumatoid arthritis patients: A quantitative study. *Clinical and Experimental Immunology*, 64, 302-310.

Youinou, P., Devauchelle-Pensec, V. & Pers, J.O. (2010) Significance of B cells and B cell clonality in sjogren's syndrome. *Arthritis and Rheumatism*, 62, 2605-2610.

Youinou, P., Papadopoulos, N.M., Katsikis, P., Pennec, Y.L., Jouquan, J., Lelong, A. & Moutsopoulos, H.M. (1988) Monoclonal immunoglobulins in the serum of patients with primary sjogren's syndrome. *Clinical and Experimental Rheumatology*, 6, 247-252.

Young, L.S. & Rickinson, A.B. (2004) Epstein-barr virus: 40 years on. *Nature Reviews.Cancer*, 4, 757-768.

Zatuchni, J., Campbell, W.N. & Zarafonetis, C.J. (1953) Pulmonary fibrosis and terminal bronchiolar (alveolar-cell) carcinoma in scleroderma. *Cancer*, 6, 1147-1158.

Zhang, Y., Holford, T.R., Leaderer, B., Zahm, S.H., Boyle, P., Morton, L.M., Zhang, B., Zou, K., Flynn, S., Tallini, G., Owens, P.H. & Zheng, T. (2004) Prior medical conditions and medication use and risk of non-hodgkin lymphoma in connecticut united states women. *Cancer Causes & Control : CCC*, 15, 419-428.

Zintzaras, E., Voulgarelis, M. & Moutsopoulos, H.M. (2005) The risk of lymphoma development in autoimmune diseases: A meta-analysis. *Archives of Internal Medicine*, 165, 2337-2344.

Part 2

Immunology of Pregnancy

6

Mechanism of Autoimmunity in Pregnancy - The Good and the Bad

Lotti Tajouri[1,2], Ekua W. Brenu[1,2],
Donald R. Staines[1,3] and Sonya M. Marshall-Gradisnik[1,2]
*[1]Population Health and Neuroimmunology Unit, Faculty of Health
Science and Medicine, Bond University, Robina,
[2]Faculty of Health Science and Medicine, Bond University, Robina,
[3]Queensland Health, Gold Coast Population Health Unit, Southport,
Australia*

1. Introduction

In humans, female's humoral and cellular immunity are actually stronger than men (Nalbandian & Kovats, 2005) and present a higher antibody serum titration than men (Giron-Gonzalez et al., 2000) which could logically and possibly explain their gender predisposition and susceptibility to autoimmunity. Holding an autoimmune disease and becoming pregnant is a serious matter for a woman and knowledge of the course of the condition during pregnancy is essential. Relational variations exist between types of autoimmuny during pregnancy and consequently proper advices from physicians are provided accordingly. In Systemic lupus erythematosus, all advices provided to the patients are meant to dissuade women from getting pregnant while being in a relapse stage of the disease and better wait for the end of the flare pathological course. As for Rheumatoid arthritis and multiple sclerosis, no real dangers are encountered while being pregnant and while the disease symptoms are expressed it still does not present life threatening risks to the gestation. In Myasthenia gravis, during gestation the risks are variable and retrospective studies show increase complications.

Logically, the baby carrying semi-allogenic antigens should prompt an autoimmune reaction from the mother. However a plethora of tolerance measures is put into action by both the mother and the foetus. Pre implantation immunological events are in place to best prepare the nidation of the foetus into the mother endometrium. There is large paucity of published scientific research studies that have attempted to understand the entire pregnancy immune profile due to low power studies, limiting longitudinal samplings and narrow immune component analysis. However, a recent study has shown a Th1 toTh2 shift with increase interleukin 10 synthesis and a decrease responses to pro-inflammatory cytokines such as TNFα, Il-1β and Il-6 during pregnancy (Denney et al., 2011). Immunological adaptations occur early in gestation and are mediated by the uterine epithelium including the fallopian tube secretion of granulocyte macrophage colony stimulating factors (GM-CSF) (Rosendaal, 1975). In addition, the trophoblast that is derived from the fertilized egg secretes GM-CSF to prepare best for the next step of implantation and formation of the placenta (Burgess et al., 1977). Post implantation, the placenta is formed to accommodate, protect and feed with key nutrients the growing foetus. The placenta is formed of different layers with the basal plate or deciduas basalis, a structure in direct contact with the endometrium, the intermediate layer being the lacunar system and finally the chorionic plate made of two leaflets, the chorionic plate and the amniotic plate. Interestingly, the content of the decidua is composed of different key factors aiming at inducing tolerance and include cells such as maternal Natural killers and regulatory T-cells. Natural killer cells are secreting lots of cytokines with immunoregulation purposes and are non cytotoxic (Chantakru et al., 2002). As for the regulatory T-cells, data showed that human chorionic gonadotropin hormone is responsible for the attraction of such cells in the placenta (Schumacher et al., 2009). It has also been proved that Treg are key determinants in murine pregnancy (Zenclussen et al., 2005) with possibly the mediation of interleukin 10 (Taylor et al., 2006 & Akdis et al., 2001). The relative proportion of immune cells found in the deciduas are as follows, 70% of natural killers (Moffet et al., 2004), 20% of macrophages (Lessin et al., 1988), around 2% of T lymphocytes (Lessin et al., 1988), 1% of dendritic cells (Gardner et al., 2003) and very minute B cell lymphocytes (Veenstra Van Nieuwenhoven et al., 2003). In addition, regulatory proteins decreasing complement action are found in the decidua basalis more precisely on the syncyciotrophoblast T-cells along with cellular membranar Fas ligands and MHC molecules. MHC molecules consist of class III MHC molecules but lack of particular HLAI and HLA II molecules including HLA-A and -B as well as HLA-DP, -DQ and –DR is noticed (Landek-Salgado et al., 2010). Interestingly the placenta is maintaining a tied tolerance status mediated by each of its functional molecular and cellular components playing a major role in this process. Mostly, any activated T-cells that would reach this mother-foetus interface border would be bound to Fas ligand on their Fas receptor condemning them to enter apoptosis (Pongcharoen et al., 2004). This apoptotic process is mediated by Fas pathway through the activation of the death induce signaling complex that ultimately activates the caspase apoptotic cascade. More importantly, regulatory T-cells accumulating in the decidua during pregnancy, dampen any pro-inflammatory that harm the foetus (Tilburgs et al., 2008).

Along with this immunosuppressive function, an immune tolerance is strongly put in place. Transient gestational lowering reactivity is set to prevent potent T-cells from reacting against the semi-allogenic foetus and previously demonstrated in animal studies (Tafuri et al., 1995). Immuno tolerance features that directly play roles on pro-inflammatory immune cells are relying on particular cells called T regulatory cells or Tregs (Kuniyasu et al., 2000). Tregs can be Th4 lymphocytes or T8 lymphocytes and are mostly found to act as immunomodulators in regions of inflammation (Gavin et al., 2002). The action is mediated by contact inhibition of non Treg cells such include subsets of T 4 and T8 lymphocytic cells. Specific markers are differentiating these subsets from regulatory to non regulatory effective T-cells (Teff) and include CD25 markers (α chain of IL-2 receptor) with the so called CD4+ CD25+ and CD8+CD25+ cells. Additional markers are also found in Tregs such as FoxP3+ marker, a repressor activator of activated T-cells such as CD4+CD25+FoxP3+ Treg cells or Cd8+ CD25+ CDFoxP3+ Treg cells. Another Treg marker is CXCR3+ seen in CD8+ CXCR3+ Treg cells. The Treg mediation in tolerance restoration can be undertaken through different mechanisms. Tolerance could be undertaken by contact interaction such as Fas- Fas ligand interaction dictating an apoptotic faith to the Teff cells (Watanabe et al, 2002). The other way Tregs are promoting tolerance to Teff cells is to inhibit Teff cytokine synthesis and subsequently their Teff cytolytic activation as well as diminishing their proliferation (Duthoit et al., 2005). Teff cells can be CD8+ or CD4+ cells with the latter being classified into two types, TH1 and TH2 both differing in action as pro-inflammatory and anti-inflammatory actions respectively. Briefly, the Th1 activation pathway consists in interferon γ inducing activation of its cell surface receptor on T cells and subsequent intracellular cascade activation. Such cascade leads to the activation of the transcription factor T-bet which function is to bind DNA responsive elements of genes within the nucleus. The main responsive elements controlled and activated belong to the genes interferon γ and IL-12 receptor β2 chain. Upon activation, further expression of these genes is undertaken and IL-12 receptor becomes widely available at higher amounts in the cellular T-cell membranar surface and therefore can be prompted to activation due to the presence of local IL-12 cytokine. IL-12 receptor actiavtion induces a second cascade that is Stat 4 dependent, with the ultimate goal to produce furthermore T-bet transcription factor. Relation between Tregs and pro-inflammatory TH1 and CD8+ T-cells demonstrate an interesting phenomenon that is build around the competition for Interleukin 2 binding. In sites of inflammation, binding of IL-2 by Tregs diminishes the availability of IL-2 to Teffs and therefore limiting their growth, function and even at early stage turning Teffs to be anergic towards antigens (Piccirillo et al., 2001). Briefly, T-cells are activated through the contact of antigen with T-cell receptor under the restriction of MHC class molecules. Such binding activates p56lck tyrosine kinase with subsequent downstream phosphorylation of proteins and activation of phospholipase C. Such phospholipase generates from phosphatidyl inositol diphosphate, two compounds; the diacyl glycerol and inositol tri-phosphate, IP3. The endoplasmic reticulum IP3 receptor is therefore activated with release of calcium in the cytosol. Such Ca2++ induces a membranar activation of the cell membrane calcium release activated calcium channel named CRAC and subsequently increases highly the intracellular Ca2++ concentration. High levels of Ca2++ activate caclineurin, a phosphatase that dephosphorylates the transcriptional factor NFAT (nuclear factor of activated T-cells). Such dephosphorylated NFAT translocates into the nucleus to reach responsive elements of Il-2, AP1 and NFKB enabling their expression and future function. Beside the roles of Tregs as pro-apoptotic cytolytic Teff cells inducers and Teff cells expansion inhibitors, Tregs are capable to modulate the inflammatory 'soup' and pattern observed in inflammation sites. Such action of Tregs is mediated by their synthesis and secretion of both TGFβ and interleukin 10. A higher content of Il-10 is maintained due to Teffs response to TGFβ action and secondly by Il-10 action on dictating Teffs to respond with higher affinity to TGFβ. In addition, the constant increase of progesterone in gestation, which is peaking at the third trimester, is responsible for the activation of particular subsets of T-cells called γδ T-cells. Upon binding to its receptor, progesterone activates γδ T-cells to secrete Il-10 and progesterone induced blocking factor (PIBF) that result in the inhibition of natural killer cells (Barakonyi et al., 1999). In addition, these cells synthesise TGFβ that enhances the mother's T-cell tolerance for the foetus (Mincheva-Nilsson et al., 1992).

2. Autoimmunity and pregnancy

Women are more prevalent to autoimmunity and 3 to 5% will be affected by such disorders. During pregnancy, clinical course of several autoimmune disease are expressed with variable degrees. Some range from higher remission of signs and symptoms while others are being increased in exacerbations. These influences observed in Pregnancy denote a complex interaction between the pathophysiological course of the disease and the physiological adaptations during pregnancy. Presence of a wide spectrum of auto-antibodies correlates with the parturient pathophysiological course. In some autoimmune diseases, the risk of transient neonatal illness could be observed and can range from low risk as in myasthenia gravis to relatively higher as in Lupus. Self tolerance mechanisms at the cellular and genetic levels are modulated during pregnancy by these autoimmune diseases. Such modulation might reside at different levels and include, allelic variation with the HLA loci and expression, physiological adaptations during pregnancy (hormones) and alteration towards the host immunity or the foetal antigens (paternal HLAs), cytokine profile during pregnancy, HLA from foetus (HLA-G), structural interface integrity between foetus and mother, status of intrinsic and extrinsic controls preventing autoimmunity. We aim in this review at discussing the immunological events that surround pregnancy and autoimmunity especially by focusing on Systemic lupus erythematosus, Rheumatoid arthritis, Myasthenia gravis and Multiple sclerosis.

2.1 Systemic Lupus Erythematosus
2.1.1 Pathophysiology of SLE
Systemic lupus erythematosus (SLE) is an autoimmune disease mainly affecting the connective tissue that consequently demonstrating a plethora of systemic effects mostly observed in individuals of African-Asian origin. A staggering 9:1 ratio females to males is noted with a peak age of onset in young woman between 25 and 35 years of age. More than 98% of SLE patients are positive for the antinuclear auto-antibody (ANA), a marker of the disease. Other auto-antibodies are used to better refine the diagnosis of SLE and include anti cytoplasmic and anti DNA antibodies. The pathology shows a diverse range of symptoms affecting several organs ranging from common cutaneous lesions, serous membrane alteration and intermittent joints debilitations. More precisely, facial malar rashes, arthralgia, polyathritis, pleurisy, pericarditis are experienced along with other symptoms like Raynand's phenomenon and fever. The etiology of this complex disease is unknown but several hypotheses have been raised. Cellular release of antigens from apoptotic and necrotic cells is raised that will trigger macrophage phagocytosis and subsequent antigen presentation, under MHC class II, of such autoantigens to both T and B-cells. Intracellular and extracellular signaling are thought to be dysregulated such as the so called interferon signature, a cytokine profile under scrutiny as links with IRF5 has been shown to be associated with SLE (Graham et al., 2006). CD19 positive B-cells are of high attention in research as several auto-antibodies are pathogenic in the disease such as the anti nuclear antibodies (Madaio et al., 2003).

The genetics of SLE has pinpointed several chromosomal loci with interestingly the 1q23-24 region also called the pentraxin locus, a region harboring some key candidates including the CRP4 allele gene and the PDCD1 gene. A single nucleotide polymorphism in the PDCD1 gene was found to disrupt an intronic enhancer that prevents the gene from further activation with subsequent apoptotic process alterations. Other hypotheses have been investigated such as the possible occupational exposure or environmental effects but with no direct significant links to the disease. An interesting phenomenon though is well documented with the attention on precipitating factors. Such precipitating factors seen in SLE are the intake of oral estrogen contraceptives and hormonal replacement therapies (HRT) (Sanchez-Guerrero et al., 1997). Several studies including a nurse health study for oral contraceptive use have shown an increase of 1.9 time SLE manifestations compared to non users (Sanchez-Guerrero et al., 1995) and similar effect have been demonstrated with HRT (Cooper et al., 2002). In addition a lot of evidence is showing that the SLE manifestations are correlated with ovarian cycle alterations (Shabanova et al., 2008). A clear link is seen between hormonal changes and SLE therefore higher vigilance is sought for SLE women willing to become pregnant.

2.1.2 Modulation effects of pregnancy in SLE mothers

Pregnancy presents as a life experience where mother's hormonal levels are evolutionally and physiologically adapting to host the baby. Careful monitoring is undertaken as different gestational outcome scenarios are observed, with some being unpredictable, due to recurrence of flares and possible life threatening issues affecting both the mother and the child. Such dangers ranges from intra-uterine growth retardations in 30% of cases (Meyer Oliver, 2003), preterm birth with 25-30% of cases to miscarriages and foetal death. Co-morbidity is most likely to be observed in SLE patients with increase manifestation of the disease in the third trimester of gestation. Lots of evidence show detrimental effects to the kidney such as lupus nephritis, and ateroslcerotic pathophysiological establishments (Roman et al., 2003 and Asanuma et al., 2003) all to which can be further aggravated with other common pregnancy experienced problems like seen with preeclampsia occurrence. Death of the mother can be observed with common SLE risks due to high elevations of pulmonary hypertension. In 37% of SLE pregnant patients, mild increased of pulmonary arterial hypertension can be seen (Johnson et al., 2004). Such monitoring requires the use of several tests, serum antibodies, choice of specific medication, compliance with hydroxychloroquine, as well as the monitoring of SLE disease activity index (SLEDAI) measuring the flaring panel observed in SLE patients. Interestingly, SLE patients would have positive benefits and gains to start their gestation in period of remission before conception. An otherwise preconception with active disease otherwise shows increased flares with particularly renal disease associated problems (Moroni et al., 2002). In addition, lower birth weigths and high number of caesarian deliveries are encountered in proliferative nephritis cohorts. Foetal loss in SLE is a major problem with several studies attempting to link this fatal outcome to molecular triggering factors. The Hughes syndrome is a phospholipid induced pregnancy syndrome commonly named the antiphospholipid syndrome. Such syndrome is part of the coagulopathy diseases and SLE pregnant women are commonly tested for the presence of lupus anticoagulant factor, an anti phospholipid factor named anti-cardiolipin. This immunoglobulin G anti-cardiolipin antibody targets the apoprotein H or beta 2 glycoprotein 1. Such antibody prevents the glycoprotein from undertaking its possible known function as an inhibitor of the intrinsic coagulation cascade, an inhibition required and mediated by the release of complement molecules, C3 and C5 from the liver. As a consequence, SLE mothers with increase anti-ApoH denote a procoagulant pattern with detrimental foetal loss as an outcome. Interestingly, with treatment regimens of aspirin and heparin intakes, levels of live birth rates from SLE pregnant patients is now around 80% (Clark et al., 2007 and Girardi et al., 2004). Several markers for the disease have been found to better classify and understand the pathological course.

Efforts of the research community have helped in the discovery of a series of serum markers for SLE such as adipokine, a cell to cell signaling protein secreted by the adipose tissue (De Sanctis et al., 2009), CD40L or CD154 found in T-cell surface (De Sanctis et al., 2009 b) and the poly-reactive immunoglobulin M from B-cells (Zhang et al., 2009). All these markers denote an intense cell to cell communication and intense modulatory involvement of the immune system. Both arms of the immunity system are involved in SLE and particular attentions are drawn to further unravel the pathophysiological mechanism in SLE patient's immunity. SLE immune dysregulation involves a role to T-cell activation (Fernandez et al., 2009), B-cell signaling (Liu et al., 2009 and Peng, 2009) along with altered chemokine patterns (Youinou et al., 2009 and Wittmann et al., 2009) with IL-6 playing a role in polyarthritis and joint damage (Fonseca et al., 2009) and as mentioned previously an interferon signature (Finke et al., 2009).

The complex cascade of T-cell activation from the T-cell receptor (TCR) the consequently increase in intracellular content of Ca2++ and NFAT mediated IL-2 Transcriptional activation is an important immune component in SLE. In SLE, such pathway of activation is altered and seems to be associated with the calcium processing. ER calcium content not being an issue, a lot of attention was given to CRAC and studies have shown altered efficiency in this Ca2+ channel. Evidence has also shown that in SLE patients a Ca+ alteration was observed and linked to an upstream mitochondrial dysregulation. Evidence of high membrane hyperpolarisation (MHP) of the inner membrane of the mitochondrial has been pinpointed in SLE T-cells with subsequent ATP decreasing synthesis and failure to regenerate glutathione reduced forms, a anti oxidant molecule. Such dysregulation seems to be as well the cause of the unbalance fate observed in SLE T-cells deaths. Instead of progressing to a program cell death, with the common FAS pathway and death inducing signaling complex cascade, SLE T-cells instead enter necrosis. As both ATP and reduced glutathione pools are low, apoptosis is prevented and as such unbalance of quality cell death tends to develop into two main consequences. First, necrosis is favored and induces inflammation whereas apoptotic bodies do not. Secondly, in SLE, such overall dysregulation of calcium (katsiari et al., 2002), ATP formation (Perl et al., 2004) and low antioxidant capacity profile (Wang et al., 2010) is in favor to auto-reactive T-cells.

A strong correlation has been found between CXCL10 and SLE disease (Kong et al., 2009). CXCL10 is the interferon inducible factor, chemokine (C-X-C motif) ligand 10 also known as IP10 that acts on the receptor CXCR3. Interestingly, the gene coding for such receptor is the unique chemokine receptor found in chromosome X. This is in clear contrast to all other chemokine receptor genes, suggesting unique functions for CXCR3 and the ligand CXCL10 in possibly the role in SLE immunity. In sites of inflammation, a subset of B-cells with high expression of the marker CD19, a co-receptor of the B-cell receptor and known to be implicated in auto-immuniy, shows elevated CXCR3 levels (Nicholas et al., 2007). More challenges are met during pregnancy where placental tissues and the new born semi-allogenic foetal cells are brought together along with SLE (Doria et al., 2008). High consequences were recently tabulated in pregnant women with SLE with approximately 25% of women presenting with disease exacerbations (Lockshin et al., 1989).

2.2 Myasthenia and pregnancy
2.2.1 Pathophysiology of myasthenia gravis
Besides T-cells, breakdown of self tolerance in autoimmune diseases can be associated with humoral B-cell mediated immunity producing pathological auto-antibodies contributing to tissue damage as seen in myasthenia gravis (MG). MG is an autoimmune disease affecting predominantly women with clinical muscle fatigability with patients suffering from degrees

of weakness at various body systems. Under approximately 40 years of age, women are prevalent but after 50 years of age, incidence is then lesser in women than men. (Grob et al., 2008). The disease is categorised into two clinical presentations with on one hand, the ocular MG affecting of the levator and extra ocular palpebrae skeletal muscles with common diplopia and ptosis and in the other hand, generalised MG affecting other skeletal muscles. Interestingly, the disease can occur as relapsing remitting and the onset of symptomatology is varying from acute to subacute. Auto-antibodies target different antigens including the acetylcholine receptor (AchR) and, in most intense disease presentation, target the muscle specific muscle protein named MuSK (Padua et al., 2006). AchR and MusK seropositivity lead to neuromuscular dysfunctions. In the case of anti AChR, the antibodies trigger neutralisation of AChR function (Drachman et al., 1982), as well as antibody dependent complement activation with membrane attack complex formation (Engel et al., 1987) and finally antibody cross link with the ACHR leading to the destruction of AChR. The early onset MG is also associated with the possible occurrence of other autoimmune insults most commonly against the thyroid (Christensen, 1995). In early onset MG, the thymus gland is enlarged and patients present with multiple auto-antibodies. However, late onset MG is not associated with enlarged thymus. Association of HLA markers with individual type of MG onset has been undertaken and data showed that the early onset MG is associated with HLA-B8 and DR3 (Compston et al., 1980) whereas late onset MG is associated with HLA B7 and DR2 (Maggi et al., 1991). Immunologically the thymus is a primary lymphoid organ with a highly responsible function to maturate T-cells. T-cells that were produced in the bone marrow enter the thymus to become thymocytes to undergo a subsequent series of selection. The whole thymus is built to this process with a well vascularised content, clusters of different types of cells including antigen presenting cells such as macrophages, dendritic cells and parenchymal epithelial cells. When maturation of thymocytes is terminated, an efferent drainage successfully drains these cells into mediastinal lymph nodes. This selection is aiming at positively selecting immature T-cells which T-cell receptor would recognise MHC molecules. In the other hand, the negative selection aims at discarding the T-cells that would react to autoantigens presented by APCs. A failure in undertaking the removal of autoimmune T-cells is thought to be the problem occurring in MG disease. Certain T-cells, Th4 or CD4 + were investigated for their possible cell mediated autoimmune dysregulations. Interestingly though, both patients and free of disease normal individuals do have autoimmune T-cells targeting AChR (Schluep et al., 1987). Using experimental autoimmune **myasthenia** gravis (EAMG) animal models with Th1 deficient cells, researchers have shown actually that such animals have susceptibility to autoimmunity (Balasa et al., 1997). In this latter study, the focus was to distinguish between wild type and EAMG interferon gamma knockout mice. Result showed that EAMG knockout mice had no weakness to their muscles and were resistance to MG. However, the level of proliferation of AChR primed lymph nodes was still proliferating as normally observed in wild type mice. As interferon gamma is the primary pro-inflammatory stimulator of TH1 cells with downstream activation of the T-bet transcription factor inducing further interferon gamma transcription, MG autoimmunity induced solely with Th1 cannot be explaining the entire course of the disease. Even other types of autoimmunity such as in multiple sclerosis experimental allergic encephalomyelitis animals, observation of both interferon gamma deficient mice and T-bet knockout mice did not protect these autoimmunity disorders (Ferber et al., 1996). In Balasa et al. study, lymphogenic changes using mice with intact thymus were investigated but researchers focus is also turned into directly thymectomized animals. The thymic tissue is also harboring regulatory T-cells CD4+ CD25+ cells or Tregs that are anergic to antigen presentation (Crispin et al., 2003). These cells act as suppressors of effective autoimmune T-cells as demonstrated in Tregs deficient animal studies showing increase signs of autoimmunity disorders (Sakaguchi et al., 1995). Particular markers on the surface of Tregs are responsible for the immunological self tolerance function of Treg and include CD80, CD28, CD40 and CTLA4 with the later being a strong negative regulator of T-cell activity. Other subsets of cells called CD4+ CD25+ CD103+ are showing furthermore potentials in self tolerance and suppressive functional features in comparison to CD4+ CD25+ T-cells.

2.2.2 Modulation effects of pregnancy in Myasthenia gravis mothers

T-cells detain estrogen receptors on their membrane and studies have shown a high correlation between estrogens and disease detrimental activity. Interestingly, estrogens induce an expansion of specific Th1 effector cells with subsequent MG autoimmunity and increase of anti AChR antibodies (Delpy et al., 2005). In normal pregnancy, Tregs mediate immune tolerance (Guerin et al., 2009) and data previous data show that in early pregnancy estrogens do act on these CD4+ CD25+ T-cells to mediate indeed immunosuppression and higher immune tolerance. Such effect is relayed by progesterone during the rest of the gestation (Mao et al., 2010). Such positive effect might resign in the difference between CD4+ CD25+ and CD4+ CD25- T-cells. Differential gene expression of these two subsets showed higher expression levels of CTLA4, galactin, CD103, TNFRSF18, TNFRSF4 and the glucocorticoid induced TNF receptor called GITR (McHugh et al., 2002) in CD4+ CD25+ cells. Interestingly, inhibition of GITR abrogates regulatory T-cell activity precipitating autoimmunity. In addition, GITR can be activated by progesterone receptor (Nelson et al., 1999 and Kanamaru et al., 2004) and possibly progesterone acts on Treg cells by upregulating GITR among other effects. Interestingly, in studies experimenting EAMG animals, the treatment of analogs of myasthenogenic peptides notably demonstrated a decrease in lymph node proliferation as well as a decrease of INFγ involving the action of CD8+ Tregs (Ben-David et al., 2007).

Newborn can develop neonatal MG and is observed in around 10 % of mother holding the burden of the disease (Beekman etal., 1997). This acquisition is mediated by the passage from the mother to the foetus of immunoglobulin G anti acetylcholine receptors. In large majority, babies do not pursue the course of neonatal MG and few weeks following their birth, neonatal MG naturally undergo full resolution.

2.3 Rheumatoid arthritis and pregnancy
2.3.1 Pathophysiology of rheumatoid arthritis

Rheumatoid arthritis is a severe chronic inflammatory disease of relatively high prevalence that primarily affects the joints via a systemic autoimmune reaction. While its aetiology remains unknown, many cell populations contribute to the inflammatory response in the synovium, leading to joint erosions, joint deformation and loss of function. Histological features often include proliferation of synovial cells, plasma and lymphoid cell infiltration, neovascularisation, macrophage accumulation and typical palisading structure of the cell lining hyperblasting synovial membranes. One particular hallmark used in diagnosis of RA is the rheumatoid factor (RF) and the particular association with HLA-DR4. Common cytokine abnormalities in RA include an increase in tumor necrosis factor alpha (TNFα) and interleukin-1β (IL-1β) with subsequent induction of metalloproteinases (MMPs) degrading the synovial matrix (Dayer et al., 2001). Gene expression studies sampling synovial tissue have highlighted the heterogeneous nature of the disease and suggest the existence and contribution of multiple pathogenic pathways (van der Pouw Kraan et al. 2003). As tissue biopsies are invasive, alternative and clinically more practical studies of gene expression changes in peripheral blood mononuclear cells (PBMC) from patients with RA have been reported (Olsen et al., 2004 & Edwards et al., 2007), with a recent study highlighting that 10 differentially regulated transcripts in RA patient PBMC mapped to chromosome region 6p21.3, the major histocompatibility (MHC) locus III (Edwards et al., 2007). In addition to the cellular involvement, Rheumatoid arthritis is an auto-antibody disorder that will ultimately affect the joints. Antibodies like IgM and IgA are known to target the Fc fragments of IgG but in addition targeted citrullinated antigens are found in RA patients but are not exclusive to these patients. The autoimmune attack mainly is associated with elevated amounts of Tumor necrosis factor (Feldmann et al., 1996) and elevation of specific joint cells (found in both cartilage and synovium). The synovium contains macrophage like synovial cells and fibroblast like synovial cells. In RA, the joint macrophage like cells are known to secrete a large panel of pro-inflammatory cytokines whereas the fibroblast like cells are showing invasive the cartilage (Muller-Ladner et al., 1996) and are responsible, at some extent, to joint destruction with osteoclastic activity (Tolboom et al., 2005). Interestingly, inhibiting and preventing osteoclast induce destruction of the joints is not associated cessation of the overall localised pro-inflammatory profile (Cohen et al., 2008). Common therapeutic agents used in treating RA include disease-modifying anti-rheumatic drugs (DMARDs), such as methotrexate, non steroidal anti-inflammatory drugs (NSAIDs), corticosteroids and Tumor Necrosis Factor (TNF) inhibitors which inhibit the pro-inflammatory activity of TNF, identified as a key mediator in the inflammatory response. Despite the improvement of joint function in 60-80% of patients with TNF inhibitors and methotrexate combination therapy, a remaining 20-40% of patients do not respond to this treatment (Baton et al., 2000 & Keystone et al., 2004 & Maini et al., 2004).

2.3.2 Modulation effects of pregnancy in Rheumatoid Arthritis mothers

In pregnancy, RA signs are improved in more than 76% of cases (Pope et al., 1983) but beneficial signs disappear postpartum for approximately 6 to 8 months post delivery. These gestational ameliorations seem to be independent of cortisol rises in pregnancy and independent to administration of different exogenous estrogen levels (Van den Brink et al., 1992). Of note, twenty five percent of RA pregnant women have continuing active arthritis. Interestingly two reports reported that pregnancy decreases by two fold in RA when compared to nulliparous RA women (Spector et al., 1990 & Hazes et al., 1990). During pregnancy, important tolerance occurs in RA. Auto-reactive B cells in RA are somewhat down-regulated since serum levels of alloantibodies remain the same while improvement in the severity is observed (Elenkov et al., 1997). Autoantibodies such as ANA have been reported to decrease in RA pregnancy (Ostensen et al., 1983) as well as the rheumatoic factor, RF (Pope et al., 1983). Interstingly, the disparity between the foetus and the mother seems to be positive for the pregnancy course in RA (Nelson et al, 1993). The impact of the disease on pregnancy and outcomes of RA to gestation seem to show no adverse effects with RA women falling pregnant and giving birth with no life threatening consequences. However, postpartum flares are high and possibly aggravated due to high correlated levels of prolactin postpartum (Zrour et al., 2010). The influence of pregnancy on RA disease is still unknown and no explannations to date are given for the reasons for observing either remission or none of RA during pregnancy. As for the remissions, attention is dedicated to the maternofetal HLA incompatibility but investigations is generating contrasting reports (Brennan et al., 2000). As for what is possibly occuring in RA and pregancy, a hormonal conditioning mediated by estradiol and progesterone contribute to a shift from TH1 to Th2 immune profile (Ekerfelt et al., 1997) and suppression of both autoreactive T cells and NK cells (Otensen & Villiger, 2002).

2.4 Multiple Sclerosis and pregnancy
2.4.1 Pathophysiology of Multiple Sclerosis

MS is a neurological debilitating disorder that affects particularly Caucasians in their second to fourth decades of their life (Weinshenker BG, 1998). MS was characterised for the first time, by Dr Jean Martin Charcot in 1868 from the hospital "Salpêtrière", in Paris who reported the presence of multiple plaques in the central nervous system (CNS) of a deceased patient. Despite the progress of research in the last 150 years the aetiology of MS remains still unknown.

The disorder is well documented for its neuroinflammatory course and symptoms. The disease has particular hallmarks and is more prevalent in women, and symptoms appear typically between 20 and 40 years of age (Weinshenker BG, 1998). Females account for approximately 60% of MS cases (Weinshenker BG et al., 1994). There are several forms of MS, characterised by the degree of symptomatic debilitation over time: Benign MS (B-MS), Relapsing Remitting MS (RR-MS), Secondary Progressive (SP-MS), Progressive-Relapsing MS (PR-MS), Primary Progressive MS (PP-MS). MS plaques appear as lesions in the normal white matter (NWM) and occasionally in the gray matter (Peterson et al., 2001). Lesions are restricted to the CNS and are not present in the peripheral nervous system (PNS). Plaques are classified into three main types: acute (A), chronic active (CA) and chronic silent (CS) MS lesions. Acute MS lesions are not well-demarcated (oedematous) and are filled with macrophages commonly containing myelin debris. Additionally, these lesions contain hypertrophic astrocytes but no fibrous astrogliosis with an abundance of demyelinated axons. This plaque-type is characterised by the presence of perivascular lymphocytic infiltration and damaged of the blood brain barrier (BBB) (Gay et al., 1991). Chronic active MS lesions, are the second type and do contain a well-demarcated margin. In this case the centre of the plaque is lacking in lymphocyte activity. Instead macrophages reside in a margin which contains the debris of myelin degeneration. These macrophages are microglia in origin. The centre of a CA plaque is astrogliotic, with a generally absence of myelin. However, in this case the centre of CA lesions is characterised by signs of remyelination.

In contrast to both CA and A lesions, CS MS lesions have a highly demarcated margin with a fibrous centre with no inflammatory component. Remyelination can occur in the centre and within the margin. These plaques appear circular and differ from other forms of demyelination (eg. Balo's syndrome). Balo's syndrome, is characterised by alternate rings of degeneration and regeneration (or intact myelin)(Moore et al., 1985). MS also has an autoimmune component, characterised by infiltration in the CNS of activated T-cells that are auto-reactive to myelin white matter proteins. MS is also more prevalent at higher latitudes of the globe (Hernan et al., 1999), suggesting a strong environmental influence; while disease susceptibility has a strong genetic link, as evidenced by numerous twin studies (Mumford et al., 1994). Symptoms include limb weakness, sensory loss, visual alterations and bladder dysfunction, and the appearance of lesions or plaques that are disseminated in time and space. Multiple sclerosis is an autoimmune disease of the central nervous system, characterized by zones of demyelination and inflammatory plaques.

The genetic of MS has been extensively researched and a major focus in comparison to other autoimmune diseases. Studies appreciating the concordance of twins have shown a six time increase in risk in monozygoting than among dizogotic twins (Sadovnick et al, 1993).

2.4.1.1 The Major Histocompatibility Complex (MHC) and Multiple Sclerosis

The MHC Locus on Chromosome 6p has been linked to the pathogenenesis of MS with the fundamental basis of this association being established as a strong association with HLA-DRB1*15 of the class II gene *HLA-DRB1*(Fogdell et al., 1995). In addition to the problem in exploring possible etiological reasons behind MS, epistatic interaction across alleles are taking place that even are mors of a risky as seen with *HLA-DRB1*08*, on interaction with *HLA-DRB1*15*. A number of genes have been implicated in MS pathophysiology and were discovered throughout both immunological and genetic studies. One of the most consistent findings has been an association of specific major histocompatibility class II haplotypes in MS (Kellar-Wood et al., 1995). The MHC region in 6p21.3, includes MHC I, II and III. As all evidences are supporting an autoimmune basis for MS, the MHC locus is the focus of a lot of research attention as the genes in this locus are involved in antigen presentation. Class I and class II are involved in antigen presentation to CD8 and CD4 lymphocytes respectively. Class I has a region containing HLA loci (HLA A, B, C, E, F, G) known to be altered in normal pregnancy especially at the placental border between the foetus and the mother. Association between MS and molecules on the chromosome 6p21 is variable to the type of population studied. Northern European populations affected with MS do show an association with Class II DR15 and DQ6 phenotypes in (Hillert, 1994). In the other hand, Asians with MS are associated with DPB1 (Ito et al., 1998).

The MHC Class II locus is composed of genes coding for proteins LMP2 (proteasome subunit, beta type, 9) and LMP7 (proteasome subunit, beta type, 7), two protein being integrative of the proteasome complex. Normally, viral proteins or cellular proteins are turned into small peptides by the proteasome. These fragmented petides are then entering the reticulum endoplasmic (RE) binding with new synthesised MHC class I molecules. Both molecules are then deposited to the surface cell where the peptide is then presented to vigilant immune cells. The translocation into the RE is facilitated by the transporter 1, ATP-binding cassette (TAP) 1 and 2 which are coded by genes in the MHC Class II region. Studies attempted to demonstrate a probable association between TAP1 and TAP2 locus polymorphisms but data showed no association with MS (Vandevyver et al., 1994). However, the same study revealed though a differential level of gene expression of these two genes between affected and non-affected tissues. Interestingly, a lot of attention was brought into a region 100kb telomeric to HLA F. This locus harbors the myelin oligodendrocyte glycoprotein (MOG), another potential candidate gene in multiple sclerosis as it plays an important role in myelin sheath maintenance and immunogenicity. Experiments using antisera raised against MOG would activate a downstream signaling pathway resulting in the degradation of microtubules and disruption of myelin basic protein (MBP) (Johns et al., 1999). This pathway is also triggered by antibodies of a marker of myelin-producing cells, the galactolipid galactocerebroside, that was illustrated in glioma cells (Joshi et al., 1992), with possibly engaging a second messenger (most likely Inositol Phosphate 3) activating a voltage Ca^{2+} channel (Joshi et al., 1998) that ultimately results into in an increase of intracellular calcium and microtubule disruption.

In the Class III MHC region, candidate genes possibly implicated in MS pathology include the steroid enzyme 21-hydroxylase gene (CYP21A2) and heat shock proteins (HSP): HSP70-1 and HSP70-2. In addition, MHC class III region contains genes coding for complement molecules of the immune system and interestingly the tumour necrosis factor genes (TNFα and TNFβ). In Multiple sclerosis, TNFα has been shown to be toxic to oligodendrocytes and myelin (Wingerchuk et al., 1997). In MS plaques, TNFβ is present and is at the origin of tissue repair (De Groot et al., 1999). Some studies have investigated TNFα polymorphisms (Wingerchuk et al., 1997) however no association was found with MS except in HLA-DR2+ MS patients compared with HLA-DR2- individuals (Oturai et al., 1999). Studies investigating Caucasians of European descent have shown that class II HLA alleles are more strongly associated with the HLA-DR2 haplotype in MS (Haines et al., 1998).

Noteworthy a predominant immunological hallmark of multiple sclerosis is the important clonal expansion of class I MHC T8 lymphocytes observed in MS (Gay et al., 1997).

2.4.1.2 Immunological mechanism involved in MS

The immune system response is comprised of two immune systems: humoral and cellular. In the case of MS, both systems apply resulting in CNS inflammation coupled with degeneration in myelin sheath. A plethora of cells may be involved in this disorder including microglial cells (macrophages of the CNS), B and T lymphocytes, natural killer cells and peripheral macrophages (Li et al., 1993). Their activities are coupled with the secretion of activating signals such as cytokines and interleukines that upon production affect surrounding cells. It has been reported that auto-reactive T-cells exist in the peripheral blood from both MS affected and healthy individuals (Lindert et al., 1999). In order to reach the CNS, the immune cells have to cross through the BBB but only activated T-cells can penetrate this fence. However, it has been reported that in MS the BBB undergoes a breakdown resulting in facilitated passage of immune cells (McDonald et al., 1992). The activation of T-cells is supposed to be due to a misguided immune response secondary to cross recognition of epitopes shared between a microbial pathogen and a putative antigen in the CNS (Wucherpfennig et al., 1995). These CNS-antigen specific T-cells transmigrate through the endothelial BBB by secreting and expressing adhesion molecules such as selectins and integrins (Monteyne et al., 1997). The T-cells occupy the CNS in regions where further events take place. Furthermore, once they have occupied the CNS, the T-cells stimulate the entry of further immune cells such as peripheral macrophages. Passage of macrophages in the CNS is facilitated by the T-cell induced BBB disruption due to secretion of activated matrix metalloproteases (MMPs). In the cerebrospinal fluid of MS patients, a high gelatinase (MMP9) concentration has been found (Rosenberg et al., 1996). Gelatinase B breaks down the BBB and its inhibition, by serine protease inhibitors, shows a protective effect on the MS animal model, EAE Lewis rats (Brosnan et al., 1980). In the parenchymal of the CNS, T-cells are reactivated with the myelin antigen proximity and secrete a vast group of pro-inflammatory agents such as interferon gamma (INFγ), tumour necrosing factor alpha and beta (TNFα and TNFβ), interleukin 2 (IL-2) (Olsson et al., 1995). IL-2 is an autocrine interleukin triggering a T-cell auto-activation loop process. On both astrocytes and microglial cells, those inflammatory mediators trigger an up-regulation of MHC class II molecules. The increase of MHC class II molecules at the surface of these cells improves the amount of antigen presenting cells. Moreover, microglia as well as T lymphocytes are developing a proliferating process in response of INFγ action (Martino et al., 1995 & Grau et al., 1997). Interestingly, T-bet knockout mice show resistance to autoimmunity (Bettelli et al., 2004).

Activated astrocytes trigger an up-regulation of adhesion molecules at the surface of the BBB (Weiss et al., 1998). Chemo-attractants are produced such as the monocyte chemo-attractant protein 1 (MCP-1) (Van Der Voon et al., 1999) that chemically orientate peripheral phagocytes towards the BBB. The BBB endothelium is thus facilitated for further influx of inflammatory cells such as macrophages. Even macrophages disrupt the BBB with the secretion of neurotoxins (Brosnan et al., 1981). Secondly, activated astrocytes are able to excrete more pro-inflammatory molecules that turn the local CNS microglia (CNS resident macrophages) into ameboid microglia, a more active macrophage state. The activated astrocytes excrete factors such as GM-CSF (granulocyte monocyte-colony stimulating factor) whose role is to induce the proliferation of the ameboid cells.

The local microglia plays an important role in local antigen presentation in the CNS of EAE animals (Bauer et al., 1994) allowing an immune response. The microglia is expressing B7 (Dangond et al., 1997) and vascular cell adhesion molecule (VCAM-1). These two molecules bind CD28 and the very late antigen 4 (VLA4) respectively, on the surface of T-cells (Chabot et al., 1997) and these molecular interactions affect T-cell activation. Complement receptors (CR1 and CR2) are also found and are molecules that allow the binding of complement coated targets to phagocytosis. Complement activation constitutes the major component mechanism of humoral immunity. Contact with complement permits a better activation of the microglia but also the release of TNFα and interleukins (IL-1 and IL-6) (Rajan et al., 1996). Microglia express receptors for Fc fragments of immunoglobulins (Ulvestad et al., 1994) and completes an association action with B-lymphocytes. Those B-lymphocytes, fewer in numbers, can pass the damaged BBB and produce antibodies against myelin proteins (Gerritse et al., 1994). The antibodies are observed, after a lumbo-puncture, in CSF from MS patients appearing as oligoclonal bands in agarose gel electrophoresis. T-cell infiltration in the CNS not only induces microglial activation but also triggers the recruitment of high numbers of macrophages (Hulkower et al., 1993).

Besides inflammation, demyelination is the second most characteristic feature of MS pathology. Both microglia and macrophages are capable of ingesting myelin in EAE animals (Rinner et al., 1995). However, oligodendrocytes do not express MHC calls II molecules so CD4+T-cells cannot have a direct effect. Studies have shown that both complement and immunoglobulins are detected on oligodendrocytes and microglia in MS brain but none of the studies have ever shown the complement system alone (Fabry et al., 1994). Oligodendrocytes are damaged via antibody cell mediated cytotoxicity (ADCC) triggered by microglia, macrophages with the help of T4+, B-cells and complements molecules (Ozawa et al., 1994). The macrophages act as APCs via the major histocompatibility molecule class II. Their activities are indicators of ongoing demyelination activity (Li et al., 1993). Furthermore, the interaction of B-cells with T4 cells (CD40-CD40L) turns the B-lymphocytes into APCs, which in consequence increase the myelinotoxic activity. Antibodies to CD 40 ligand (CD 40L) can prevent the MS like disease in EAE animals (Boon et al., 2001). MBP-specific CD8+ T-cells are detected in MS plaques and have been shown to be cytotoxic in vitro on HLA-A2 not HLA-A3 transfected oligodendrocyte cell lines in the presence of MBP peptide 110-118 (Jurewicz et al., 1998).

2.4.2 Modulation effects of pregnancy in Multiple Sclerosis mothers

A first and remarkable large prospective study was undertaken to monitor MS and pregnancy relation and finally counseling MS pregnant women for their venture into pregnancy (Confavreux et al, 1998). MS disease does not affect the outcome of pregnancy and interestingly from the first to the successive trimesters of gestation, a decrease in exacerbation rates is observed with at the third trimester a decrease of 87.5% of relapse rates (Confavreux et al., 1998). This gestational decrease in symptomatology is directly observed with a decrease of MS MRI abnormalities in the CNS in MS pregnant women (Van Walderveen et al., 1994). Most interestingly MS patients entering pregnancy even show a reduced MS progressive course and severity in comparison to controls (Runmarker et al., 1995 & Verdru et al., 1994). No differences in rates of caesarians are seen in MS (Mueller et al., 2002). A lot of attention is driven towards obvious gestational steroids such as estrogens and progesterone. Previous studies have shown the autoimmune protection of estrogens which action decrease TNF-α secretion from microglial cells (Dimayuga et al., 2005) and the neurosteroid enhancement effects of progesterone on myelin formation (Jung-Testas et al., 1999). Progesterone has been shown to act on myelination in the peripheral nervous system with marked remyelination following cryo-lesions in mouse sciatic nerves (Koenig et al., 2000). Progesterone acts on its receptor, progesterone receptor (PGR), a receptor localized in Chromosome 11q12, a locus with denotes slight association in MS susceptibility in Australia (Ban et al, 2003). In animals, progesterone shows remarkable actions as a neuro-protector agent (Singh et al., 2008). Activation of the PR by progesterone exerts immunosuppressive roles by directly inhibiting a subunit of NF-κB, a well known intermediate of the pro-inflammatory molecule TNF alpha action (Kalkhoven et al., 1996). In addition, it has been demonstrated that progesterone exerts a protective role on damage brain tissues (Cutler et al., 2007) especially in Traumatic Brain Injuries (TBI) (VanLandingham et al., 2007).

A very interesting study has been undertaken to assess the immunogenic activity occurring in MS pregnancy (Saraste et al., 2007). Natural killer cells and B and T-cells populations with both CD4+ and CD8 + T-cells were all assessed during pregnancy in MS with staggering results showing a decrease from first to third trimester of nearly 40% of NK count in blood of MS patients to then increase by 53% by three months postpartum. In healthy pregnant women a same trend of decrease in NK population is observed (Saraste et al., 2007). This fluctuation of such important innate immunity cellular component is obviously strongly altered by pregnancy and accomplished seen in MS women. Steroids such as progesterone were investigated to establish their roles on NK cells and it has been shown that progesterone induces apoptosis of mature peripheral blood natural killers CD16+ CD56 dim (Arruvito et al., 2008). In Saraste et al. study, an important hallmark demonstrated though a grand difference in CD4+/CD8+ ratios in MS pregnant women versus healthy pregnant women. In From the first to third trimester, MS pregnant women have a CD4+/CD8+ ratio of 1.9 that increase to 2.7 in the third trimester whereas healthy pregnant women showed an inverse trend from 2.4 to 1.6. Authors attempted to give an explanation by seeing such trend as either an increase in T regulatory T-cells or the act that T-cells were prevented from reaching the CNS in pregnancy.

In contrary to gestational time, post partum MS condition is associated with an increase of relapse rate (Bernardi et al., 1991) to resume back to baseline values approximately three months post partum (Roullet et al.,1993). Breast feeding is not affecting the postpartum relapse rate frequency and could be encouraged by the physician except if particular drug treatments are in use (Nelson et al., 1988).

3. Conclusion

The following review was aimed at understanding the interactive relation of the physiological gestational adaptations in coexistence with particular autoimmune diseases. Discussion focused on four diseases that include SLE, MS, MG and RA. Such relation is of no doubt a very complicating process that progressively starts to unravel. Thanks to the overall international research on both the pathogenic mechanism of autoimmunity and enhancement of gestational immunity understanding, new hypothesises and more importantly more insights are found. A powerful physiological protective process occurs in pregnancy, a process strong enough to demonstrate decrease symptomatology in MS, RA and MG pregnancies. In the other hand, SLE pregnancies do not follow such trend and even is showing further aggravation. Mothers are facing a double challenge by undertaking all physiological adaptations of their pregnancy and going through these autoimmune diseases. Steroid hormones play an important role and attempt to orchestrate the foeto-maternal immunological cross communication. In addition regulatory T cells are the direct biological 'diplomats' that taking act on immune-modulating this complex biological enigma.

4. References

Akdis CA, Blaser K. Mechanisms of interleukin-10-mediated immune suppression. Immunology. 2001 Jun;103(2):131-6. Review.

Asanuma Y, Oeser A, Shintani AK, Turner E, Olsen N, Fazio S, Linton MF, Raggi P, Stein CM. Premature coronary-artery atherosclerosis in systemic lupus erythematosus. N Engl J Med. 2003 Dec 18;349(25):2407-15.

Ashley Moffett, Lesley Regan, Peter Braude. Natural killer cells, miscarriage, and infertility. BMJ. 2004 NOV;329.

Balasa B, Deng C, Lee J, Bradley LM, Dalton DK, Christadoss P, Sarvetnick N. Interferon gamma (IFN-gamma) is necessary for the genesis of acetylcholine receptor-induced clinical experimental autoimmune myasthenia gravis in mice. J Exp Med. 1997 Aug 4;186(3):385-91.

Ban M, Sawcer SJ, Heard RN, Bennetts BH, Adams S, Booth D, Perich V, Setakis E, Compston A, Stewart GJ. A genome-wide screen for linkage disequilibrium in Australian HLA-DRB1*1501 positive multiple sclerosis patients. J Neuroimmunol. 2003;143(1-2):60-4.

Barakonyi A, Polgar B, Szekeres-Bartho J. The role of gamma/delta T-cell receptor-positive cells in pregnancy: part II. Am J Reprod Immunol. 1999 Aug;42(2):83-7.

Barcellos LF, Thomson G, Carrington M, Schafer J, Begovich AB, Lin P, Xu XH, Min BQ, Marti D, Klitz W. Chromosome 19 single-locus and multilocus haplotype associations with multiple sclerosis. Evidence of a new susceptibility locus in Caucasian and Chinese patients. JAMA. 1997;278(15):1256-61.

Bauer J, Sminia T, Wouterlood FG, Dijkstra CD. Phagocytic activity of macrophages and microglial cells during the course of acute and chronic relapsing experimental autoimmune encephalomyelitis. J Neurosci Res. 1994;38(4):365-75.

Beekman R, Kuks JB, Oosterhuis HJ. Myasthenia gravis: diagnosis and follow-up of 100 consecutive patients. J Neurol. 1997 Feb;244(2):112-8.

Ben-David H, Sharabi A, Dayan M, Sela M, Mozes E.The role of CD8+CD28 regulatory cells in suppressing myasthenia gravis-associated responses by a dual altered peptide ligand. Proc Natl Acad Sci U S A. 2007 Oct 30;104(44):17459-64.

Bernardi S, Grasso MG, Bertollini R, Orzi F, Fieschi C. The influence of pregnancy on relapses in multiple sclerosis: a cohort study. Acta Neurol Scand. 1991 Nov;84(5):403-6.

Bettelli E, Sullivan B, Szabo SJ, Sobel RA, Glimcher LH, Kuchroo VK. Loss of T-bet, but not STAT1, prevents the development of experimental autoimmune encephalomyelitis. J Exp Med. 2004 Jul 5;200(1):79-87.

Mueller BA, Zhang J, Critchlow CW. Birth outcomes and need for hospitalization after delivery among women with multiple sclerosis.. Am J Obstet Gynecol. 2002 Mar;186(3):446-52.

Boon L, Brok HP, Bauer J, Ortiz-Buijsse A, Schellekens MM, Ramdien-Murli S, Blezer E, van Meurs M, Ceuppens J, de Boer M, Hart BA, Laman JD. Prevention of experimental autoimmune encephalomyelitis in the common marmoset (Callithrix jacchus) using a chimeric antagonist monoclonal antibody against human CD40 is associated with altered B cell responses. J Immunol. 2001;167(5):2942-9.

Brennan P, Barrett J, Fiddler M, et al. Maternal-fetal HLA incompatibility and the course of inflammatory arthritis during pregnancy. J Rheumatol 2000;27:2843-8

Brosnan CF, Bornstein MB, Bloom BR. The effects of macrophage depletion on the clinical and pathologic expression of experimental allergic encephalomyelitis. J Immunol. 1981;126(2):614-20.

Brosnan CF, Cammer W, Norton WT, Bloom BR. Proteinase inhibitors suppress the development of experimental allergic encephalomyelitis. Nature. 1980;285(5762):235-7.

Burgess AW, Wilson EM, Metcalf D. Stimulation by human placental conditioned medium of hemopoietic colony formation by human marrow cells. Blood. 1977 Apr;49(4):573-83.

Chabot S, Williams G, Yong VW. Microglial production of TNF-alpha is induced by activated T lymphocytes. Involvement of VLA-4 and inhibition by interferonbeta-1b. J Clin Invest. 1997;100(3):604-12.

Chantakru S, Miller C, Roach LE, Kuziel WA, Maeda N, Wang WC, Evans SS, Croy BA. Contributions from self-renewal and trafficking to the uterine NK cell population of early pregnancy. J Immunol. 2002 Jan 1;168(1):22-8.

Christensen PB, Jensen TS, Tsiropoulos I, Sørensen T, Kjaer M, Højer-Pedersen E, Rasmussen MJ, Lehfeldt E. Associated autoimmune diseases in myasthenia gravis. A population-based study. Acta Neurol Scand. 1995 Mar;91(3):192-5.

Clark CA, Spitzer KA, Crowther MA, Nadler JN, Laskin MD, Waks JA, Laskin CA. Incidence of postpartum thrombosis and preterm delivery in women with antiphospholipid antibodies and recurrent pregnancy loss. J Rheumatol. 2007 May;34(5):992-6.

Cohen SB, Cohen MD, Cush JJ, Fleischmann RM, Mease PJ, Schiff MH, Simon LS, Weaver AL. Unresolved issues in identifying and overcoming inadequate response in rheumatoid arthritis: weighing the evidence. J Rheumatol Suppl. 2008 Feb;81:4-30; quiz 31-4. Review.

Compston DA, Vincent A, Newsom-Davis J, Batchelor JR. Clinical, pathological, HLA antigen and immunological evidence for disease heterogeneity in myasthenia gravis. Brain. 1980 Sep;103(3):579-601.

Confavreux C, Hutchinson M, Hours MM, Cortinovis-Tourniaire P, Moreau T. Rate of pregnancy-related relapse in multiple sclerosis. Pregnancy in Multiple Sclerosis Group. N Engl J Med. 1998 Jul 30;339(5):285-91.

Cooper GS, Dooley MA, Treadwell EL, St Clair EW, Gilkeson GS. Hormonal and reproductive risk factors for development of systemic lupus erythematosus: results of a population-based, case-control study. Arthritis Rheum. 2002 Jul;46(7):1830-9.

Crispin JC, Martínez A, Alcocer-Varela J. Quantification of regulatory T cells in patients with systemic lupus erythematosus. J Autoimmun. 2003 Nov;21(3):273-6.

Culton DA, Nicholas MW, Bunch DO, Zhen QL, Kepler TB, Dooley MA, Mohan C, Nachman PH, Clarke SH. Similar CD19 dys-regulation in two autoantibody-associated autoimmune diseases suggests a shared mechanism of B-cell tolerance loss. J Clin Immunol. 2007 Jan;27(1):53-68.

Cutler SM, Cekic M, Miller DM, Wali B, VanLandingham JW, Stein DG. Progesterone improves acute recovery after traumatic brain injury in the aged rat. J Neurotrauma. 2007 Sep;24(9):1475-86.

Dangond F, Windhagen A, Groves CJ, Hafler DA. Constitutive expression of costimulatory molecules by human microglia and its relevance to CNS autoimmunity. J Neuroimmunol. 1997;76(1-2):132-8.

Dayer JM, Feige U, Edwards CK 3rd, Burger D. Anti-interleukin-1 therapy in rheumatic diseases. Curr Opin Rheumatol. 2001 May;13(3):170-6. Review.

De Groot CJ, Montagne L, Barten AD, Sminia P, Van Der Valk P. Expression of transforming growth factor (TGF)-beta1, -beta2, and -beta3 isoforms and TGF-beta type I and type II receptors in multiple sclerosis lesions and human adult astrocyte cultures. J Neuropathol Exp Neurol. 1999;58(2):174-87.

De Sanctis JB, Garmendia JV, Chaurio R, Zabaleta M, Rivas L. Total and biologically active CD154 in patients with SLE. Autoimmunity. 2009 May;42(4):263-5.

De Sanctis JB, Zabaleta M, Bianco NE, Garmendia JV, Rivas L. Serum adipokine levels in patients with systemic lupus erythematosus. Autoimmunity. 2009 May;42(4):272-4.

Delpy L, Douin-Echinard V, Garidou L, Bruand C, Saoudi A, Guéry JC. Estrogen enhances susceptibility to experimental autoimmune myasthenia gravis by promoting type 1-polarized immune responses. J Immunol. 2005 Oct 15;175(8):5050-7.

Denney JM, Nelson EL, Wadhwa PD, Waters TP, Mathew L, Chung EK, Goldenberg RL, Culhane JF. Longitudinal modulation of immune system cytokine profile during pregnancy. Cytokine. 2011 Feb;53(2):170-7.

Dimayuga FO, Reed JL, Carnero GA, Wang C, Dimayuga ER, Dimayuga VM, Perger A, Wilson ME, Keller JN, Bruce-Keller AJ. Estrogen and brain inflammation: effects on microglial expression of MHC, costimulatory molecules and cytokines. J Neuroimmunol. 2005 Apr;161(1-2):123-36.

Doria A, Tincani A, Lockshin M. Challenges of lupus pregnancies. Rheumatology (Oxford). 2008 Jun;47 Suppl 3:iii9-12. Review.

Drachman DB, Adams RN, Josifek LF, Self SG. Functional activities of autoantibodies to acetylcholine receptors and the clinical severity of myasthenia gravis. N Engl J Med. 1982 Sep 23;307(13):769-75.

Duthoit CT, Mekala DJ, Alli RS, Geiger TL. Uncoupling of IL-2 signaling from cell cycle progression in naive CD4+ T cells by regulatory CD4+CD25+ T lymphocytes. J Immunol. 2005 Jan 1;174(1):155-63.

Dyer CA, Benjamins JA. The structure and function of myelin oligodendrocyte glycoprotein. J Neurochem. 1992;72(1):1-9.

Edwards CJ, Feldman JL, Beech J, Shields KM, Stover JA, Trepicchio WL, Larsen G, Foxwell BM, Brennan FM, Feldmann M, Pittman DD. Molecular profile of peripheral blood mononuclear cells from patients with rheumatoid arthritis. Mol Med. 2007 Jan-Feb;13(1-2):40-58.

Ekerfelt C, Matthiesen L, Berg G, Ernerudh J. Paternal leukocytes selectively increase secretion of Il-4 in peripheral blood during normal pregnancies: Demonstrated by a novel one-way MLC measuring cytokine secretion. Am J Reprod Immunol 1997;38:320 -326.

Elenkov IJ, Hoffman J, Wilder RL. Does differential neuroendocrine control of cytokine production govern the expression of autoimmune diseases in pregnancy and the postpartum period? Mol Med Today. 1997 Sep;3(9):379-83.

Engel AG, Arahata K. The membrane attack complex of complement at the endplate in myasthenia gravis. Ann N Y Acad Sci. 1987;505:326-32.

Fabry Z, Raine CS, Hart MN. Nervous tissue as an immune compartment: the dialect of the immune response in the CNS. Immunol Today. 1994;15(5):218-24.

Feldmann M. What is the mechanism of action of anti-tumour necrosis factor-alpha antibody in rheumatoid arthritis? Int Arch Allergy Immunol. 1996 Dec;111(4):362-5. Review.

Ferber IA, Brocke S, Taylor-Edwards C, Ridgway W, Dinisco C, Steinman L, Dalton D, Fathman CG. Mice with a disrupted IFN-gamma gene are susceptible to the induction of experimental autoimmune encephalomyelitis (EAE). J Immunol. 1996 Jan 1;156(1):5-7.

Fernandez D, Bonilla E, Phillips P, Perl A. Signaling abnormalities in systemic lupus erythematosus as potential drug targets. Endocr Metab Immune Disord Drug Targets. 2006 Dec;6(4):305-11. Review.

Finke D, Eloranta ML, Rönnblom L. Endogenous type I interferon inducers in autoimmune diseases. Autoimmunity. 2009 May;42(4):349-52. Review.

Fogdell-Hahn A, Ligers A, Gronning M, Hillert J, Olerup O. Multiple sclerosis: a modifying influence of HLA class I genes in an HLA class II associated autoimmune disease. Tissue Antigens. 2000;55(2):140-8.

Fonseca JE, Santos MJ, Canhão H, Choy E. Interleukin-6 as a key player in systemic inflammation and joint destruction. Autoimmun Rev. 2009 Jun;8(7):538-42. Review.

Gardner L, Moffett A. Dendritic cells in the human decidua. Biol Reprod. 2003 Oct;69(4):1438-46.

Gay D, Esiri M. Blood-brain barrier damage in acute multiple sclerosis plaques. An immunocytological study. Brain. 1991;114(Pt 1B):557-72.

Gay FW, Drye TJ, Dick GW, Esiri MM. The application of multifactorial cluster analysis in the staging of plaques in early multiple sclerosis. Identification and characterization of the primary demyelinating lesion. Brain. 1997;120 (Pt 8):1461-83.

Gerritse K, Deen C, Fasbender M, Ravid R, Boersma W, Claassen E. The involvement of specific anti myelin basic protein antibody-forming cells in multiple sclerosis immunopathology. J Neuroimmunol. 1994;49(1-2):153-9.

Girardi G, Redecha P, Salmon JE. Heparin prevents antiphospholipid antibody-induced fetal loss by inhibiting complement activation. Nat Med. 2004 Nov;10(11):1222-6.

Girón-González JA, Moral FJ, Elvira J, García-Gil D, Guerrero F, Gavilán I, Escobar L. Consistent production of a higher TH1:TH2 cytokine ratio by stimulated T cells in men compared with women. Eur J Endocrinol. 2000 Jul;143(1):31-6.

Graham RR, Kozyrev SV, Baechler EC, Reddy MV, Plenge RM, Bauer JW, Ortmann WA, Koeuth T, González Escribano MF; Argentine and Spanish Collaborative Groups, Pons-Estel B, Petri M, Daly M, Gregersen PK, Martín J, Altshuler D, Behrens TW, Alarcón-Riquelme ME. A common haplotype of interferon regulatory factor 5 (IRF5) regulates splicing and expression and is associated with increased risk of systemic lupus erythematosus. Nat Genet. 2006 May;38(5):550-5.

Grau V, Herbst B, van der Meide PH, Steiniger B. Activation of microglial and endothelial cells in the rat brain after treatment with interferon-gamma in vivo. Glia. 1997;19(3):181-9.

Guerin LR, Prins JR, Robertson SA. Regulatory T-cells and immune tolerance in pregnancy: a new target for infertility treatment? Hum Reprod Update. 2009 Sep-Oct;15(5):517-35.

Haines JL, Terwedow HA, Burgess K, Pericak-Vance MA, Rimmler JB, Martin ER, Oksenberg JR, Lincoln R, Hazes JM, Dijkmans BA, Vandenbroucke JP, de Vries RR, Cats A. Pregnancy and the risk of developing rheumatoid arthritis. Arthritis Rheum. 1990 Dec;33(12):1770-5.

Hernan MA, Olek MJ, Ascherio A. Geographic variation of MS incidence in two prospective studies of US women. Neurology. 1999;53(8):1711-8.

Hillert J. Human leukocyte antigen studies in multiple sclerosis. Ann Neurol. 1994;36(l):15-7.

Hulkower K, Brosnan CF, Aquino DA, Cammer W, Kulshrestha S, Guida MP, Rapoport DA, Berman JW. Expression of CSF-1, c-fms, and MCP-1 in the central nervous system of rats with experimental allergic encephalomyelitis. J Immunol. 1993;150(6):2525-33.

Ito H, Yamasaki K, Kawano Y, Horiuchi I, Yun C, Nishimura Y, Kira J. HLA-DP-associated susceptibility to the optico-spinal form of multiple sclerosis in the Japanese. Tissue Antigens. 1998 Aug;52(2):179-82.

Johns TG, Bernard CC. The structure and function of myelin oligodendrocyte glycoprotein. J Neurochem. 1999;72(1): 1-9.

Johnson SR, Gladman DD, Urowitz MB, Ibañez D, Granton JT. Pulmonary hypertension in systemic lupus. Lupus. 2004;13(7):506-9.

Joshi PG, Mishra S. A novel type of Ca^{2+} channel in U-87 MG cells activated by anti-galactocerebroside. Life Sci. 1998;62(5): 469-77.

Joshi PG, Mishra S. Galactocerebroside mediates Ca^{2+} signaling in cultured glioma cells. Brain Res. 1992;597(1):108-13.

Jung-Testas I, Do Thi A, Koenig H, Désarnaud F, Shazand K, Schumacher M, Baulieu EE. Progesterone as a neurosteroid: synthesis and actions in rat glial cells. J Steroid Biochem Mol Biol. 1999 Apr-Jun;69(1-6):97-107. Review.

Jurewicz A, Biddison WE, Antel JP. MHC class I-restricted lysis of human oligodendrocytes by myelin basic protein peptide-specific CD8 T lymphocytes. J Immunol. 1998;160(6):3056-9.

Kalkhoven E, Wissink S, van der Saag PT, van der Burg B. Negative interaction between the RelA(p65) subunit of NF-kappaB and the progesterone receptor. J Biol Chem. 1996 Mar 15;271(11):6217-24.

Kanamaru F, Youngnak P, Hashiguchi M, Nishioka T, Takahashi T, Sakaguchi S, Ishikawa I, Azuma M. Costimulation via glucocorticoid-induced TNF receptor in both conventional and CD25+ regulatory CD4+ T cells. J Immunol. 2004 Jun 15;172(12):7306-14.

Kariuki SN, Kirou KA, MacDermott EJ, Barillas-Arias L, Crow MK, Niewold TB. Cutting edge: autoimmune disease risk variant of STAT4 confers increased sensitivity to IFN-alpha in lupus patients in vivo. J. Immunol. 2009;182:34–38.

Katsiari CG, Liossis SN, Dimopoulos AM, Charalambopoulo DV, Mavrikakis M, Sfikakis PP. CD40L overexpression on T cells and monocytes from patients with systemic lupus erythematosus is resistant to calcineurin inhibition. Lupus. 2002;11(6):370-8.

Kellar-Wood HF, Wood NW, Holmans P, Clayton D, Robertson N, Compston DA. Multiple sclerosis and the HLA-D region: linkage and association studies. J Neuroimmunol. 1995;58(2):183-90.

Keystone EC, Kavanaugh AF, Sharp JT, Tannenbaum H, Hua Y, Teoh LS, Fischkoff SA, Chartash EK. Radiographic, clinical, and functional outcomes of treatment with adalimumab (a human anti-tumor necrosis factor monoclonal antibody) in patients with active rheumatoid arthritis receiving concomitant methotrexate therapy: a randomized, placebo-controlled, 52-week trial. Arthritis Rheum. 2004 May;50(5):1400-11.

Koenig HL, Gong WH, Pelissier P. Role of progesterone in peripheral nerve repair. Rev Reprod. 2000 Sep;5(3):189-99. Review.

Kong KO, Tan AW, Thong BY, Lian TY, Cheng YK, Teh CL, Koh ET, Chng HH, Law WG, Lau TC, Leong KP, Leung BP, Howe HS. Enhanced expression of interferon-inducible protein-10 correlates with disease activity and clinical manifestations in systemic lupus erythematosus. Clin Exp Immunol. 2009 Apr;156(1):134-40.

Kozyrev SV, Alarcon-Riquelme ME. The genetics and biology of Irf5-mediated signaling in lupus. Autoimmunity. 2007;40:591–601.

Kuniyasu Y, Takahashi T, Itoh M, Shimizu J, Toda G, Sakaguchi S. Naturally anergic and suppressive CD25(+)CD4(+) T cells as a functionally and phenotypically distinct immunoregulatory T cell subpopulation. Int Immunol. 2000 Aug;12(8):1145-55.

Landek-Salgado MA, Gutenberg A, Lupi I, Kimura H, Mariotti S, Rose NR, Caturegli P. Pregnancy, postpartum autoimmune thyroiditis, and autoimmune hypophysitis: intimate relationships. Autoimmun Rev. 2010 Jan;9(3):153-7. Review.

Lessin DL, Hunt JS, King CR, Wood GW. Antigen expression by cells near the maternal-fetal interface. Am J Reprod Immunol Microbiol. 1988 Jan;16(1):1-7.

Li H, Newcombe J, Groome NP, Cuzner ML. Characterization and distribution of phagocytic macrophages in multiple sclerosis plaques. Neuropathol Appl Neurobiol. 1993;19(3):214-23.

Lifetime course of myasthenia gravis. Grob D, Brunner N, Namba T, Pagala M. Muscle Nerve. 2008 Feb;37(2):141-9. Review.

Lindert RB, Haase CG, Brehm U, Linington C, Wekerle H, Hohlfeld R. Multiple sclerosis: B- and T-cell responses to the extracellular domain of the myelin oligodendrocyte glycoprotein. Brain. 1999;122 (Pt 11):2089-100.

Liu K, Mohan C. Altered B-cell signaling in lupus. Autoimmun Rev. 2009 Jan;8(3):214-8. Review.

Lockshin MD, Qamar T, Levy RA, Druzin ML. Pregnancy in systemic lupus erythematosus. Clin Exp Rheumatol. 1989 Sep-Oct;7 Suppl 3:S195-7. Review.

Maggi G, Casadio C, Cavallo A, Cianci R, Molinatti M, Ruffini E. Thymoma: results of 241 operated cases. Ann Thorac Surg. 1991 Jan;51(1):152-6.

Mao G, Wang J, Kang Y, Tai P, Wen J, Zou Q, Li G, Ouyang H, Xia G, Wang B. Progesterone increases systemic and local uterine proportions of CD4+CD25+ Treg cells during midterm pregnancy in mice. Endocrinology. 2010 Nov;151(11):5477-88.

Martino G, Moiola L, Brambilla E, Clementi E, Comi G, Grimaldi LM. Interferon-gamma induces T lymphocyte proliferation in multiple sclerosis via a Ca(2+)-dependent mechanism. J Neuroimmunol. 1995;62(2):169-76.

McDonald WI, Miller DH, Barnes D. The pathological evolution of multiple sclerosis. Neuropathol Appl Neurobiol. 1992;18(4):319-34.

McHugh RS, Whitters MJ, Piccirillo CA, Young DA, Shevach EM, Collins M, Byrne MC. CD4(+)CD25(+) immunoregulatory T cells: gene expression analysis reveals a functional role for the glucocorticoid-induced TNF receptor. Immunity. 2002 Feb;16(2):311-23.

Meyer O. Neonatal cutaneous lupus and congenital heart block: it's not all antibodies. Lancet. 2003 Nov 15;362(9396):1596-7.

Mincheva-Nilsson L, Hammarström S, Hammarström ML. Human decidual leukocytes from early pregnancy contain high numbers of gamma delta+ cells and show selective down-regulation of alloreactivity. J Immunol. 1992 Sep 15;149(6):2203-11.

Monteyne P, Van Laere V, Marichal R, Sindic CJ. Cytokine mRNA expression in CSF and peripheral blood mononuclear cells in multiple sclerosis: detection by RT-PCR without in vitro stimulation. J Neuroimmunol. 1997;80(1-2):137-42.

Moore GR, Neumann PE, Suzuki K, Lijtmaer HN, Traugott U, Raine CS. Balo's concentric sclerosis: new observations on lesion development. Ann Neurol. 1985;17(6):604-11.

Moroni G, Quaglini S, Banfi G, Caloni M, Finazzi S, Ambroso G, Como G, Ponticelli C. Pregnancy in lupus nephritis. Am J Kidney Dis. 2002 Oct;40(4):713-20.

Müller-Ladner U, Kriegsmann J, Franklin BN, Matsumoto S, Geiler T, Gay RE, Gay S. Synovial fibroblasts of patients with rheumatoid arthritis attach to and invade normal human cartilage when engrafted into SCID mice. Am J Pathol. 1996 Nov;149(5):1607-15.

Mumford, C J; Wood, N W; Kellar-Wood, H; Thorpe, J W; Miller, D H; Compston, D A. The British Isles survey of multiple sclerosis in twins. Neurology. 1994;44:11–15.

Nalbandian G, Kovats S. Understanding sex biases in immunity: effects of estrogen on the differentiation and function of antigen-presenting cell. Immunol Res. 2005;31(2):91-106. Review

Nelson CC, Hendy SC, Shukin RJ, Cheng H, Bruchovsky N, Koop BF, Rennie PS. Determinants of DNA sequence specificity of the androgen, progesterone, and glucocorticoid receptors: evidence for differential steroid receptor response elements. Mol Endocrinol. 1999 Dec;13(12):2090-107.

Nelson JL, Hughes KA, Smith AG, Nisperos BB, Branchaud AM, Hansen JA. Maternal-fetal disparity in HLA class II alloantigens and the pregnancy-induced amelioration of rheumatoid arthritis. N Engl J Med. 1993 Aug 12;329(7):466-71.

Nelson LM, Franklin GM, Jones MC. Risk of multiple sclerosis exacerbation during pregnancy and breast-feeding. JAMA. 1988 Jun 17;259(23):3441-3.

Arruvito L, Giulianelli S, Flores AC, Paladino N, Barboza M, Lanari C, Fainboim L. NK cells expressing a progesterone receptor are susceptible to progesterone-induced apoptosis.. J Immunol. 2008 Apr 15;180(8):5746-53.

Olsen N, Sokka T, Seehorn CL, Kraft B, Maas K, Moore J, Aune TM. A gene expression signature for recent onset rheumatoid arthritis in peripheral blood mononuclear cells. Ann Rheum Dis. 2004 Nov;63(11):1387-92.

Olsson T. Critical influences of the cytokine orchestration on the outcome of myelin antigen-specific T-cell autoimmunity in experimental autoimmune encephalomyelitis and multiple sclerosis. Immunol Rev. 1995;144:245-68.

Østensen M, Peter M Villiger PM. Immunology of pregnancy – pregnancy as a remission inducing agent in rheumatoid arthritis. Transplant Immunology 2002;9(2-4):155-160.

Ostensen M, Lundgren R, Husby G, Rekvig OP. Studies on humoral immunity in pregnancy: immunoglobulins, alloantibodies and autoantibodies in healthy pregnant women and in pregnant women with rheumatoid disease. J Clin Lab Immunol. 1983 Jul;11(3):143-7.

Oturai A, Larsen F, Ryder LP, Madsen HO, Hillert J, Fredrikson S, Sandberg-Wollheim M, Laaksonen M, Koch-Henriksen N, Sawcer S, Fugger L, Sorensen PS, Svejgaard A. Linkage and association analysis of susceptibility regions on chromosomes 5 and 6 in 106 Scandinavian sibling pair families with multiple sclerosis. Ann Neurol. 1999;46(4):612-6.

Ozawa K, Suchanek G, Breitschopf H, Bruck W, Budka H, Jellinger K, Lassmann H. Patterns of oligodendroglia pathology in multiple sclerosis. Brain. 1994;117(Pt 6):1311-22.

Padua L, Tonali P, Aprile I, Caliandro P, Bartoccioni E, Evoli A. Seronegative myasthenia gravis: comparison of neurophysiological picture in MuSK+ and MuSK- patients. Eur J Neurol. 2006 Mar;13(3):273-6.

Peng SL. Altered T and B lymphocyte signaling pathways in lupus. Autoimmun Rev. 2009 Jan;8(3):179-83. Review.

Perl A, Nagy G, Gergely P, Puskas F, Qian Y, Banki K. Apoptosis and mitochondrial dysfunction in lymphocytes of patients with systemic lupus erythematosus. Methods Mol Med. 2004;102:87-114.

Peterson JW, Bo L, Mork S, Chang A, Trapp BD. Transected neurites, apoptotic neurons, and reduced inflammation in cortical multiple sclerosis lesions.Ann Neurol. 2001;50(3):389-400.

Pongcharoen S, Searle RF, Bulmer JN. Placental Fas and Fas ligand expression in normal early, term and molar pregnancy. Placenta. 2004 Apr;25(4):321-30.

Pope RM, Yoshinoya S, Rutstein J, Persellin RH. Effect of pregnancy on immune complexes and rheumatoid factors in patients with rheumatoid arthritis. Am J Med. 1983 Jun;74(6):973-9.

Rajan AJ, Gao YL, Raine CS, Brosnan CF. A pathogenic role for gamma delta T cells in relapsing-remitting experimental allergic encephalomyelitis in the SJL mouse. J Immunol. 1996;157(2):941-9.

Rinner WA, Bauer J, Schmidts M, Lassmann H, Hickey WF. Resident microglia and hematogenous macrophages as phagocytes in adoptively transferred experimental autoimmune encephalomyelitis: an investigation using rat radiation bone marrow chimeras. Glia. 1995;14(4):257-66.

Roman MJ, Shanker BA, Davis A, Lockshin MD, Sammaritano L, Simantov R, Crow MK, Schwartz JE, Paget SA, Devereux RB, Salmon JE. Prevalence and correlates of accelerated atherosclerosis in systemic lupus erythematosus. N Engl J Med. 2003 Dec 18;349(25):2399-406. Erratum in: N Engl J Med. 2006 Oct 19;355(16):1746.

Rosenberg GA, Dencoff JE, Correa N Jr, Reiners M, Ford CC. Effect of steroids on CSF matrix metalloproteinases in multiple sclerosis: relation to blood-brain barrier injury. Neurology. 1996;46(6):1626-32.

Rosendaal M. Colony-stimulating factor (CSF) in the uterus of the pregnant mouse. J Cell Sci. 1975 Nov;19(2):411-23.

Roullet E, Verdier-Taillefer MH, Amarenco P, Gharbi G, Alperovitch A, Marteau R. Pregnancy and multiple sclerosis: a longitudinal study of 125 remittent patients. J Neurol Neurosurg Psychiatry. 1993 Oct;56(10):1062-5.

Runmarker B, Andersen O. Pregnancy is associated with a lower risk of onset and a better prognosis in multiple sclerosis. Brain. 1995 Feb;118 (Pt 1):253-61.

Sadovnick AD, Amstrong H, Rice GP, Bulman D, Hashimoto L, Paty DW, Hashimoto SA, Warren S, Hader W, Murray TJ, et al. A population-based study of multiple sclerosis in twins: update. Ann Neurol. 1993;33(3):281-5.

Sakaguchi Y, Nakamura Y, Sutani T, Tsuchihashi M, Yamano S, Hashimoto T, Dohi K, Hiasa Y, Kawai S, Okada R. Immunohistochemical study of the endomyocardial biopsy of systemic lupus erythematosus. J Cardiol. 1995 Apr;25(4):181-8.

Sanchez-Guerrero J, Karlson EW, Liang MH, Hunter DJ, Speizer FE, Colditz GA. Past use of oral contraceptives and the risk of developing systemic lupus erythematosus. Arthritis Rheum. 1997 May;40(5):804-8.

Sánchez-Guerrero J, Liang MH, Karlson EW, Hunter DJ, Colditz GA. Postmenopausal estrogen therapy and the risk for developing systemic lupus erythematosus. Ann Intern Med. 1995 Mar 15;122(6):430-3.

Saraste M, Väisänen S, Alanen A, Airas L; Finnish Multiple Sclerosis And Pregnancy Study Group. Clinical and immunologic evaluation of women with multiple sclerosis during and after pregnancy. Gend Med. 2007 Mar;4(1):45-55

Schluep M, Willcox N, Vincent A, Dhoot GK, Newsom-Davis J. Acetylcholine receptors in human thymic myoid cells in situ: an immunohistological study. Ann Neurol. 1987 Aug;22(2):212-22.

Schumacher A, Brachwitz N, Sohr S, Engeland K, Langwisch S, Dolaptchieva M, Alexander T, Taran A, Malfertheiner SF, Costa SD, Zimmermann G, Nitschke C, Volk HD, Alexander H, Gunzer M, Zenclussen AC. Human chorionic gonadotropin attracts regulatory T cells into the fetal-maternal interface during early human pregnancy. J Immunol. 2009 May 1;182(9):5488-97.

Shabanova SS, Ananieva LP, Alekberova ZS, Guzov II. Ovarian function and disease activity in patients with systemic lupus erythematosus. Clin Exp Rheumatol. 2008 May-Jun;26(3):436-41.

Shlomchik MJ, Madaio MP. Springer Semin Immunopathol. The role of antibodies and B cells in the pathogenesis of lupus nephritis. 2003 May;24(4):363-75. Review.

Spector TD. Rheumatoid arthritis. Rheum Dis Clin North Am. 1990 Aug;16(3):513-37. Review.

Tafuri A, Alferink J, Möller P, Hämmerling GJ, Arnold B. Science. T cell awareness of paternal alloantigens during pregnancy.1995 Oct 27;270(5236):630-3.

Taylor A, Verhagen J, Blaser K, Akdis M, Akdis CA. Mechanisms of immune suppression by interleukin-10 and transforming growth factor-beta: the role of T regulatory cells. Immunology. 2006 Apr;117(4):433-42. Review.

Tilburgs T, Roelen DL, van der Mast BJ, de Groot-Swings GM, Kleijburg C, Scherjon SA, Claas FH. Evidence for a selective migration of fetus-specific CD4+CD25bright regulatory T cells from the peripheral blood to the decidua in human pregnancy. J Immunol. 2008 Apr 15;180(8):5737-45.

Tolboom TC, van der Helm-Van Mil AH, Nelissen RG, Breedveld FC, Toes RE, Huizinga TW, Ulvestad E, Williams K, Vedeler C, Antel J, Nyland H, Mork S, Matre R. Reactive microglia in multiple sclerosis lesions have an increased expression of receptors for the Fc part of IgG. J Neurol Sci. 1994;121(2):125-31.

Van den Brink HR, van Wijk MJ, Bijlsma JW. Influence of steroid hormones on proliferation of peripheral blood mononuclear cells in patients with rheumatoid arthritis. Br J Rheumatol. 1992 Oct;31(10):663-7.

Van der Pouw Kraan TC, van Gaalen FA, Huizinga TW, Pieterman E, Breedveld FC, Verweij CL. Discovery of distinctive gene expression profiles in rheumatoid synovium using cDNA microarray technology: evidence for the existence of multiple pathways of tissue destruction and repair. Genes Immun. 2003 Apr;4(3):187-96.

Van Der Voorn P, Tekstra J, Beelen RH, Tensen CP, Van Der Valk P, De Groot CJ. Expression of MCP-1 by reactive astrocytes in demyelinating multiple sclerosis lesions. Am J Pathol. 1999;154(1):45-51.

Van Walderveen MA, Tas MW, Barkhof F, Polman CH, Frequin ST, Hommes OR, Valk J. Magnetic resonance evaluation of disease activity during pregnancy in multiple sclerosis. Neurology. 1994 Feb;44(2):327-9.

Vandevyver C, Raus P, Stinissen P, Philippaerts L, Cassiman JJ, Raus J. Polymorphism of the tumour necrosis factor beta gene in multiple sclerosis and rheumatoid arthritis. Eur J Immunogenet. 1994;21(5):377-82.

Veenstra van Nieuwenhoven AL, Heineman MJ, Faas MM. The immunology of successful pregnancy. Hum Reprod Update. 2003 Jul-Aug;9(4):347-57. Review.

Verdru P, Theys P, D'Hooghe MB, Carton H. Pregnancy and multiple sclerosis: the influence on long term disability. Clin Neurol Neurosurg. 1994 Feb;96(1):38-41.

Walters E, Rider V, Abdou NI, Greenwell C, Svojanovsky S, Smith P, Kimler BF. Estradiol targets T cell signaling pathways in human systemic lupus. Clin Immunol. 2009 Dec;133(3):428-36.

Wang G, Pierangeli SS, Papalardo E, Ansari GA, Khan MF. Markers of oxidative and nitrosative stress in systemic lupus erythematosus: correlation with disease activity. Arthritis Rheum. 2010 Jul;62(7):2064-72.

Watanabe T, Yoshida M, Shirai Y, Yamori M, Yagita H, Itoh T, Chiba T, Kita T, Wakatsuki Y. Administration of an antigen at a high dose generates regulatory CD4+ T cells expressing CD95 ligand and secreting IL-4 in the liver. J Immunol. 2002 Mar 1;168(5):2188-99.

Weinshenker BG, Santrach P, Bissonet AS, McDonnell SK, Schaid D, Moore SB, Rodriguez M. Major histocompatibility complex class II alleles and the course and outcome of MS: a population-based study Neurology 1998;51(3):742-7.

Weinshenker BG. Natural history of multiple sclerosis. Ann Neurol. 1994;36 Suppl:S6-11.

Weiss JM, Downie SA, Lyman WD, Berman JW. Astrocyte-derived monocyte-chemoattractant protein-1 directs the transmigration of leukocytes across a model of the human blood-brain barrier. J Immunol. 1998;161(12):6896-903.

Wingerchuk D, Liu Q, Sobell J, Sommer S, Weinshenker BG. A population-based case-control study of the tumour necrosis factor alpha-308 polymorphism in multiple sclerosis. Neurology. 1997;49(2): 626-8.

Wittmann L, Sensky T, Meder L, Michel B, Stoll T, Büchi S. Suffering and posttraumatic growth in women with systemic lupus erythematosus (SLE): a qualitative/ quantitative case study. Psychosomatics. 2009 Jul-Aug;50(4):362-74.

Wucherpfennig KW, Strominger JL. Molecular mimicry in T cell-mediated autoimmunity: viral peptides activate human T cell clones specific for myelin basic protein. Cell. 1995;80(5):695-705.

Youinou P, Taher TE, Pers JO, Mageed RA, Renaudineau Y. B lymphocyte cytokines and rheumatic autoimmune disease. Arthritis Rheum. 2009 Jul;60(7):1873-80. Review.

Zenclussen AC, Gerlof K, Zenclussen ML, Ritschel S, Zambon Bertoja A, Fest S, Hontsu S, Ueha S, Matsushima K, Leber J, Volk HD. Regulatory T cells induce a privileged tolerant microenvironment at the fetal-maternal interface. Eur J Immunol. 2006 Jan;36(1):82-94.

Zhang DY, Banatao DR, Gatto N, Goodkin DE, Hauser SL. Linkage of the MHC to familial multiple sclerosis suggests genetic heterogeneity. Hum. Mol. Genet. 1998;7(8):1229-1234.

Zhang J, Jacobi AM, Wang T, Berlin R, Volpe BT, Diamond B. Polyreactive autoantibodies in systemic lupus erythematosus have pathogenic potential. J Autoimmun. 2009 Nov-Dec;33(3-4):270-4.

Zrour SH, Boumiza R, Sakly N, Mannai R, Korbaa W, Younes M, Bejia I, Touzi M, Bergaoui N. The impact of pregnancy on rheumatoid arthritis outcome: the role of maternofetal HLA class II disparity. Joint Bone Spine. 2010 Jan;77(1):36-40.

7

T Lymphocyte Characteristics and Immune Tolerance During Human Pregnancy

Gergely Toldi, András Treszl and Barna Vásárhelyi
Research Group of Pediatrics and Nephrology, Hungarian Academy of Sciences
Hungary

1. Introduction

To ensure a fruitful and healthy pregnancy, every maternal organ system needs to adapt to the novel physiological needs raised by the developing fetus. The maternal immune system is no exception. Since the conceptus is half of foreign origins, presenting paternal antigens, it is considered a semi-allograft to maternal immunity. Therefore, an immune tolerance must develop to avoid immunological rejection of the fetus. In the normal course of pregnancy, the mother extends her 'definition of self' for 40 weeks on the foreign antigens of the fetus, and the conceptus is accepted by the mother's immune system. The impairment of this tolerance and the development of an abnormal immune response directed at the fetus play a major role in adverse pregnancy outcomes, including spontaneous abortion, preterm labour and preeclampsia. In recurrent abortion and preeclampsia, abnormal maternal immune reactions have an autoimmune character, and the disorders resemble many features typically seen in autoimmune diseases, or in association with autoimmune reactions. Although this does not mean that recurrent abortion or preeclampsia should be considered autoimmune conditions, it still suggests that abnormal autoimmune processes play an important role in their pathogenesis. In this regard, preeclampsia mimics autoimmune responses observed in both allograft rejection and graft-versus-host disease.

Several aspects of the development of the pregnancy-specific immune tolerance have been described recently. Initially, the contact between maternal and fetal cells is taking place on a local level and is restricted to the decidua, but during the second trimester of pregnancy, it is extended to the entire body of the mother. Both the innate and adaptive arms of immunity are involved in these events. In this chapter we will focus on the role of T lymphocytes, the adaptive cellular elements of the immune system. We will discuss the characteristic alterations of T lymphocyte subsets in prevalence and functionality in healthy and pathologic development of the immune tolerance in human pregnancy.

2. Th1 and Th2 cells

T helper (Th) lymphocytes are traditionally classified into the Th1 and Th2 subsets based on their cytokine production pattern (Romagnani, 1991). The most important cytokines produced by Th1 cells are interleukin-2 (IL-2), tumor necrosis factor-α (TNF-α) and interferon-γ (IFN-γ). Considered to be the main effectors of phagocyte-induced host defense, these cells are highly protective against infections sustained by intracellular agents. On the other hand, Th2 cells produce IL-4, which stimulates IgE and IgG1 antibody production, IL-5, which promotes the growth and differentiation of eosinophils, and IL-10 and IL-13, which together with IL-4 inhibit macrophage functions. The Th2 subset is mainly responsible for phagocyte-independent host defense, for example against helminthic infections.

For many years, it was hypothesized that normal pregnancy induces a shift from Th1 immunity towards Th2 immunity. However, it has been demonstrated recently that the levels of particular Th1 cytokines are raised, instead of lowered in normal pregnancy compared with the non-pregnant state (Challis et al., 2009). Current findings indicate that gravidity is both a pro-inflammatory and an anti-inflammatory condition, depending upon the stage of gestation. Grossly, pregnancy has three distinct immunological phases. The events of implantation and the first trimester require a strong inflammatory response to ensure the adequate remodelling of the uterine epithelium and the removal of cellular debris following the implantation of the blastocyst. Therefore, healthy pregnancy cannot be regarded as merely a state of relative immunosuppression, as once thought. On the contrary, by means of various cytokines, successful implantation is dependent upon the active contribution of the maternal immune system to stimulate adequate invasion of the trophoblastic tissue into the maternal uterine wall. Thus, the first trimester of pregnancy is hallmarked by pro-inflammatory events. The second immunological phase of gravidity consists of the second and third trimesters. This is the period of fetal growth and development, when an anti-inflammatory state is established. Finally, delivery represents the third immunological phase of pregnancy, when pro-inflammatory events dominate again and promote uterinal contractions to deliver the fetus and the placenta (Mor & Cardenas, 2010).

IFN-γ appears to be a key cytokine in the regulation of pregnancy related inflammatory events. Under pathologic conditions with insufficient immune tolerance such as in preeclampsia, IFN-γ production is significantly increased compared with healthy pregnancy (Piccinni, 2010). In mice, it was reported that IL-4, IL-5 and IL-10 are detectable at the fetomaternal interface during all periods of gestation, whereas the presence of IFN-γ is transient, being detectable only in the first period (Lin et al., 1993; Wegmann et al., 1993). Although decidual NK cells are able to produce IFN-γ (Ashkar et al., 1998), they do not have a central role in fetal allograft rejection, since they do not express receptors specific for antigens and thus are not sensitive for the presence of paternal alloantigens. The significance of local Th2-type cytokine production in the decidua has been observed in humans as well. Piccinni et al. measured cytokine production in decidual CD4 cells isolated from women with recurrent spontaneous abortions. Compared with women with a normal pregnancy, the decidual CD4 cells from women with abortion show a defect in IL-4 and IL-10 production (Piccinni et al., 1998).

The antigens of the developing fetus are present at two interfaces as pregnancy progresses. The first interface is found between the invasive extravillous cytotrophoblast and maternal immune cells in the decidua. This local, tissue interface is of importance for immune adaptation during implantation. The second interface is that between the syncytiotrophoblast and the immune cells in maternal blood. This systemic interface is established at about the 10th gestational week and becomes increasingly important in the second half of pregnancy (Sargent et al., 2006a). Two contrary requirements influence the extent of invasion by fetal extravillous cytotrophoblast cells in the maternal decidua: the anchorage of the placenta to ensure fetal nutrition and the protection of the uterine wall against over-invasion (von Rango, 2008). If, due to excessive immunological tolerance and acceptance of trophoblast cells, the uterine wall is over-invaded, pathologic conditions, such as placenta accreta, increta or percreta might develop (Bulmer, 1992). If the adequate invasion of the uterinal spiral arterioles by extravillous cytotrophoblasts does not occur, this sets up the conditions for placental hypoxia and oxidative stress that eventually triggers a maternal systemic inflammatory response, leading to clinical manifestations of preeclampsia (von Rango, 2008).

This disorder is characterized by hypertension, proteinuria, edema and endothelial dysfunction generally evolving in the third trimester of pregnancy; however, it may also occur earlier. Although preeclampsia is quite common (i.e. it affects about 5-8% of all pregnancies globally), its clear cause and the mechanisms leading to immune dysfunction remain to be elucidated. Preeclampsia is estimated to be responsible for about 70,000 maternal deaths each year worldwide (Walker, 2000). HELLP syndrome (consisting of hemolysis, elevated liver enzymes, low platelet count) and eclampsia are other manifestations of the same disorder. Although these conditions are generally coupled with a number of other symptoms (including headaches, abdominal pain, nausea, vomiting, abnormal vision, dyspnoe, anxiety, mental confusion, seizures), these manifestations are not necessarily more serious than preeclampsia. Besides a maternal systemic inflammatory response, signs of systemic vasoconstriction may also be observed in the mother in these pregnancy-associated disorders (Baumwell & Karumanchi, 2007).

In preeclampsia, the anti-inflammatory state during the second and third trimesters develops insufficiently (Saito et al., 2007). An excessive maternal systemic inflammation is considered to be a dominant component in the pathogenesis of this pregnancy-specific disorder, since its important feature is the absence of Th2 skewness and thus the predominance of pro-inflammatory cytokines. Saito et al. reported on their observations regarding higher prevalence of IFN-γ and lower prevalence of IL-4-producing CD4 lymphocytes among peripheral blood mononuclear cells (PBMCs) of preeclamptic women compared with healthy pregnant women. Furthermore, the percentage of Th1 and Th2 cells and the Th1/Th2 ratio correlated with IFN-γ and IL-4 secretion levels (Saito et al., 1999a). In another study, this group observed increased production of IL-2, IFN-γ and TNF-α by PBMCs in preeclampsia and, interestingly, a positive correlation between mean blood pressure and Th1 cytokines (Saito et al., 1999b). The shift to a predominant Th1-type immunity in preeclampsia is reinforced by other experiments on intracellular cytokine measurements in T and NK cells, as well as by the assessment of cytokine secretion levels of PBMCs isolated from preeclamptic patients. (Azizieh et al., 2005; Darmochwal-Kolarz et al., 2002; Rein et al., 2002).

3. The influence of galectin-1 on the Th1/Th2 cell ratio

Previous studies demonstrated that soluble factors may also play a role in the development of the Th2 shift characteristic for healthy pregnancy. Such a factor is galectin-1, also produced by peripheral lymphocytes. Galectin-1, a 14 kDa protein, is a β-galactoside-binding mammalian lectin. Within the immune system, it is expressed by activated T, B and NK cells as well as macrophages (Blaser et al., 1998; Koopman et al., 2003; Rabinovich et al., 1998; Zuniga et al., 2001). Galectin-1 exerts immunoregulatory effects through various mechanisms. By binding to the cell surface glycoproteins, it inhibits T cell proliferation and induces apoptosis of activated Th1, Th17 and CD8 cells (Blaser et al., 1998; Perillo et al., 1995; Toscano et al., 2007). Galectin-1 has been demonstrated in vitro to inhibit T cell adhesion to the extracellular matrix and to abrogate the secretion of proinflammatory cytokines (Rabinovich et al., 1999a). Furthermore, in vivo administration of galectin-1 in experimental models of autoimmunity skewed the balance toward a Th2-dominant cytokine profile (Rabinovich et al., 1999b; Toscano et al., 2006). Recent data show that galectin-1 promotes fetomaternal tolerance, since treatment with recombinant galectin-1 prevented fetal loss in an abortion-prone mouse model. The protective effect of galectin-1 was abrogated in regulatory T cell (Treg) depleted mice (Blois et al., 2007). Garin et al. showed that Tregs selectively up-regulate galectin-1 expression (Garin et al., 2007). Experiments using galectin-1 homozygous null mutant mice showed a reduced regulatory activity in Tregs and the blockage of galectin-1 binding diminished the inhibitory effects of human and mouse Treg cells (Rabinovich et al., 1998). These findings suggest that Tregs expressing galectin-1 may also support the acceptance of the fetus by maternal immune cells.

In a recent study, we measured circulating galectin-1 and anti-galectin-1 autoantibody levels, as well as intracellular galectin-1 expression of unstimulated peripheral blood T and NK cells in healthy pregnancy and preeclampsia (Molvarec et al., 2011). Our findings indicate that the majority of CD4+ and CD8+ T cells and NK cells express intracellular galectin-1 in healthy pregnant women, while only a small fraction of them do so in healthy non-pregnant women. In preeclampsia, the proportion of galectin-1-expressing peripheral T and NK cells was markedly decreased compared with healthy pregnancy. However, circulating levels of galectin-1 and anti-galectin-1 autoantibodies were not altered in preeclamptic patients as compared to healthy pregnant women, nor were related to the proportions of galectin-1-expressing peripheral blood lymphocytes in any of the study groups.

While Th1 and Th17 cells are susceptible to galectin-1-induced cell death, Th2 cells are protected from galectin-1 due to the differential sialylation of their cell surface glycoproteins. Indeed, galectin-1-deficient mice were shown to develop greater Th1 and Th17 responses (Toscano et al., 2007). Therefore, it is tempting to speculate that decreased production of galectin-1 by circulating T and NK cells might contribute to the development of the pro-inflammatory Th1 and Th17 immune responses, which are characteristic features of preeclampsia (Saito et al., 1999b; Toldi et al., 2011a).

4. Regulatory T cells

The recent discovery of a distinct T helper lymphocyte subset, referred to as Th17 cells, led to the transformation of the Th1/Th2 paradigm of immunity into a four-component model. This novel viewpoint incorporates Th1, Th2, Th17 and regulatory T cells (Tregs) as elements of a complex and mutually interacting network in the establishment of pregnancy-specific immune tolerance. Indeed, besides the imbalance of Th1 and Th2 cells, alterations of the prevalence of Th17 and Treg cells have been suggested to be of importance in the pathogenesis of adverse pregnancy outcomes (Saito, 2010).

Tregs are important regulators of tolerance induction. During pregnancy, a systemic expansion of Tregs specific for paternally derived cells can be observed already at very early stages, indicating that their function is to protect paternally derived cells from immune rejection (Mjösberg et al., 2007). The prevalence of Tregs expands in the periphery and these cells are also present at significant numbers at the fetomaternal interface, preferentially in the maternal decidua. Sasaki et al. were the first to describe an increase in the CD4+ CD25+ Treg cell prevalence in decidual tissue in early human pregnancy (Sasaki et al., 2004). This was supported by the works of Heikkinen et al. and Somerset et al. who observed an increase in the population of CD4+ CD25+ circulating Treg cells in early pregnancy and described a peak of this population during the second trimester and a subsequent gradual decrease to levels slightly higher than non-pregnant levels during the postpartum period (Heikkinen et al., 2004; Somerset et al., 2004). The tolerogenic impact of Tregs needs permanent antigen presentation without inflammatory co-stimulation. This explains the transient nature of the fetal tolerance and the fact that, especially during the first weeks of pregnancy, inflammatory infection of the mother may compromise pregnancy outcome. An expansion of Tregs in the decidua in healthy pregnant women accompanied by a low occurrence of Th17 cells was recently confirmed by Mjösberg et al. (Mjösberg et al., 2009). Furthermore, these authors propose that Tregs may be in charge of controlling the Th1 activity found locally in healthy early pregnancy.

Decreased Treg cell numbers during pregnancy are associated with immunological rejection of the fetus (Zenclussen, 2006). Sasaki et al. reported that spontaneous abortion cases are associated with lower systemic Treg levels when compared to normally developing pregnancies (Sasaki et al., 2004). A number of groups including ours demonstrated that the prevalence of peripheral Tregs is lower in preeclampsia compared with healthy pregnancy (Darmochwal-Kolarz et al., 2007; Sasaki et al., 2007; Steinborn et al., 2008; Toldi et al., 2008). Furthermore, Sasaki et al. reported that the prevalence of Tregs is lower not only in peripheral blood samples but also in deciduas of preeclamptic patients compared with healthy pregnant women (Sasaki et al., 2007).

Tregs function in a delicate cellular network that includes inducer (myeloid and lymphoid dendritic cells) and target cells (CD4 and CD8 cells, NK cells and NKT cells) of Tregs (Fig. 1). Besides the peripheral prevalence of Tregs, we also characterized the prevalence of inducers and cellular targets of this T cell subset in preeclampsia and healthy pregnancy in the third trimester. We made efforts to find out whether the alteration of the number of Treg inducers is associated with the decreased number of Tregs. According to a previous study, the ratio of these cells is skewed toward the myeloid dendritic cells in the third trimester of preeclamptic pregnancy (Darmochwal-Kolarz et al., 2003). Theoretically, this may contribute to low Treg prevalence due to the lower Treg inducer capacity of myeloid dendritic cells than that of lymphoid dendritic cells (Ito et al., 2007). In our patients, however, the prevalence and ratio of myeloid and lymphoid dendritic cells did not differ, possibly indicating that dendritic cells are not responsible for low Treg numbers, at least in this stage of pregnancy. The lack of association may support the contribution of non-cellular factors, including pro-inflammatory cytokines such as TNF-α which has a direct inhibitory effect on suppressive Treg function in vitro (Valencia et al., 2006). TNF-α and other pro-inflammatory cytokine levels (such as IFN-γ, IL-6 and IL-12) are reportedly increased in PE (Rusterholz et al., 2007). Lower Treg numbers are not reflected in the proportion of NK, NK-T and activated CD4 and CD8 cells, at least at this stage of pregnancy. This does not exclude, however, that the function (such as the cytokine production pattern) of these cells is modified due to altered Treg numbers.

Steinborn et al. further analyzed the prevalence of Tregs using various markers to identify this subset. Their analysis revealed two distinct Treg subsets that differed with regard to their FoxP3 and CD25 expression: CD4+ CD25+ FoxP3high+ and CD4+ CD25high+ FoxP3+ cells. When monitoring the two populations during healthy pregnancy and preeclampsia, they found a strong increase in the percentage of the CD4+ CD25+ FoxP3high+ Treg

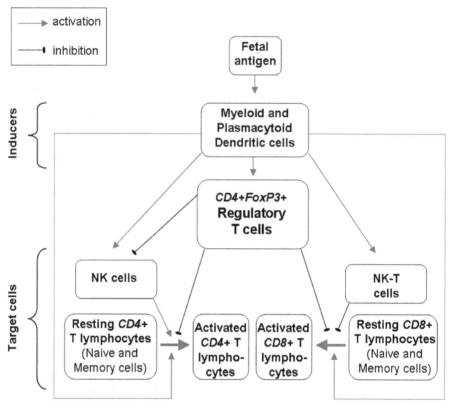

(Based on Toldi et al., 2008.)

Fig. 1. The cellular network of regulatory T cells (Tregs). Tregs are in connection with inducer and target cells through various mechanisms of activation and inhibition.

population during the first and second trimesters, while in the third trimester, this Treg subset decreased gradually until term. The prevalence of CD4+ CD25+ FoxP3high+ Tregs correlated with suppressive capacity: Treg cells obtained from healthy pregnant women during the first and second trimester showed a two-fold higher suppressive activity than cells obtained in the third trimester or at term. The same correlation was true for patients affected by preeclampsia. The significantly diminished percentage of CD4+ CD25+ FoxP3high+ Tregs correlated with low suppressive capacity. In contrast to healthy pregnancy, the percentage of CD4+ CD25high+ FoxP3+ Treg cells was found to be increased in the circulation of preeclamptic women. In healthy pregnant women these cells expanded during the first trimester and reached maximum levels in the second trimester. Therefore, in preeclamptic women the population of CD4+ CD25high+ FoxP3+ Treg cells was particularly apparent, while the population of CD4+ CD25+ FoxP3high+ Tregs was significantly decreased. The authors proposed that CD4+ CD25+ FoxP3high+ and CD4+ CD25high+ FoxP3+ cell populations represent distinct Treg subsets, and that abnormalities in the balance of these subsets are associated with the presence of preeclampsia (Steinborn et al., 2008).

5. The role of regulatory T cells in the process of tolerance induction

Preeclampsia occurs more frequently in the first conception (Dekker & Sibai, 1998). However, preeclampsia appears to be a problem of primipaternity rather than primigravidity, since epidemiological data indicate that when the conception is with a new partner in multiparous mothers, the risk increases to the level seen in the first pregnancy (Robillard et al., 1993; Trupin et al., 1996). The symptoms of preeclampsia regress rapidly after delivery, suggesting that the exposure of the maternal immune system to the fetus and placenta, expressing paternal alloantigens, are of central importance in the pathogenesis.

In donated spermatozoa, semen exposure does not occur and the fetus is a semi-allograft to the mother. The risk of preeclampsia in donated spermatozoa is very high (18.2%) (Salha et al., 1999), suggesting that semen exposure reduces the risk of preeclampsia. Soluble MHC class I antigens in the seminal fluid are taken up by vaginal and uterine epithelial cells, and these antigens might induce tolerance to cells expressing paternally derived MHC class I antigens. Indeed, semen triggers an influx of antigen-presenting cells into the female reproductive tract (Robertson et al., 2003). Usually, the fetus is a semi-allograft to the maternal host. The risk of preeclampsia is also increased in complete allograft-pregnant cases. In ovum donation, the antigens of the fetus are derived from the husband and the donor woman. Exposure to the husband's semen is appropriately present. The risk of preeclampsia in ovum donation cases is high (16%), suggesting that the allografted fetus is a greater challenge for the maternal immune system, and is a risk factor for preeclampsia (Salha et al., 1999). In donated embryo transfer cases, the fetus is an allograft and semen exposure is not present. In this case, this risk of preeclampsia is even higher (33%), probably due to an additive effect of the allografted fetus and the absence of sperm exposure.

Regulatory T cells, which induce tolerance to paternal antigens, may explain these epidemiological findings. Darmochwal-Kolarz et al. demonstrated that the levels of CD4+ CD45RO+ and CD8+ CD25+ cells are increased in preeclampsia, suggesting the activation of CD4+ and CD8+ T lymphocytes. It seems possible that the activation of T lymphocytes is associated with the deficiency of Tregs (Darmochwal-Kolarz etal., 2007). Before the first pregnancy, Treg cell numbers may increase due to seminal priming. Koelman et al. reported that soluble MHC class I antigens are present in the seminal fluid. It is well known that continuous oral exposure to antigens induces tolerance, called 'oral tolerance'. Similarly, a continuous vaginal exposure to paternal soluble MHC class I antigens may induce tolerance to these antigens (Koelman et al., 2000). Robertson et al. suggest that insemination activates the maternal immune system and leads to hypo-responsiveness in T cells reactive with paternal alloantigens in mice (Robertson et al., 2003). This idea is supported by the epidemiological finding that condom users have a high risk for preeclampsia (Klonoff-Cohen et al., 1989).

The prevalence of Tregs is low in the mother before pregnancy (Fig. 2). This minor population of T cells, which reacts to paternal antigens and induces tolerance to them, expands after conception. When a threshold of prevalence is reached, sufficient immune tolerance to paternal antigens is achieved to ensure a healthy development of pregnancy. If the prevalence of Tregs does not reach the threshold, the risk for the development of preeclampsia is high. Subsequently, Tregs increase to a maximum in the second trimester of pregnancy and gradually decrease in the third trimester (Somerset et al., 2004). This finding is related to the clinical observation that the symptoms of preeclampsia generally appear in the third trimester, after 24 weeks of gestation. After delivery, the prevalence of Tregs may

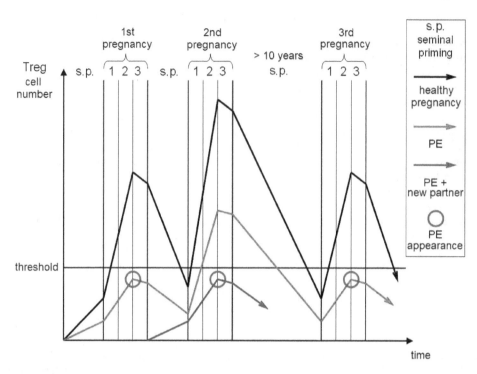

Fig. 2. Alterations of maternal regulatory T cell (Treg) numbers during pregnancy. The prevalence of Tregs is low before pregnancy. When a threshold of Treg prevalence is reached during healthy pregnancy (black curve), the symptoms of preeclampsia do not develop. This is aided by seminal priming. If the prevalence of Tregs does not reach the threshold, the risk of preeclampsia is high (green curve). After the conception of a second pregnancy with the same partner, the number of Tregs increases more rapidly compared with the first pregnancy, independently from the initial prevalence of Tregs during the first pregnancy. However, in a second pregnancy with a new partner, the risk for developing preeclampsia is similar to that in the first pregnancy (blue curve). An increasing interval (> 10 years) between the second and third deliveries was associated with an increasing risk of preeclampsia, and a lower prevalence of Tregs.

rapidly decrease and at the beginning of a second pregnancy, there may be only a low number of Tregs present. Seminal priming may keep the number of these cells to a certain level (Fig. 2). After the conception of a second pregnancy with the same partner, the number of Tregs increases more rapidly compared with the first pregnancy, independently from the initial prevalence of Tregs (and the presence or lack of preeclampsia) during the first pregnancy. However, in a second pregnancy with a new partner, Tregs which induce tolerance to the new partner's antigens may be very rare. Therefore, the risk for developing preeclampsia is similar to that in the first pregnancy.

Skjaerven et al. reported that preeclampsia occurred in 3.9% of first pregnancies, 1.7% of second pregnancies, and 1.8% of third pregnancies when mothers had the same partner. Furthermore, an increasing interval between the second and third deliveries was associated with an increasing risk of preeclampsia. When more than 10 years had passed after the previous delivery, the frequency rose to 3.0%. They also showed that a paternal change was not associated with an increased risk of preeclampsia after adjustment for the interval between births (Skjaerven et al., 2002). These findings might be explained by the population of Tregs. Tregs may gradually decrease and reach very low levels when more than 10 years have passed after the last delivery. A low level of these tolerance-inducing T cells may be maintained by seminal priming. However, in a subsequent pregnancy, some pregnant women may not be able to achieve adequate tolerance, resulting in an increased risk of preeclampsia.

6. Th17 cells

CD4+ IL-17+ (Th17) cells, this recently identified subpopulation of CD4 lymphocytes, originate from a developmental lineage that is distinct from both Th1 and Th2 cells. Th17 cells produce IL-17 and other pro-inflammatory cytokines. IL-17 has an important role in the development of autoimmune disorders and in the induction and maintenance of chronic inflammation (Basso et al., 2009). The effect of Th17 cells on the inflammatory balance is opposed by Tregs. Th17 cells and Tregs originate from the same developmental lineage, distinct from both Th1 and Th2 cells. An exclusive dichotomy was observed in their generation: either Th17 or Treg cells develop from the ancestor cells depending on whether they are activated in the presence of transforming growth factor-β (TGF-β) or TGF-β plus inflammatory cytokines (Basso et al., 2009).

In addition to their distinct role in the regulation of the inflammatory status, Th1, Th2, Th17 and Treg cells mutually influence one another through the production of different cytokines. For instance, an increase in the Th17/Treg cell ratio may contribute to a shift towards the Th1 direction because IL-17 induces the production of other pro-inflammatory cytokines, such as that of IFN-γ (Afzali et al., 2007), while the inhibitory effect of Tregs on Th1 cells is decreased at the same time.

In a previous study, Santner-Nanan et al. found that, besides a higher prevalence of Tregs, the percentage of Th17 cells is significantly decreased in the third trimester of healthy pregnancy compared with non-pregnant controls and preeclamptic patients. Consequently, the Th17/Treg cell ratio was significantly decreased in healthy but not in preeclamptic pregnancies. Thus, preeclampsia is associated with the absence of normal systemic skewing away from IL-17 production towards FoxP3 expression. Additionally, preeclamptic women had significantly higher levels of soluble endoglin, an inhibitor of TGF-β receptor signaling, which may bias towards IL-17 production (Santner-Nanan et al., 2009).

In accordance with the above data, we also found that simultaneously with higher than normal Th17 numbers, the prevalence of Tregs is lower in PE, resulting in an elevated Th17/Treg ratio compared with uncomplicated pregnancy. The altered ratio of Th17/Treg cells may contribute to the shift towards the Th1 direction in preeclampsia. However, we could not detect a correlation between the prevalence of Th17 and Th1 cells (using the cell surface marker, CXCR3 for the identification of the latter subset). Thus, the effect of Th17 cells and IL-17 on the inflammatory status is more likely to be exerted in a direct manner rather than through the modulation of the Th1/Th2 balance in preeclampsia (Toldi et al., 2011a).

The alterations of Th17 cells have been observed in other pregnancy-related disorders as well, suggesting that the balance of Th17 cells and Tregs and not only that of Th1 and Th2 cells has crucial effects on the inflammatory status in human pregnancy. Ito et al. recently demonstrated the importance of IL-17-producing cells in the pathomechanism of preterm labour (Ito et al., 2010). Nakashima et al. found that the prevalence of decidual IL-17-producing cells is significantly higher in inevitable abortion cases (but not in missed abortion) than in normal pregnancy, indicating that these cells might be involved in the induction of inflammation in the late stage of abortion, but not in the early stage (Nakashima et al., 2010). In another study, Wang et al. showed that the prevalence of Th17 cells in the peripheral blood and decidua is increased in unexplained recurrent spontaneous abortion patients (Wang et al., 2010). They observed that the expression of a Th17-associated factor, RAR-related orphan receptor gamma (ROR-γ or RORc), is also higher in peripheral blood lymphocytes and decidua of these patients. In a recent study, Jianjun et al. found that the mRNA level of this factor in PBMCs and decidua is elevated in preeclamptic patients when compared with healthy pregnant women (Jianjun et al., 2010). Therefore, the increased expression of this transcription factor may partly be responsible for the increased prevalence of Th17 cells in peripheral blood of preeclamptic patients.

7. IL-17-producing CD8 and NK cells

Although IL-17 was first identified in CD4 cells, later on other immune cells, including CD8 and NK cells, were also shown to produce this cytokine (Passos et al., 2010; Shin et al., 1999). Emerging evidence suggests that these IL-17-producing lymphocyte subsets, especially NK cells, largely contribute to the inflammatory status during pregnancy. Sargent et al. proposed that the innate rather than the adaptive immune system controls immune regulation during human pregnancy, and that NK cells are of central importance to this process (Sargent et al., 2006b; Sargent et al., 2007). The aberrant activation of NK cells both systematically and locally in the placenta may be of major interest in the malfunction of immune tolerance and the pathogenesis of pregnancy-associated disorders.

In our previously unpublished investigation, we measured the peripheral prevalence of IL-17-producing cells in the CD4, CD8 and NK subsets and that of the IL-17 producing CD4, CD8 and NK cells in the overall lymphocyte population. We took peripheral blood samples from 24 healthy non-pregnant and 23 healthy pregnant age-matched women (with a median of 32 and 33 years, respectively), in the third trimester of pregnancy (with a median of 31 weeks of gestation). Non-pregnant women were in the early follicular phase of the menstrual cycle (between cycle days 3 and 5), and none of them received hormonal contraception. Informed consent was obtained from all participating subjects. We separated the mononuclear cells from the samples and performed cell surface marker and intracellular cytokine staining. Finally, samples were measured on a flow cytometer.

The prevalence of Th17 cells was lower among healthy pregnant compared with healthy non-pregnant women (2.8 [2.4-3.1] % vs. 3.2 [2.9-3.5] %). The prevalence of CD8+ IL-17+ (Tc17) cells among CD8 lymphocytes was higher in healthy pregnant than in healthy non-pregnant samples (4.8 [3.6-6.2] % vs. 2.4 [1.7-3.7] %). The frequency of CD56+ IL-17+ (IL-17-producing NK) cells was lower in healthy pregnant than in healthy non-pregnant samples (1.0 [0.6-1.2] % vs. 1.6 [1.1-2.5] %).

We further analyzed the frequency of IL-17-producing CD4, CD8 and NK lymphocytes. After the initial assessment of the Th17, Tc17 and IL-17-producing NK cell prevalence among CD4, CD8 and NK cells, respectively (Fig. 3, graphs a-c), we also determined the prevalence of these subsets among the overall lymphocyte population (Fig. 3, graphs d-f) along with the frequency of CD4+ IL-17-, CD8+ IL-17- and CD56+ IL-17- cells among the overall lymphocyte population (Fig. 3, graphs g-i).

Our findings revealed two different mechanisms explaining the differing alterations observed in the prevalence of Th17 and Tc17 cells in the study groups. The alteration of CD4+ IL-17+ cell prevalence in the overall lymphocyte subset (Fig. 3, graph d) followed that seen among CD4 cells (Fig. 3, graph a), as the frequency of CD4+ IL-17- cells was comparable in both study groups (Fig. 3, graph g). Therefore, the prevalence of Th17 (CD4+ IL-17+) cells show absolute alterations, since Th17 cell numbers are altered not only in the CD4 subset, but also in the overall lymphocyte population. In contrast, Tc17 cell frequencies do not show significant difference if assessed among the overall lymphocyte population (Fig. 3, graph e); only the prevalence of CD8+ IL-17- cells differs between the study groups

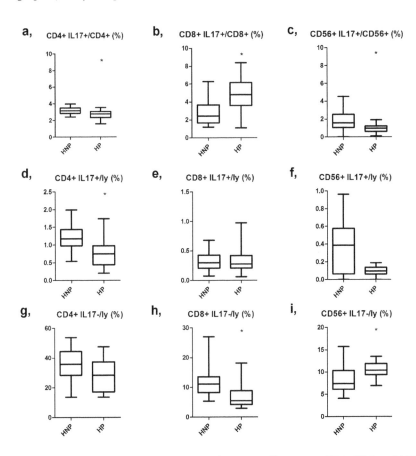

Fig. 3. Box-plots representing the prevalence of IL-17+ cells among CD4, CD8 and NK (CD56+) cells (graphs a-c) and in the overall lymphocyte population (ly) (graphs d-f), as well as the prevalence of IL-17- cells in the overall lymphocyte population (ly) (graphs g-i) in healthy non-pregnant (HNP) and healthy pregnant (HP) women. Horizontal line: median, box: interquartile range, whisker: range. * p values less than 0.05 were regarded significant.

(Fig. 3, graph h) and the direction of IL-17- cell alteration is the opposite of that seen at Tc17 cell prevalence in the CD8 subset (Fig. 3, graph b). Therefore, the prevalence of Tc17 cells does not show absolute alterations, only relative ones, as a consequence of different CD8+ IL-17- cell frequencies in the study groups. The alteration of IL-17-producing NK cell prevalences among parent populations showed similar tendencies to that observed in case of CD4 cells.

Of note, existing data are not consistent concerning the alterations of CD4 and CD8 cell frequencies during pregnancy. Tallon et al. found that CD4 cell numbers decrease in the second and third trimesters, while CD8 cells decrease during the third trimester (Tallon et al., 1984). Another study demonstrated that peripheral blood CD8 cells decreased during the first trimester, while CD4 cells decreased in the third trimester, with both populations increasing to non-pregnant values four months postpartum (Watanabe et al., 1997). The investigations by Kühnert et al. found no significant changes in the percentage CD4 and CD8 lymphocytes, nor in the CD4/CD8 ratio at any stage of pregnancy or postpartum.

Based on our results, the apparent increase in Tc17 cell prevalence in healthy pregnancy compared with non-pregnant controls appears to be the consequence of decreased CD8+ IL-17- cell frequency in this group, resulting in a higher proportion of Tc17 cells in the CD8 subset. Since Tc17 cells have been described to have a lower cytotoxic activity in comparison with CD8+ IL-17- cells (Huber et al., 2009), the decrease in the latter subset and a relative increase in Tc17 prevalence may be regarded as part of the immunosuppressive mechanisms characterizing healthy pregnancy.

In preeclampsia, our results show that in addition to CD4 cells, the prevalence of CD8 and NK cells that express IL-17 is also higher compared with healthy pregnant women. IL-17 production by these lymphocyte subsets might contribute to the development of a systemic pro-inflammatory environment in PE (Toldi et al., 2011a).

8. Lymphocyte activation kinetics

Previous studies demonstrated that not only the prevalence of T lymphocyte subsets, but also their functionality is altered during pregnancy. For instance, calcium handling of T cells differs in healthy pregnancy and in the non-pregnant state. Previous reports indicate a sustained increase of basal intracellular calcium level in lymphocytes of healthy pregnant and preeclamptic women compared with non-pregnant women, with the highest levels in preeclampsia (Hojo et al., 1999; Thway et al., 2004; von Dadelszen et al., 1999). The availability of cytoplasmic free calcium has an important role in controlling the level of lymphocyte activation. We hypothesized that the elements of calcium handling of activated T lymphocytes, including lymphocyte potassium channels, may be affected in healthy pregnancy and preeclampsia compared to the non-pregnant state. Voltage-gated Kv1.3 channels along with calcium-dependent IKCa1 channels play a key role in the regulation of intracellular calcium homeostasis as they counterbalance the increase of cytoplasmic free calcium content in the course of lymphocyte activation. These channels grant the efflux of potassium from the cytoplasm, thus maintaining an electrochemical potential gradient needed for further calcium entry. Specific inhibition of these channels results in a diminished calcium influx into lymphocytes and a lower level of lymphocyte activation (Panyi et al., 2006). Our group characterized the activation-elicited calcium influx in the Th1, Th2, CD4 and CD8 lymphocyte subsets in healthy pregnant, preeclamptic and non-pregnant women and tested its alteration upon the inhibition of Kv1.3 and IKCa1 potassium channels (Toldi et al., 2011b).

Until recently, primarily single-cell techniques were applied to study the process of lymphocyte activation, and no reliable high-throughput method was available to investigate lymphocyte activation kinetics in more than one lymphocyte subsets simultaneously. The use of single-cell techniques are limited by the fact that they are not suitable for the description of kinetic processes in a complex cellular milieu that contains different types of interacting immune cells. For this purpose, we developed a novel, flow cytometry-based approach that enabled us to monitor lymphocyte activation simultaneously in different lymphocyte subtypes.

For our measurements, we collected peripheral blood samples from healthy pregnant, preeclamptic and non-pregnant women. PBMCs were separated by a standard density gradient centrifugation. PBMCs were then incubated with conjugated anti-human surface marker monoclonal antibodies (CD4, CD8, CXCR3 for Th1 cells, CCR4 for Th2 cells) to identify lymphocyte subsets and were loaded with calcium sensitive Fluo-3 and Fura Red dyes to monitor alterations of the cytoplasmic free calcium level. PBMCs were divided into three vials. One vial was treated with margatoxin (MGTX), a selective blocker of the Kv1.3 channel. Another vial was treated with a triarylmethane compound (TRAM), a specific inhibitor of the IKCa1 channel. The third vial was used as control. Measurements were initiated directly after the addition of 20 µg of phytohemagglutinin (PHA) as an unspecific activating stimulus. Cell fluorescence data were measured and recorded for 10 minutes in a kinetic manner on flow cytometer.

Data acquired from the measurements were evaluated by fitting a double-logistic function for each recording (Kaposi et al., 2008). This function is used to describe measurements that have an increasing and a decreasing intensity as time passes. The software also calculates parameter values describing each function, such as the Maximum value (Max), the Time to reach maximum value (t_{max}), and the Area Under the Curve (AUC). These parameters represent different characteristics of lymphocyte calcium influx kinetics. The Maximum value represents the peak value of the calcium influx curve upon lymphocyte activation, thus it reflects the maximal amount of cytoplasmic free calcium in the course of activation. The Time to reach maximum value describes how soon the peak value of the calcium influx curve is reached. The Area Under the Curve describes the full amount of cytoplasmic free calcium during the whole period of lymphocyte activation and thus the magnitude of the elicited calcium response in general.

Our results indicate that calcium influx kinetics in activated T lymphocytes markedly differs in healthy pregnancy compared with the non-pregnant state: AUC values of the calcium response are lower in healthy pregnancy in the Th1, CD4 and CD8 lymphocyte subsets (Fig. 4). Based on this observation, it is reasonable to assume that the physiological immune tolerance towards fetal antigens in pregnancy is partly attributed to a lower calcium response. This hypothesis is further supported by the particular role of the impaired function of Th1 and CD8 lymphocyte subsets in maternal immune tolerance. On contrary to Th1 cells, the activation induced calcium response of the Th2 subset is not decreased compared with the non-pregnant state. The decreased activation of the Th1 subset (reflected by low AUC values in our study) and the lack of decrease in Th2 cells may partly be responsible for the well established Th2 skewness in healthy pregnancy.

Unlike in healthy pregnancy, we could not detect a difference in the AUC values of calcium influx kinetics of Th1 and CD8 cells in preeclampsia compared to non-pregnant women (Fig. 4). The absence of calcium influx characteristics specific for healthy pregnancy suggests that

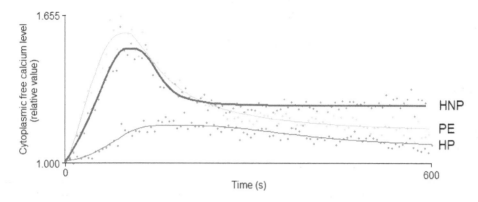

Fig. 4. Calcium influx kinetics of peripheral Th1 lymphocytes isolated from healthy non-pregnant (HNP), healthy pregnant (HP) and preeclamptic (PE) women (without lymphocyte potassium channel inhibitor treatment). Calcium influx is lower in healthy pregnancy compared with the non-pregnant state and preeclampsia.

this element may associate with the impaired maternal immune tolerance present in preeclampsia, since the calcium influx kinetics is comparable to that seen in non-pregnant samples. Indeed, the maintained activation properties of Th1 lymphocytes in preeclamptic patients may contribute to the lack of Th2 dominance associated with normal pregnancy. Similarly to the Th1 subset, CD8 cells in preeclampsia are also characterized by the lack of suppressed activation kinetics. Thus the decrease of cytotoxic activity observed in healthy pregnancy (Malinowski et al., 1994) is not present in preeclampsia. Interestingly, t_{max} values were decreased in Th2 and CD4 cells in preeclampsia compared with healthy pregnancy. This finding may indicate an increased reactivity of lymphocytes in preeclampsia, possibly reflecting an elevated responsiveness of T lymphocytes due to the ongoing maternal systemic inflammation.

Since Kv1.3 and IKCa1 potassium channels significantly influence the calcium response elicited upon lymphocyte activation, we tested their expression and function in healthy pregnancy and preeclampsia. According to comparable fluorescence values of the samples stained with specific antibodies against Kv1.3 channels, their expression is not altered in any of the investigated T lymphocyte subsets. Therefore, the differences detected between calcium influx of non-pregnant, healthy pregnant and preeclamptic lymphocytes upon treatment with specific inhibitors of the potassium channels is probably due to the altered function, and not to the altered expression of these channels.

Our results suggest that the overall lymphocyte population and particularly the CD4 subset are sensitive to MGTX and TRAM inhibition in each investigated study group, indicating that both Kv1.3 and IKCa1 channels play an important regulatory role in calcium influx. This is reflected by the decrease of the AUC and Max values compared with the respective samples where no inhibitors were applied. However, the sensitivity of calcium influx measured in other lymphocyte subsets shows clear variability. It is of particular interest that calcium influx of Th2 lymphocytes in healthy pregnancy was insensitive to potassium channel inhibition, while calcium influx decreased significantly in non-pregnant samples upon treatment with the specific channel blockers. Of note, Th2 lymphocytes in preeclampsia presented with non-pregnant-like characteristics, and were also sensitive to MGTX and TRAM treatment. Since the regulatory function of Kv1.3 and IKCa1 channels on calcium influx appears to be limited in healthy pregnant samples (as the inhibition of these channels did not result in a decrease of the AUC and Max values), it is tempting to speculate that this may be an element contributing to the Th2 shift present in healthy pregnancy, but absent in preeclampsia. This hypothesis may be supported by reports suggesting that the shape of calcium influx influenced by potassium channel functions may determine the cytokine production profile of helper T lymphocytes (Dolmetsch et al., 1998; Fanger et al., 2000).

Interestingly, other differences were also observed between healthy pregnancy and preeclampsia. While calcium influx in CD8 and Th1 lymphocytes was resistant to potassium channel inhibition in preeclamptic samples, that of healthy pregnant lymphocytes was sensitive. Similarly to Th2 cells, while it is unclear whether the resistance of Th1 lymphocytes to potassium channel inhibition is reflected in their function, the insensitivity of the Th1 subset to the inhibition of regulatory lymphocyte potassium channels in preeclampsia may be linked to the Th1 skewness.

Our findings suggest that there is a characteristic pattern of calcium influx in T lymphocytes and its sensitivity to potassium channel inhibition in normal pregnancy that is missing in preeclampsia. This raises the notion that T lymphocyte calcium handling may have a role in the development of the pregnancy-specific immune tolerance.

9. The association between preeclampsia and autoimmunity

Considering the immunological alterations described in preeclampsia, one may notice characteristic similarities in the etiology shared with autoimmune disorders. As a result of the impaired immune tolerance, preeclampsia is distinguished by many features typically seen in autoimmune diseases, or in association with autoimmune reactions. This does not mean that preeclampsia should be considered an autoimmune condition. However, it does suggest that abnormal autoimmune processes play an important part in the pathogenesis of preeclampsia. An interpretation of preeclampsia can be found in analogies to organ rejection after allograft transplantation and in graft-versus-host disease (GVHD); like preeclampsia, these conditions are also characterized by a multitude of systemic symptoms. The similarities with acute organ rejection and GVHD are paralleled by the notion that if a 100% allograft can elicit autoimmune responses during organ transplantation, one should not be surprised that a 50:50 autograft-allograft can do the same thing. This recognition may lead to better clinical approaches to preeclampsia and thereby to better diagnosis and treatment (Gleicher, 2007).

The clinical relationship between autoimmune diseases and pregnancy is unique. No other diseases are characterized by an exacerbation pattern that is particularly pronounced in the peripartum and postpartum periods (Gleicher et al., 1993). A recently recognized example is peripartum cardiomyopathy, with disease flares from late pregnancy up to approximately three months postpartum (Ansari et al., 2002). Preeclampsia is also characterized by a peripartal exacerbation pattern, with the majority of cases developing after 36 weeks of gestation.

Besides the cellular abnormalities already discussed, autoantibody abnormalities have also been reported in association with preeclampsia. So far, a number of autoantibodies have been implicated in the pathogenesis (Branch et al., 1994; Milliez et al., 1990; Rappaport et al.,

1990; Yamamoto et al., 1993). The most important one of them appears to be an agonistic autoantibody against the angiotensin II type 1 receptor (Wallukat et al., 1999). Moreover, as in classical autoimmune diseases, more severe preeclampsia appears to result in more autoantibody abnormalities (El-Roeiy et al., 1991). Evidence suggests that classical, nonorgan-specific autoantibodies, such as antiphospholipid antibodies, are characteristic of preeclampsia, and especially in its more severe clinical expression (El-Roeiy et al., 1991; Yamamoto et al., 1993). Dekker et al. therefore recommended active laboratory surveillance for patients at risk (Dekker et al., 1995).

Both GVHD-related and classical autoimmune conditions often improve upon treatments that have been found successful also in preeclampsia and HELLP syndrome. Three examples are the treatment with corticosteroids, removal of autoantibody abnormalities via plasmapheresis, and the competitive binding of autoantibodies with intravenous immunoglobulin (Katz et al., 1990; Martin et al., 1990; Martin et al., 2006).

Considering the significant degree of bidirectional cell traffic during pregnancy, one can speculate that, in analogy to GVHD, the autoimmune phenomena, seen in association with preeclampsia, may be immune responses by fetal lymphocytes to epitopes shared by mother and fetus. Alternatively, the autoimmune response in preeclampsia could be distinct from that in GVHD, and purely autoimmune in nature. This would then represent an immune response solely against maternal self-epitopes on fetal cells that have entered the maternal circulation. A number of observations indicate that the paternal genotype is of importance in that regard. For instance, the more similar the paternal histocompatibility complex is to that of the mother, the more likely a miscarriage will occur due to increased autoantigenity (Kishore et al., 1996). The fetus is not only an allograft but also an autograft. Since one half of the fetus is maternally derived in its antigenicity, the maternal immune system also faces an unprecedented autoimmune load. At no other period in life needs the maternal immune system to be prepared for autoimmune challenges of this extent. The immunological adjustment to pregnancy, therefore, does not only involve the development of tolerance to the paternal allogenic, but also to the maternal autoimmunogenic components of the fetus.

Autoimmune phenomena are mostly seen in two periods of pregnancy: during early conception and the peripartum period. In early conception, abnormal immune activation may be coupled with pregnancy loss. Later stage presentation appears to be associated with preeclampsia. Indeed, women with early autoimmune activation, who (with treatment) do not miscarry, demonstrate a greatly increased risk for preeclampsia (Gleicher et al., 1993). This observation supports the idea of a common alloimmune or autoimmune etiology for both of these conditions. It has also been suggested that an analogy might exist not only between chronic graft rejection and preeclampsia, but also between acute graft rejection and recurrent abortion (Wilczyński, 2006).

Accepting the concept that preeclampsia is characterized by autoimmune phenomena may have benefits for better diagnosis and treatment. For example, autoimmune phenomena usually go through pre- or subclinical stages before their clinical manifestation. Laboratory markers are often already detectable at those early stages (Davidson & Diamond, 2001). If the autoimmune phenomena of preeclampsia were to follow a similar pattern, earlier diagnosis and specific treatment might become possible.

10. Conclusion

T lymphocytes play a central role in the development of the maternal immune tolerance during pregnancy. Pathologic alterations of T cells in prevalence and functionality contribute to the onset of pregnancy-related disorders, and might represent a possible future target for therapeutic intervention.

It has been recognized for many years that the prevalence of distinct T cell subpopulations are subject to a characteristic adjustment during pregnancy in order to facilitate the specific needs raised by the developing fetus. The course of this adjustment may be insufficient in pregnancy-related disorders. Recently, it has been demonstrated that not only cell numbers, but also the functionality of cells needs to go through specific alterations to help the maternal immune system in acquisition of the pregnancy-specific tolerance. As an example, we have demonstrated that there is a characteristic pattern of calcium influx in T lymphocytes and its sensitivity to lymphocyte potassium channel inhibition in healthy pregnancy that is missing in preeclampsia, raising the notion that T lymphocyte calcium handling may have a role in the distinctive immune status of uncomplicated pregnancy. Further research needs to be carried out applying different methods to identify additional factors involved in these alterations. This approach might lead to better strategies for the prevention and treatment of adverse pregnancy outcomes, facilitating the development and maintenance of immune tolerance needed for healthy pregnancy.

11. Acknowledgement

The preparation of this chapter was supported by grants OTKA 76316 and ETT 05-180/2009.

12. References

Afzali, B., Lombardi, G., Lechler, R.I., Lord, G.M. (2007). The role of T helper 17 (Th17) and regulatory T cells (Treg) in human organ transplantation and autoimmune disease. *Clin Exp Immunol,* Vol.148, No.1, (April 2007), pp. 32-46

Ansari, A.A., Fett, J.D., Carraway, R.E., Mayne, A.E., Onlamoon, N., Sundstrom, J.B. (2002). Autoimmune mechanisms as the basis of human peripartum cardiomyopathy. *Clin Rev Allergy Immunol,* Vol.23, No.3, (December 2002), pp. 301-324

Ashkar, A.A., Di Santo, J.P., Croy, B.A. (1998). Interferon gamma contributes to initiation of uterine vascular modification, decidual integrity, and uterine natural killer cell maturation during normal murine pregnancy. *J Exp Med,* Vol.192, No.2, (July 2000), pp. 259-270

Azizieh, F., Raghupathy, R., Makhseed, M. (2005). Maternal cytokine production patterns in women with pre-eclampsia. *Am J Reprod Immunol,* Vol.54, No.1, (July 2005), pp. 30-37

Basso, A.S., Cheroutre, H., Mucida, D. (2009). More stories on Th17 cells. *Cell Res,* Vol.19, No.4, (April 2009), 399-411

Baumwell, S., Karumanchi, S.A. (2007). Pre-eclampsia: clinical manifestations and molecular mechanisms. *Nephron Clin Pract,* Vol.106, No.2, (June 2007), pp. c72-81

Blaser, C., Kaufmann, M., Müller, C., Zimmermann, C., Wells, V., Mallucci, L., Pircher, H. (1998). Beta-galactoside-binding protein secreted by activated T cells inhibits antigen-induced proliferation of T cells. *Eur J Immunol,* Vol.28, No.8, (August 1998), pp. 2311-2319

Blois, S.M., Ilarregui J.M., Tometten, M., Garcia, M., Orsal, A.S., Cordo-Russo, R., Toscano, M.A., Bianco, G.A., Kobelt, P., Handjiski, B., Tirado, I., Markert, U.R., Klapp, B.F., Poirier, F., Szekeres-Bartho, J., Rabinovich, G.A., Arck, P.C. (2007). A pivotal role for galectin-1 in fetomaternal tolerance. *Nat Med*, Vol.13, No.12, (December 2007), pp. 1450-1457

Branch, D.W., Mitchell, M.D., Miller, E., Palinski, W., Witztum, J.L. (1994). Pre-eclampsia and serum antibodies to oxidised low-density lipoprotein. *Lancet*, Vol.343, No.8898, (March 1994), pp. 645-646

Bulmer, J.N. (1992). Immune aspects of pathology of the placental bed contributing to pregnancy pathology. *Baillieres Clin Obstet Gynaecol*, Vol.6, No.3, (September 1992), pp. 461-488

Challis, J.R., Lockwood, C.J., Myatt, L., Norman, J.E., Strauss, J.F. 3rd, Petraglia, F. (2009). Inflammation and pregnancy. *Reprod Sci*, Vol.16, No.2, (February 2009), pp. 206-215

Darmochwal-Kolarz, D., Rolinski, J., Leszczynska-Goarzelak, B., Oleszczuk, J. (2002). The expressions of intracellular cytokines in the lymphocytes of preeclamptic patients. *Am J Reprod Immunol*, Vol.48, No.6, (December 2002), pp. 381-386

Darmochwal-Kolarz, D., Rolinski, J., Tabarkiewicz, J., Leszczynska-Gorzelak, B., Buczkowski, J., Wojas, K., Oleszczuk, J. (2003). Myeloid and lymphoid dendritic cells in normal pregnancy and preeclampsia. *Clin Exp Immunol*, Vol.132, No.2, (May 2003), pp. 339-344

Darmochwal-Kolarz, D., Saito, S., Rolinski, J., Tabarkiewicz, J., Kolarz, B., Leszczynska-Gorzelak, B., Oleszczuk, J. (2007). Activated T lymphocytes in pre-eclampsia. *Am J Reprod Immunol*, Vol.58, No.1, (July 2007), pp. 39-45

Davidson, A., Diamond, B. (2001). Autoimmune diseases. *N Engl J Med*, Vol.345, No.5, (August 2001), pp. 340-350

Dekker, G.A., de Vries, J.I., Doelitzsch, P.M., Huijgens, P.C., von Blomberg, B.M., Jakobs, C., van Geijn, H.P. (1995). Underlying disorders associated with severe early-onset preeclampsia. *Am J Obstet Gynecol*, Vol.173, No.4, (October 1995), pp. 1042-1048

Dekker, G.A., Sibai, B.M., (1998). Etiology and pathogenesis of preeclampsia: current concepts. *Am J Obstet Gynecol*, Vol.179, No.5, (November 1998), pp. 1359-1375

Dolmetsch, R.E., Xu, K., Lewis, R.S. (1998). Calcium oscillations increase the efficiency and specificity of gene expression. *Nature*, Vol.392, No.6679, (April 1998), pp. 933-936

El-Roeiy, A., Myers, S.A., Gleicher, N. (1991). The relationship between autoantibodies and intrauterine growth retardation in hypertensive disorders of pregnancy. *Am J Obstet Gynecol*, Vol.164, No.5 Pt 1, (May 1991), pp. 1253-1261

Fanger, C.M., Neben, A.L., Cahalan, M.D. (2000). Differential Ca2+ influx, KCa channel activity, and Ca2+ clearance distinguish Th1 and Th2 lymphocytes. *J Immunol*, Vol.164, No.3, (February 2000), pp. 1153-1160

Garin, M.I., Chu, C.C., Golshayan, D., Cernuda-Morollón, E., Wait, R., Lechler, R.I. (2007). Galectin-1: a key effector of regulation mediated by CD4+CD25+ T cells. *Blood*, Vol.109, No.5, (March 2007), pp. 2058-2065

Gleicher, N., Pratt, D., Dudkiewicz, A. (1993). What do we really know about autoantibody abnormalities and reproductive failure: a critical review. *Autoimmunity*, Vol.16, No.2, (February 1993), pp. 115-140

Gleicher, N. (2007). Why much of the pathophysiology of preeclampsia-eclampsia must be of an autoimmune nature. *Am J Obstet Gynecol*, Vol.196, No.1, (January 2007), pp. 5.e1-7

Heikkinen, J., Möttönen, M., Alanen, A., Lassila, O. (2004). Phenotypic characterization of regulatory T cells in the human decidua. *Clin Exp Immunol*, Vol.136, No.2, (May 2004), pp. 373-378

Hojo, M., Suthanthiran, M., Helseth, G., August, P. (1999). Lymphocyte intracellular free calcium concentration is increased in preeclampsia. *Am J Obstet Gynecol*, Vol.180, No.5, (May 1999), 209-214

Huber, M., Heink, S., Grothe, H., Guralnik, A., Reinhard, K., Elflein, K., Hünig, T., Mittrücker, H.W., Brüstle, A., Kamradt, T., Lohoff, M. (2009). A Th17-like developmental process leads to CD8(+) Tc17 cells with reduced cytotoxic activity. *Eur J Immunol*, Vol.39, No.7, (July 2009), pp. 1716-1725

Ito, T., Yang, M., Wang, Y.H., Lande, R., Gregorio, J., Perng, O.A., Qin, X.F., Liu, Y.J., Gilliet, M. (2007). Plasmacytoid dendritic cells prime IL-10-producing T regulatory cells by inducible costimulator ligand. *J Exp Med*, Vol.204, No.1, (January 2007), pp. 105-115

Ito, M., Nakashima, A., Hidaka, T., Okabe, M., Bac, N.D., Ina, S., Yoneda, S., Shiozaki, A., Sumi, S., Tsuneyama, K., Nikaido, T., Saito, S. (2010). A role for IL-17 in induction of an inflammation at the fetomaternal interface in preterm labour. *J Reprod Immunol*, Vol.84, No.1, (January 2010), pp. 75-85

Jianjun, Z., Yali, H., Zhiqun, W., Mingming, Z., Xia, Z. (2010). Imbalance of T-cell transcription factors contributes to the Th1 type immunity predominant in preeclampsia. *Am J Reprod Immunol*, Vol.63, No.1, (January 2010), pp. 38-45

Kaposi, A.S., Veress, G., Vásárhelyi, B., Macardle, P., Bailey, S., Tulassay, T., Treszl, A. (2008). Cytometry-acquired calcium-flux data analysis in activated lymphocytes. *Cytometry A*, Vol.73, No.3, (March 2008), pp. 246-253

Katz, V.L., Thorp, J.M. Jr, Watson, W.J., Fowler, L., Heine, R.P. (1990). Human immunoglobulin therapy for preeclampsia associated with lupus anticoagulant and anticardiolipin antibody. *Obstet Gynecol*, Vol.76, No.5 Pt 2, (November 1990), pp. 986-988

Kishore, R., Agarwal, S., Halder, A., Das, V., Shukla, B.R., Agarwal, S.S. (1996). HLA sharing, anti-paternal cytotoxic antibodies and MLR blocking factors in women with recurrent spontaneous abortion. *J Obstet Gynaecol Res*, Vol.22, No.2, (April 1996), pp. 177-183

Klonoff-Cohen, H.S., Savitz, D.A., Cefalo, R.C., McCann, M.F. (1989). An epidemiologic study of contraception and preeclampsia. *JAMA*, Vol.262, No.22, (December 1989), pp. 3143-3147

Koelman, C.A., Coumans, A.B., Nijman, H.W., Doxiadis, I.I., Dekker, G.A., Claas, F.H. (2000). Correlation between oral sex and a low incidence of preeclampsia: a role for soluble HLA in seminal fluid? *J Reprod Immunol*, Vol.46, No.2, (March 2000), pp. 155-166

Koopman, L.A., Kopcow, H.D., Rybalov, B., Boyson, J.E., Orange, J.S., Schatz, F., Masch, R., Lockwood, C.J., Schachter, A.D., Park, P.J., Strominger, J.L. (2003). Human decidual natural killer cells are a unique NK cell subset with immunomodulatory potential. *J Exp Med*, Vol.198, No.8, (October 2003), pp. 1201-1212

Kühnert, M., Strohmeier, R., Stegmüller, M., Halberstadt, E. (1998). Changes in lymphocyte subsets during normal pregnancy. *Eur J Obstet Gynecol Reprod Biol*, Vol.76, No.2, (February 1998), pp. 147-151

Lin, H., Mosmann, T.R., Guilbert, L., Tuntipopipat, S., Wegmann, T.G. (1993). Synthesis of T helper 2-type cytokines at maternal–fetal interface. *J Immunol*, Vol.151, No.9, (November 1993), pp. 4562-4573

Malinowski, A., Szpakowski, M., Tchórzewski, H., Zeman, K., Pawlowicz, P., Wozniak, P. (1994). T lymphocyte subpopulations and lymphocyte proliferative activity in normal and pre-eclamptic pregnancy. *Eur J Obstet Gynecol Reprod Biol*, Vol.53, No.1, (January 1994), pp. 27-31

Martin, J.N. Jr, Files, J.C., Blake, P.G., Norman, P.H., Martin, R.W., Hess, L.W., Morrison, J.C., Wiser, W.L. (1990). Plasma exchange for preeclampsia. I. Postpartum use for persistently severe preeclampsia-eclampsia with HELLP syndrome. *Am J Obstet Gynecol*, Vol.162, No.1, (January 1990), pp. 126-137

Martin, J.N. Jr, Rose, C.H., Briery, C.M. (2006). Understanding and managing HELLP syndrome: the integral role of aggressive glucocorticosteroids for mother and child. *Am J Obstet Gynecol*, Vol.195, No.4, (October 2006), pp. 914-934

Milliez, J., Lelong, F., Bayani, N., Jannet, D., El Medjadji, M., Latrous, H., Hammami, M., Paniel, B.J. (1991). The prevalence of autoantibodies during third trimester pregnancy complicated by hypertension or idiopathic fetal growth retardation. *Am J Obstet Gynecol*, Vol.165, No.1, (July 1991), pp. 51-56

Mjösberg, J., Berg, G., Ernerudh, J., Ekerfelt, C. (2007). CD4+ CD25+ regulatory T cells in human pregnancy: development of a Treg-MLC-ELISPOT suppression assay and indications of paternal specific Tregs. *Immunology*, Vol.120, No.4, (April 2007), pp. 456-466

Mjösberg, J., Berg, G., Jenmalm, M.C., Ernerudh, J. (2010). FOXP3+ regulatory T cells and T helper 1, T helper 2, and T helper 17 cells in human early pregnancy decidua. *Biol Reprod*, Vol.82, No.4, (April 2010), pp. 698-705

Molvarec, A., Blois, S.M., Stenczer, B., Toldi, G., Tirado-Gonzalez, I., Ito, M., Shima, T., Yoneda, S., Vásárhelyi, B., Rigó, J. Jr, Saito, S. (2011). Peripheral blood galectin-1-expressing T and natural killer cells in normal pregnancy and preeclampsia. *Clin Immunol*, (February 2011), in press

Mor, G., Cardenas, I. (2010). The immune system in pregnancy: a unique complexity. *Am J Reprod Immunol*, Vol.63, No.6, (June 2010), pp. 425-433

Nakashima, A., Ito, M., Shima, T., Bac, N.D., Hidaka, T., Saito, S. (2010). Accumulation of IL-17-positive cells in decidua of inevitable abortion cases. *Am J Reprod Immunol*, Vol.64, No.1, (July 2010), pp. 4-11

Panyi, G., Possani, L.D., Rodríguez de la Vega, R.C., Gáspár, R., Varga, Z. (2006). K+ channel blockers: novel tools to inhibit T cell activation leading to specific immunosuppression. *Curr Pharm Des*, Vol.12, No.18, (December 2006), pp. 2199-2220

Passos, S.T., Silver, J.S., O'Hara, A.C., Sehy, D., Stumhofer, J.S., Hunter, C.A. (2010). IL-6 promotes NK cell production of IL-17 during toxoplasmosis. *J Immunol*, Vol.184, No.4, (February 2010), pp. 1776-1783

Perillo, N.L., Pace, K.E., Seilhamer, J.J., Baum, L.G. (1995). Apoptosis of T cells mediated by galectin-1. *Nature*, Vol.378, No.6558, (December 1995), pp. 736-739

Piccinni, M.P., Beloni, L., Livi, C., Maggi, E., Scarselli, G.F., Romagnani, S., (1998). Defective production of both leukemia inhibitory factor and type 2 T-helper cytokines by decidual T cells in unexplained recurrent abortions. *Nat Med*, Vol.4, No.9, (September 1998), pp. 1020-1024

Piccinni, M.P. (2010). T cell tolerance towards the fetal allograft. *J Reprod Immunol*, Vol.85, No.1, (May 2010), pp. 71-75

Rabinovich, G.A., Iglesias, M.M., Modesti, N.M., Castagna, L.F., Wolfenstein-Todel, C., Riera, C.M., Sotomayor, C.E. (1998). Activated rat macrophages produce a galectin-1-like protein that induces apoptosis of T cells: biochemical and functional characterization. *J Immunol*, Vol.160, No.10, (May 1998), pp. 4831-4840

Rabinovich, G.A., Ariel, A., Hershkoviz, R., Hirabayashi, J., Kasai, K.I., Lider, O. (1999a). Specific inhibition of T-cell adhesion to extracellular matrix and proinflammatory cytokine secretion by human recombinant galectin-1. *Immunology*, Vol.97, No.1, (May 1999), pp. 100-106

Rabinovich, G.A., Daly, G., Dreja, H., Tailor, H., Riera, C.M., Hirabayashi, J., Chernajovsky, Y. (1999b). Recombinant galectin-1 and its genetic delivery suppress collagen-induced arthritis via T cell apoptosis. *J Exp Med*, Vol.190, No.3, (August 1999), pp. 385-398

Rappaport, V.J., Hirata, G., Yap, H.K., Jordan, S.C. (1990). Anti-vascular endothelial cell antibodies in severe preeclampsia. *Am J Obstet Gynecol*, Vol.162, No.1, (January 1990), pp. 138-146

Rein, D.T., Schondorf, T., Gohring, U.J., Kurbacher, C.M., Pinto, I., Breidenbach, M., Mallmann, P., Kolhagen, H., Engel, H. (2002). Cytokine expression in peripheral blood lymphocytes indicates a switch to T(HELPER) cells in patients with preeclampsia. *J Reprod Immunol*, Vol.54, No.1-2, (March 2002), pp. 133-142

Robillard, P.Y., Hulsey, T.C., Alexander, G.R., Keenan, A., de Caunes, F., Papiernik, E. (1993). Paternity patterns and risk of preeclampsia in the last pregnancy in multiparae. *J Reprod Immunol*, Vol.24, No.1, (May 1993), pp. 1-12

Robertson, S.A., Bromfield, J.J., Tremellen, K.P. (2003). Seminal 'priming' for protection from pre-eclampsia – a unifying hypothesis. *J Reprod Immunol*, Vol.59, No.2, (August 2003), pp. 253-265

Romagnani, S. (1991). Human Th1 and Th2: doubt no more. *Immunol Today*, Vol.12, No.8, (August 1991), pp. 256-257

Rusterholz, C., Hahn, S., Holzgreve, W. (2007). Role of placentally produced inflammatory and regulatory cytokines in pregnancy and the etiology of preeclampsia. *Semin Immunopathol*, Vol.29, No.2, (June 2007), pp. 151-162

Saito, S., Sakai, M., Sasaki, Y., Tanebe, K., Tsuda, H., Michimata, T. (1999a). Quantitative analysis of peripheral blood Th0, Th1, Th2 and the Th1:Th2 cell ratio during normal human pregnancy and preeclampsia. *Clin Exp Immunol*, Vol.117, No.3, (September 1999), pp. 550-555

Saito, S., Umekage, H., Sakamoto, Y., Sakai, M., Tanebe, K., Sasaki, Y., Morikawa, H. (1999b). Increased T-helper-1-type immunity and decreased T-helper-2-type immunity in patients with preeclampsia. *Am J Reprod Immunol*, Vol.41, No.5, (May 1999), pp. 297-306

Saito, S., Shiozaki, A., Nakashima, A., Sakai, M., Sasaki, Y. (2007). The role of the immune system in preeclampsia. *Mol Aspects Med*, Vol.28, No.2, (April 2007), pp. 192-209

Saito, S. (2010). Th17 cells and regulatory T cells: new light on pathophysiology of preeclampsia. *Immunol Cell Biol*, Vol.88, No.6, (August 2010), pp. 615-617

Salha, O., Sharma, V., Dada, T., Nugent, D., Rutherford, A.J., Tomlinson, A.J., Philips, S., Allgar, V., Walker, J.J. (1999). The influence of donated gametes on the incidence of hypertensive disorders of pregnancy. *Hum Reprod,* Vol.14, No.9, (September 1999), pp. 2268-2273

Santner-Nanan, B., Peek, M.J., Khanam, R., Richarts, L., Zhu, E., Fazekas de St Groth, B., Nanan, R. (2009). Systemic increase in the ratio between Foxp3+ and IL-17-producing CD4+ T cells in healthy pregnancy but not in preeclampsia. *J Immunol,* Vol.183, No.11, (December 2009), pp. 7023-7030

Sargent, I.L., Borzychowski, A.M., Redman, C.W. (2006a). Immunoregulation in normal pregnancy and pre-eclampsia: an overview. *Reprod Biomed Online,* Vol.13, No.5, (November 2006), pp. 680-686

Sargent, I.L., Borzychowski, A.M., Redman, C.W. (2006b). NK cells and human pregnancy--an inflammatory view. *Trends Immunol,* Vol.27, No.9, (September 2006), pp. 399-404

Sargent, I.L., Borzychowski, A.M., Redman, C.W. (2007). NK cells and preeclampsia. *J Reprod Immunol,* Vol.76, No.1-2, (December 2007), pp. 40-44

Sasaki, Y., Sakai, M., Miyazaki, S., Higuma, S., Shiozaki, A., Saito, S. (2004). Decidual and peripheral blood CD4+CD25+ regulatory T cells in early pregnancy subjects and spontaneous abortion cases. *Mol Hum Reprod,* Vol.10, No.5, (May 2004), pp. 347-353

Sasaki, Y., Darmochwal-Kolarz, D., Suzuki, D., Sakai, M., Ito, M., Shima, T., Shiozaki, A., Rolinski, J., Saito, S. (2007). Proportion of peripheral blood and decidual CD4(+) CD25(bright) regulatory T cells in preeclampsia. *Clin Exp Immunol,* Vol.149, No.1, (July 2007), pp. 139-145

Shin, H.C., Benbernou, N., Esnault, S., Guenounou, M. (1999). Expression of IL-17 in human memory CD45RO+ T lymphocytes and its regulation by protein kinase A pathway. *Cytokine,* Vol.11, No.4, (April 1999), pp. 257-266

Skjaerven, R., Wilcox, A.J., Lie, R.T. (2002). The interval between pregnancies and the risk of preeclampsia. *N Engl J Med,* Vol.346, No.1, (January 2002), pp. 33-38

Somerset, D.A., Zheng, Y., Kilby, M.D., Sansom, D.M., Drayson, M.T. (2004). Normal human pregnancy is associated with an elevation in the immune suppressive CD25+ CD4+ regulatory T-cell subset. *Immunology,* Vol.112, No.1, (May 2004), pp. 38-43

Steinborn, A., Haensch, G.M., Mahnke, K., Schmitt, E., Toermer, A., Meuer, S., Sohn, C. (2008). Distinct subsets of regulatory T cells during pregnancy: is the imbalance of these subsets involved in the pathogenesis of preeclampsia? *Clin Immunol,* Vol.129, No.3, (December 2008), pp. 401-412

Tallon, D.F., Corcoran, D.J., O'Dwyer, E.M., Greally, J.F. (1984). Circulating lymphocyte subpopulations in pregnancy: a longitudinal study. *J Immunol,* Vol.132, No.4, (April 1984), pp. 1784-1787

Thway, T.M., Shlykov, S.G., Day, M.C., Sanborn, B.M., Gilstrap, L.C. 3rd, Xia, Y., Kellems, R.E. (2004). Antibodies from preeclamptic patients stimulate increased intracellular Ca2+ mobilization through angiotensin receptor activation. *Circulation,* Vol.110, No.12, (September 2004), pp. 1612-1619

Toldi, G., Svec, P., Vásárhelyi, B., Mészáros, G., Rigó, J., Tulassay, T., Treszl, A. (2008). Decreased number of FoxP3+ regulatory T cells in preeclampsia. *Acta Obstet Gynecol Scand,* Vol.87, No.11, (November 2008), pp. 1229-1233

Toldi, G., Rigó, J. Jr, Stenczer, B., Vásárhelyi, B., Molvarec, A. (2011a). Increased prevalence of IL-17-producing peripheral blood lymphocytes in preeclampsia. *Am J Reprod Immunol*, (February 2011), in press

Toldi, G., Stenczer, B., Treszl, A., Kollár, S., Molvarec, A., Tulassay, T., Rigó, J., Vásárhelyi, B. (2011b). Lymphocyte calcium influx characteristics and their modulation by Kv1.3 and IKCa1 channel inhibitors in healthy pregnancy and preeclampsia. *Am J Reprod Immunol*, Vol.65, No.2, (February 2011), pp. 154-163

Toscano, M.A., Commodaro, A.G., Ilarregui, J.M., Bianco, G.A., Liberman, A., Serra, H.M., Hirabayashi, J., Rizzo, L.V., Rabinovich, G.A. (2006). Galectin-1 suppresses autoimmune retinal disease by promoting concomitant Th2- and T regulatory-mediated anti-inflammatory responses. *J Immunol*, Vol.176, No.10, (May 2006), pp. 6323-6332

Toscano, M.A., Bianco, G.A., Ilarregui, J.M., Croci, D.O., Correale, J., Hernandez, J.D., Zwirner, N.W., Poirier, F., Riley, E.M., Baum, L.G., Rabinovich, G.A. (2007). Differential glycosylation of TH1, TH2 and TH-17 effector cells selectively regulates susceptibility to cell death. *Nat Immunol*, Vol.8, No.8, (August 2007), pp. 825-834

Trupin, L.S., Simon, L.P., Eskenazi, B. (1996). Change in paternity: a risk factor for preeclampsia in multiparas. *Epidemiology*, Vol.7, No.3, (May 1996), pp. 240-244

Valencia, X., Stephens, G., Goldbach-Mansky, R., Wilson, M., Shevach, E.M., Lipsky, P.E. (2006). TNF downmodulates the function of human CD4+CD25hi T-regulatory cells. *Blood*, Vol.108, No.1, (July 2006), pp. 253-261

von Dadelszen, P., Wilkins, T., Redman, C.W. (1999). Maternal peripheral blood leukocytes in normal and pre-eclamptic pregnancies. *Br J Obstet Gynaecol*, Vol.106, No.6, (June 1999), pp. 576-581

von Rango, U. (2008). Fetal tolerance in human pregnancy--a crucial balance between acceptance and limitation of trophoblast invasion. *Immunol Lett*, Vol.115, No.1, (January 2008), pp. 21-32

Walker, J.J. (2000). Pre-eclampsia. *Lancet*, Vol.356, No.9237, (October 2000), pp. 1260-1265

Wallukat, G., Homuth, V., Fischer, T., Lindschau, C., Horstkamp, B., Jupner, A., Baur, E., Nissen, E., Vetter, K., Neichel, D., Dudenhausen, J.W., Haller, H., Luft, F.C. (1999). Patients with preeclampsia develop agonistic autoantibodies against the angiotensin AT1 receptor. *J Clin Invest*, Vol.103, No.7, (April 1999), pp. 945-952

Wang, W.J., Hao, C.F., Lin, Y., Yin, G.J., Bao, S.H., Qiu, L.H., Lin, Q.D. (2010). Increased prevalence of T helper 17 (Th17) cells in peripheral blood and decidua in unexplained recurrent spontaneous abortion patients. *J Reprod Immunol*, Vol.84 No.2, (March 2010), pp. 164-170

Watanabe, M., Iwatani, Y., Kaneda, T., Hidaka, Y., Mitsuda, N., Morimoto, Y., Amino, N. (1997). Changes in T, B, and NK lymphocyte subsets during and after normal pregnancy. *Am J Reprod Immunol*, Vol.37, No.5, (May 1997), pp. 368-377

Wegmann, T.G., Lin, H., Guilbert, L., Mossmann, T.R. (1993). Bidirectional cytokine interactions in the maternal–fetal relationship: is successful pregnancy a Th2 phenomenon? *Immunol Today*, Vol.14, No.7, (July 1993), pp. 353-356

Wilczyński, J.R. (2006). Immunological analogy between allograft rejection, recurrent abortion and pre-eclampsia - the same basic mechanism? *Hum Immunol*, Vol.67, No.7, (July 2006), pp. 492-511

Yamamoto, T., Yoshimura, S., Geshi, Y., Sasamori, Y., Okinaga, S., Kobayashi, T., Mori, H.
     (1993). Measurement of antiphospholipid antibody by ELISA using purified beta 2-
     glycoprotein I in preeclampsia. *Clin Exp Immunol*, Vol.94, No.1, (October 1993), pp.
     196-200
Zenclussen, A.C. (2006). Regulatory T cells in pregnancy. *Springer Semin Immunopathol*,
     Vol.28, No.1, (August 2006), pp. 31-39
Zuniga, E., Rabinovich, G.A., Iglesias, M.M., Gruppi, A. (2001). Regulated expression of
     galectin-1 during B-cell activation and implications for T-cell apoptosis. *J Leukoc
     Biol*, Vol.70, No.1, (July 2001), pp. 73-79

Part 3

Osteoimmunology

8

Osteoimmunology and Cancer - Clinical Implications

Evangelos Terpos, Maria Gkotzamanidou,
Dimitrios Christoulas and Meletios A. Dimopoulos
Department of Clinical Therapeutics, University of Athens School of Medicine, Athens,
Greece

1. Introduction

The skeletal and immune systems are interconnected in normal (physiologic) and pathologic conditions. Both systems are intimately coupled, as osteoclastogenesis and hematopoiesis occur in the bone marrow. Osteoclasts, macrophages, and dendritic cells also share common precursors. Furthermore, the skeletal and immune systems share various cytokines, receptors, adaptor proteins, signaling molecules, and transcription factors, thereby allowing crosstalk to occur between the various cells and their respective signal transduction pathways involved in osteoclastogenesis and hematopoiesis.

Hematopoietic stem cells are maintained in the bone marrow. Adjacent osteoblast precursors produce signals that control hematopoietic stem cell replication and differentiation. Hematopoietic stem cells may either maintain their pluripotency or differentiate into multipotential progenitor cells, which have the capacity to form common lymphoid progenitor or common myeloid precursor cells. Common lymphoid progenitor cells undergo additional differentiation to form T lymphocytes, B lymphocytes, or natural killer cells, whereas common myeloid precursor cells form all other myeloid lineages and preosteoclasts. Activated osteoclasts are formed from the fusion of preosteoclasts and multinucleated osteoclasts, the regulation of which is complex and affected by multiple factors. Multipotential stem cells differentiate into chondrocytes, adipocytes, and mesenchyme precursors; the latter undergo differentiation to form preosteoblasts and, eventually, mature matrix-producing osteoblasts. Osteoblasts may remain on the bone surface as lining cells or undergo terminal differentiation to form osteocytes, which become encased in the mineralized bone matrix [1]. The shared lineages and paracrine signaling between osteoclasts and hematopoietic cells highlight the potential for bone-targeted agents to influence the immune system.

2. Transduction signaling pathways between skeletal and immune system

The skeletal and immune systems share various signal transduction pathways, thereby allowing a complex interplay to occur between bone metabolism and immunology. Furthermore, immune system components, such as T cells, cytokines, and chemokines, can exert substantial effects on osteoclastogenesis.

2.1 Osteoclastogenesis and immune system

Osteoclastogenesis is primarily regulated via interactions between c-FMS and macrophage colony-stimulating factor, receptor activator of nuclear factor (NF)-kappaB (RANK) and RANK ligand (RANKL), and immunoglobulin (Ig)-like receptors and their ligands [2]. The role of RANK signaling in osteoclastogenesis has also been reviewed elsewhere [2-16]. Other key regulatory pathways are described below.

RANK/RANKL/osteoprotegerin signaling

Receptor activator of NF-κB ligand is a member of the tumor necrosis factor (TNF) cytokine superfamily that is expressed by osteoblasts, monocytes, neutrophils, dendritic cells, B lymphocytes, and T lymphocytes [3]. Secretion of RANKL by osteoclastogenesis-supporting cells (osteoblasts and synovial fibroblasts) occurs in response to osteoclastogenic factors such as 1,25-dihydroxyvitamin D3, prostaglandin E2, and parathyroid hormone [2]. T cells express RANKL as a type-2 membrane-bound protein and also release it in soluble form, although the function of the soluble form remains unknown [16]. Inflammatory cytokines, such as interleukin (IL)-1, IL-6, and TNF-α, also potently induce RANKL expression on osteoblasts and synovial fibroblasts, thereby stimulating RANKL signaling [2].

Receptor activator of NF-κB, the RANKL receptor, shares high homology with CD40, which is expressed on lymphocytes and, similar to RANKL, is reported to play a role in atherosclerosis and coronary artery disease [17-19]. Interaction of RANK with RANKL is inhibited by osteoprotegerin (OPG), a soluble competitor (decoy) receptor that binds to RANKL [12, 13]. Receptor activator of NF-κB lacks intrinsic enzymatic activity in its intracellular domain and transduces signals by recruiting adaptor molecules such as the TNF-receptor–associated factor (TRAF) family of proteins, especially TRAF6 [4, 5, 15]. By an unknown mechanism, RANKL binding to RANK induces trimerization of RANK and TRAF6, leading to activation of NF-κB and of mitogen-activated protein kinases such as Jun N-terminal kinase and p38 [6]. Activated RANK can also lead to stimulation of Ig-like receptor signaling.

Nuclear factor of activated t cells cytoplasmic (NFATc)-1 pathway

Expression of NFATc-1, the master regulator of osteoclast differentiation, depends on induction of the TRAF6–NF-κB and c-FOS pathways, in addition to activation of calcium signaling [20]. Nuclear factor of activated T cells cytoplasmic-1 is initially induced by TRAF6-activated NF-κB and NFATc-2. After translocation into the nucleus, NFATc-1 autoregulates its own expression by binding to the NFAT-binding site of its promoter, enabling robust induction of NFATc-1 expression [21]. Activator protein 1 and continuous activation of calcium signaling by calcineurin are crucial for NFATc-1 autoamplification [20]. Nuclear factor of activated T cells cytoplasmic-1 cooperates with other transcription factors, such as AP1, PU.1, microphthalmia-associated transcription factor, and cyclic AMP responsive-element-binding protein, to regulate various osteoclast-specific genes, including tartrate-resistant acid phosphatase, cathepsin K, calcitonin receptor, osteoclast-associated receptor, and β3-integrin [2, 20, 22-24].

2.2 Cytokines, chemokines and osteoclastogenesis

Immune cells produce a variety of proinflammatory cytokines that contribute to bone damage [25]. Tumor necrosis factor-alpha and IL-1, -3, -6, -7, -11, -15, and -17 potentiate bone loss by inducing RANKL expression on osteoblasts or by increasing osteoclast differentiation and activation. In contrast, IL-4, -5, -10, -12, -13, and -18, and interferon (IFN)-α, -β, and -γ, inhibit osteoclastogenesis by directly or indirectly blocking RANKL signaling

(Table 1). Interleukin-1 stimulates TRAF6 expression, thereby potentiating the RANKL-RANK signaling cascade and inducing mature osteoclasts to perform bone-resorbing activity. Interferon gamma down-regulates TRAF6 expression via proteosomal degradation,

Cytokine	Main producer cells	Primary target in osteoclastogenesis	Effect on osteoclastogenesis	Role in osteoimmunology
RANKL	T-cells; Osteoblasts	Osteoclast precursor cells	Activation	Induction of osteoclast differentiation
TNF-α	Macrophages; Th1 cells	Osteoclast precursor cells; mesenchymal cells	Activation	RANKL induction on mesenchymal cells, RANKL synergy, inflammation
IL-6	Th2 cells; dendritic cells	Mesenchymal cells; T cells	Activation	RANKL induction on mesenchymal cells, Th17-cell differentiation, inflammation
IL-17	Th17 cells; memory T cells	Mesenchymal cells	Activation	RANKL induction on mesenchymal cells, inflammation
IFN-γ	Th1 cells; natural killer cells	Osteoclast precursor cells	Inhibition	RANKL signaling inhibition, cellular immunity
IL-4	Th2 cells; natural killer T cells	Osteoclast precursor cells	Inhibition	RANKL signaling inhibition, humoral immunity
IL-10	Th2 cells	Osteoclast precursor cells	Inhibition	RANKL signaling inhibition, anti-inflammatory
IL-12	Macrophages; dendritic cells	T cells	Inhibition	Th1-cell differentiation, IFN-γ and GM-CSF induction
IL-18	Macrophages; dendritic cells	T cells	Inhibition	Th1-cell differentiation, IFN-γ induction
GM-CSF	Th1 cells	Osteoclast precursor cells	Inhibition	RANKL signaling inhibition, granulocyte differentiation

Abbreviations: GM-CSF, granulocyte-macrophage colony-stimulating factor; IFN, interferon; IL, interleukin; RANKL, receptor activator of nuclear factor-κB ligand; Th, T-helper; TNF, tumor necrosis factor.

Table 1. Cytokines Involved in Osteoclastogenesis

resulting in termination of osteoclast formation [26, 27]. Receptor activator of NF-κB induces expression of IFN-β in osteoclast precursor cells, and IFN-β functions as a negative-feedback regulator of osteoclast differentiation by interfering with RANKL-induced c-FOS expression [28]. Tumor necrosis factor-alpha stimulates NF-κB activation primarily via interacting with TRAF2. Although TNF-α alone cannot induce osteoclastogenesis and TNF-α overexpression cannot rescue RANKL deficiency, TNF-α combined with transforming growth factor (TGF)-β induces osteoclastogenesis even in the absence of RANK or TRAF6 [29-31]. These results suggest that TNF-α plays a pivotal role in the pathologic activation of osteoclasts associated with inflammation [2]. Osteoblast-mediated bone formation is also affected by various soluble cytokines such as TNF-α, IL-1, and IL-4 [32]. The molecular mechanisms involved in osteoblast regulation by the immune system and the pathologic significance of such regulation are less understood than in osteoclasts.

2.3 T cells and osteoclastogenesis
In general, activated T cells exert an inhibitory effect on osteoclastogenesis. The CD4+ T helper (Th) cells have traditionally been divided into 2 main subtypes — Th1 and Th2 — based on their associated cytokine profiles. The Th1 cells mainly produce IFN-γ and IL-2, and mediate cellular immunity. In contrast, Th2 cells mainly produce IL-4, IL-5, and IL-10, and mediate humoral immunity. Although T cells express RANKL, most Th1 cytokines, as well as certain Th2 cytokines (eg, IL-4 and IL-10), exert an inhibitory effect on osteoclastogenesis. However, the Th-cell subset involved in producing IL-17 (Th17 cells) is considered to be the typical osteoclastogenic Th subset. The Th17 cells express RANKL at higher levels than Th1 or Th2 cells and, as a result, may directly participate in osteoclastogenesis. In addition, Th17 cells do not produce large amounts of IFN-γ, an inhibitor of osteoclastogenesis. Furthermore, Th17 cells activate local inflammation, triggering release of proinflammatory cytokines that potentiate RANKL expression on osteoclastogenesis-supporting cells and RANKL-RANK signal transduction in osteoclast precursor cells [33]. Interleukin-17, produced by Th17 cells, induces the synthesis of matrix-degrading enzymes, such as matrix metalloproteinases, that mediate bone and cartilage degradation [34]. The effects of Th17 cells on osteoclastogenesis are balanced by regulatory T cells, which suppress osteoclast formation via a cytokine-dependent mechanism mediated by TGF-β, IFN-γ, IL-4, and IL-10 [35-37]. Therefore, the effects of T cells on osteoclastogenesis depend on the balance between positive and negative factors expressed by these cells under pathologic conditions.

3. Disruption of the skeletal and immune systems in cancer

Tumorigenesis can disrupt the skeletal and immune systems. Tumor growth and metastasis necessitate evasion of the immune system, especially phosphoantigen-targeted gamma delta T cells (γδ T cells), which can detect and destroy cancer cells. Immune system components also play other key roles in tumor development and progression. For example, tumor-associated macrophages (TAMs) are abundant in the bone microenvironment and influence multiple steps in tumor development, including growth, survival, invasion, and metastasis, as well as angiogenesis and lymphangiogenesis [38, 39]. During early metastasis of solid tumors, disseminated tumor cells (DTCs) survive in the bone marrow of patients with various tumor types. Cancers for which DTCs have been detected in patients who have not developed overt metastases include breast, colon, gastric, lung, and prostate cancers [40-46]. The hematopoietic niche in the bone marrow also provides a "harbor" for DTCs to survive despite anticancer therapies. Whether this niche also harbors cancer cells against anticancer immune defenses is unknown. However, the shared signal transduction pathways among the bone remodeling and immune system machineries in this common microenvironment suggest that activation of this vicious cycle of tumor growth and osteolytic bone destruction could also lead to localized immunosuppression or recruitment of metastasis-supporting TAMs, an unfortunate juxtaposition of osteoimmunology effects. Later in the disease course, interactions between malignant cells and bone may result in a vicious cycle of bone destruction and cancer growth (the "seed and soil theory") [47]. The effects of cancer on bone can result in skeletal-related events (SREs) that include pathologic fracture, spinal cord compression, hypercalcemia of malignancy, and the need for radiotherapy. Furthermore, some cancers such as myeloma can exert additional deleterious effects on bone metabolism via inducing osteolysis, systemic bone loss, and suppression of new bone formation throughout the skeleton [48, 49].

3.1 Osteoclastogenesis and cancer cell growth and metastases

Osteoclast-mediated osteolysis results in release of growth factors in the bone microenvironment that facilitate cancer growth and metastases. Bone-derived cytokines provide a chemotactic stimulus for directed tumor cell migration [50]. Recent studies established that RANKL is a chemoattractant that increases migration and invasion of RANK-positive cancer cells (bone tropism) [51, 52]. In preclinical models, bone resorption by bone cell cultures stimulated proliferation of various tumor cell types, including breast cancer that possessed bone-metastasizing properties [53]. In animal models, cancer cells located immediately adjacent to bone surfaces had significantly greater proliferation rates compared with those distant from bone, suggesting a mitogenic effect within the bone microenvironment [54]. Furthermore, in an animal model wherein bone resorption was stimulated by tumor cells, the proliferation rate of metastatic cancer cells was increased in bone but not in other tissues [55].

3.2 Cancer cell biology and bone resorption

Cancer cells stimulate osteoclast-mediated osteolysis via several mechanisms. Cancer cells may express RANKL and RANK, up-regulate RANKL expression by other osteoimmune cell types, down-regulate OPG expression, and stimulate release of factors that activate RANKL-RANK signaling in osteoclasts [56]. Expression of RANKL has been detected in prostate cancer cells [57] and multiple myeloma (MM) cells [58, 59], and RANKL expression by MM cells correlated with the propensity to cause bone destruction [58]. Although breast cancer cells do not typically express RANKL [60, 61], they can up-regulate RANKL expression by osteoblasts [60, 61] and bone marrow stromal cells [61, 62]. Prostate cancer cells can up-regulate RANKL expression in osteoblasts [63], and MM cells up-regulate RANKL expression in bone marrow stromal cells [64], endothelial cells [65], and T cells [66]. Several studies also reported expression of functional RANK by breast cancer, prostate, and melanoma cell lines [51, 52]. Breast cancer cells and MM cells down-regulate OPG production by osteoblasts and bone marrow stromal cells [60, 64]. Multiple myeloma cells express the heparin sulfate proteoglycan, syndecan, on their surface, which sequesters and degrades heparin-binding proteins including OPG [67]. Notably, the RANKL-OPG balance is disturbed in severe osteolytic pathologies in favor of RANKL, with large quantities of OPG being released within the tumor microenvironment to counterbalance high RANKL concentrations [64, 68].

Bisphosphonate	Cancer type	Patients, N	Reduction of SREs	Reduction of pain	Acute-phase reaction	Survival benefit
Clodronate [70]	Multiple myeloma	350	Yes	Yes	No	NE
Clodronate [72]	Multiple myeloma	536	Yes	Yes	No	+/−[a]
Clodronate [74]	Breast cancer	173	Yes	Yes	No	No
Clodronate [75]	Prostate cancer	819	NR	NR	No	Yes
Pamidronate [76]	Multiple myeloma	392	Yes	Yes	Yes	+/−[b]
Ibandronate [77]	Multiple myeloma	198	No	No	+/−	No
Zoledronic acid [78]	Multiple myeloma or breast cancer	1,648	Yes	Yes	Yes	Yes
Zoledronic acid [79]	Breast cancer	228	Yes	Yes	Yes	NE
Zoledronic acid [80]	Lung cancer and other solid tumors	773	Yes	NE	Yes	No
Zoledronic acid [81]	Hormone-refractory prostate cancer	122	Yes	Yes	Yes	NE
Denosumab [82]	Breast cancer	2,046	Yes	NE	Yes	NE

Abbreviations: NE, not evaluated; NR, not reported; SREs, skeletal-related events.
[a]In a post hoc analysis, patients without vertebral fracture at study entry survived significantly longer on clodronate therapy (median survival was 23 months longer compared with patients receiving placebo).
[b]Survival of patients with more advanced disease was significantly increased in the pamidronate group (median survival of 21 vs 14 months, $P = .041$).

Table 2. Efficacy of Bone-Targeted Agents in Patients With Bone Metastases

4. Bone-targeted therapies and immune system in cancer

4.1 Early generation bisphosphonates

In general, early generation bisphosphonates do not appear to activate the immune system against cancer cells. However, clodronate combined with IL-2 stimulated proliferation of γδ T cells in the absence of other cellular components in peripheral blood mononuclear cell (PBMC) cultures (wherein nitrogen-containing bisphosphonates have been tested), and clodronate-treated γδ T cells exhibited higher cytotoxic activity against neuroblastoma cells compared with untreated control cells [69]. There are currently no data on whether these effects can result in meaningful anticancer activities in in vivo models. Clodronate has shown efficacy in preventing SREs in patients with bone metastases from MM [70-73] and breast cancer [74], and was recently reported to significantly prolong survival in men with bone metastases from prostate cancer [75] (Table 2) [70, 72, 74-82]. Results from trials in the adjuvant breast cancer setting were inconsistent, and provided some evidence to suggest that clodronate can delay not only metastasis to bone but also to visceral sites.

4.2 Nitrogen-containing bisphosphonates

Nitrogen-containing bisphosphonates, such as zoledronic acid (ZOL) and pamidronate, cause immune system activation against cancer cells via activating γδ T cells [83, 84]. By blocking G-protein signaling, these agents prevent differentiation of monocytes into osteoclasts, inhibit osteoclast recruitment and maturation, induce osteoclast apoptosis, and inhibit adhesion of osteoclasts to bone [85].

Pamidronate therapy is associated with SRE reductions in patients with bone metastases from MM [76]. Although there was no overall difference in survival between pamidronate- and placebo-treated patients, pamidronate prolonged survival among patients who had received more than 1 previous antimyeloma regimen (14 vs 21 months; $P = .041$; N = 392) [86]. Although evidence is limited, pamidronate has demonstrated effects on the immune system that may result in anticancer activity. Treatment with pamidronate induced expansion of γδ T cells in PBMC cultures from healthy donors, and pamidronate-activated γδ T cells produced immunostimulatory cytokines and exhibited specific cytotoxicity against lymphoma and myeloma cell lines. Furthermore, pamidronate-treated bone marrow cultures from patients with MM exhibited reduced plasma cell survival compared with untreated cultures, especially in pamidronate-treated cultures, in which activation of bone marrow γδ T cells was evident (14 of 24 patients) [87].

Administration of ibandronate to patients with advanced MM failed to reduce bone morbidity or prolong survival [77]. Ibandronate also produced a lesser reduction in markers of bone resorption and disease activity, including N-telopeptide of type I collagen (NTX), IL-6, and β2-microglobulin, compared with pamidronate [88]. However, ibandronate has demonstrated efficacy in the reduction of skeletal complications in other tumor types such as breast cancer [89].

Numerous studies established that zoledronic acid (ZOL) exhibits consistent efficacy in delaying and preventing SREs in patients with malignant bone disease from MM [78, 90, 91] and various solid tumors including breast [79], lung [80, 92], and prostate cancers [81]. In a 25-month randomized trial comparing ZOL with pamidronate in patients with bone lesions from MM or breast cancer (N = 1,648), a 15-minute infusion of 4 mg ZOL was at least as effective as a 2-hour infusion of 90 mg pamidronate at reducing the risk of SRE complications in the overall population [78]. Similarly, treating patients with lung cancer and other solid tumors with ZOL resulted in fewer patients developing SREs (ZOL 8 mg reduced to 4 mg = 36%, placebo = 46%; P = .023; N = 773) [80]. Administration of ZOL to men with hormone-refractory metastatic prostate cancer also reduced the proportion of patients with SREs (38% vs 49%; P = .028 vs placebo; N = 122) [81].

A recent study also demonstrated that ZOL may elicit anticancer effects associated with immune system stimulation. Zoledronic acid activated γδ T cells in vitro, and administration of ZOL to patients with prostate cancer resulted in the activation of γδ T cells in peripheral blood after the first infusion. Moreover, after the first ZOL infusion, serum prostate-specific antigen (PSA) levels were reduced in 3 of 11 evaluable patients, and PSA velocity was reduced in 5 of 10 evaluable patients [93]. These results suggest that ZOL-activated γδ T cells may be associated with the induction of an anticancer response in patients with prostate cancer.

Numerous in vitro studies established that ZOL directly and indirectly inhibits multiple steps involved in the processes of cancer development and progression. In addition, ZOL stimulates cancer cell apoptosis and expansion of γδ T cells, which play an important role in immune surveillance against neoplasia [94]. Preclinical studies reported that ZOL elicits anticancer activity in various cancer types and exhibits synergy with cytotoxic agents [95-100]. Four separate studies reported that ZOL reduced the persistence of DTCs in the bone marrow of patients with breast cancer [101-104]. In the clinical setting, adding ZOL to standard anticancer therapy improved clinical outcomes in early breast cancer. Administration of ZOL combined with adjuvant endocrine therapy to premenopausal women improved disease-free survival (hazard ratio [HR] = 0.64; P = .01) compared with endocrine therapy alone in the ABCSG-12 trial (N = 1,803) [105]. Similarly, ZOL plus neoadjuvant chemotherapy reduced residual invasive tumor size by 44% compared with chemotherapy in an exploratory subgroup from the AZURE trial (P = .006; n = 205) [106]. A multivariate analysis adjusted for potential prognostic factors in addition to neoadjuvant treatment group demonstrated that patients treated with ZOL plus neoadjuvant chemotherapy had a 2-fold greater complete pathologic response rate (breast and axilla) compared with patients treated with chemotherapy alone (odds ratio = 2.2; P = .1457). In the ZO-FAST (N = 1,065; median follow-up = 48 months; HR = 0.59; P = .0176) and Z-FAST (N = 602; median follow-up = 61 months; P = .6283) studies in postmenopausal women receiving adjuvant letrozole, immediate addition of ZOL reduced disease recurrence [107, 108]. In contrast with ABCSG-12, which had disease-free survival as a primary endpoint, ZO-FAST and Z-FAST were not designed or powered to evaluate disease recurrence (primary endpoints were bone loss); however, these studies demonstrated that upfront administration of ZOL resulted in improved disease-free survival among women with breast cancer. Subset analyses of the phase III clinical studies revealed that ZOL significantly prolonged survival compared with placebo among patients with high baseline NTX levels. Benefits were independent of SRE prevention, and multiple anticancer mechanisms, some of which involved immune system activation, may have contributed [109, 110]. Additionally, ZOL elicited anticancer responses in patients with MM, bladder cancer, lung cancer, or advanced solid tumors [111-114]. The Medical Research Council (MRC) Myeloma IX trial demonstrated that, after median follow-up of 3.7 years, ZOL significantly improved overall survival (by 5.5 months; 16% reduction in risk of death; P = .0118) and progression-free survival (by 2 months; 12% reduction in risk of disease progression; P = .0179) versus clodronate in patients with newly diagnosed MM (N = 1,960 evaluable patients) [111]. The survival benefit associated with ZOL was maintained in analyses adjusting for the potential effects of SREs on survival (P = .0178 vs clodronate), again supporting anticancer mechanisms for ZOL, which may involve positive effects on anticancer immune responses [111].

4.3 Anti-RANKL agents

Denosumab is a fully human IgG2 monoclonal antibody that binds to RANKL with high affinity and specificity, thereby inhibiting osteoclastogenesis. The effects of denosumab on bone remodeling have been evaluated in patients with postmenopausal osteoporosis, rheumatoid arthritis, and various cancers [115-118]. Limited safety data from the advanced cancer setting have been released. However, results from phase III studies in bone-loss settings suggested that adverse immunologic effects might occur. The FREEDOM trial, a phase III clinical study of 7,868 healthy postmenopausal women with osteoporosis, demonstrated that denosumab reduced the risk of new vertebral fractures by 68% compared with placebo ($P < .001$) [117]. A number of recent studies also demonstrated that denosumab can prevent SREs among patients with bone metastases from breast cancer, prostate cancer, other solid tumors, or MM. Denosumab was superior to ZOL in delaying time to first on-study SRE (HR = 0.82; $P = .01$ superiority), and time to first and subsequent on-study SREs (rate ratio = 0.77; $P = .001$) in 2,046 patients with advanced breast cancer [82], and in delaying time to first on-study SRE in patients with advanced castration-resistant prostate cancer (CRPC) (HR = 0.82; $P = .008$ superiority; N = 1,901) [119]. Median time to first on-study SRE was 20.7 months for denosumab versus 17.1 months for ZOL [119]. However, a significantly greater proportion of denosumab-treated patients experienced increased PSA levels compared with ZOL-treated patients (3.8% vs 2.0%, respectively; $P < .05$) [119]. Based on these results, it is possible that RANKL inhibition may impair immunosurveillance. Denosumab was non-inferior to ZOL in delaying time to first SRE in 1,776 patients with other advanced solid tumors or MM (HR = 0.84; $P = .0007$) [115]. Denosumab demonstrated antitumor activity in a phase II trial in 37 patients with benign giant-cell tumor (GCT) of bone, a tumor type that overexpresses RANKL and is associated with increased osteoclastic activity [120]. Given the low metastatic potential of GCT, the results observed in this patient population may not translate to patients with malignancies wherein the pathophysiology is distinct from that of GCT. Anticancer activity of blocking RANKL has been recently described in mouse models. RANKL inhibition was acting directly on hormone-induced mammary epithelium at early stages in tumorigenesis, and the permissive contribution of progesterone to increased mammary cancer incidence was due to RANKL-dependent proliferative changes in the mammary epithelium [121]. Based on these data, we assume that denosumab may have an anticancer activity; however, this has not yet been demonstrated in the clinical setting. Signaling via the RANKL-RANK pathway is involved in B-cell and T-cell differentiation and in survival of dendritic cells. As a result, concerns have been raised regarding possible immunosuppression with RANKL inhibitors. Recent clinical studies suggest that increased infection risk may be associated with denosumab therapy. The incidence of skin infections requiring hospitalization (cellulitis: 0.3% vs < 0.1% for placebo; $P = .002$) and endocarditis (3 patients vs 0 for placebo) was increased among postmenopausal women with osteoporosis who received denosumab therapy (FREEDOM) [115, 117]. A meta-analysis of 10,329 patients with osteopenia or osteoporosis also reported an increased risk of serious infections (odds ratio = 4.54 for denosumab vs placebo; $P = .03$) [122]. Serious infections were reported in 2.3% of denosumab-treated patients with early stage breast cancer compared with 0.8% of placebo-treated patients (P = not reported [NR];

N = 249; HALT-BC trial) [123]. Similarly, serious infections occurred at a higher incidence among denosumab-treated patients with androgen-dependent prostate cancer (5.9% vs 4.6% for placebo; P = NR; N = 1,468; HALT-PC trial) [124]. Urinary-tract infections also occurred more frequently among denosumab-treated patients with prostate cancer-related bone metastases (15% vs 6% for bisphosphonates; P = NR; N = 49) [125].

Denosumab is specific for human and certain nonhuman primate RANKL, and fails to inactivate rodent RANKL. Consequently, no carcinogenicity studies have been performed with denosumab because of the absence of an appropriate animal model. However, safety analyses from clinical trials of denosumab to prevent bone loss in patients receiving hormone-ablation therapy (HALT) for early stage breast or prostate cancer suggest that the potential for cancer progression may be increased with denosumab therapy. Among 1,456 patients with androgen-dependent prostate cancer in HALT-PC, 8.2% (n = 60) of denosumab-treated patients and 5.5% (n = 40) of placebo-treated patients experienced metastatic events (P = NR) [115]. Similarly, metastatic events were reported in 7% (n = 9) of denosumab-treated patients compared with 4.2% (n = 5) of placebo-treated patients with breast cancer in HALT-BC (P = NR; N = 249) [115]. Indeed, given the significantly increased rates of PSA progression in patients with CRPC and the significantly reduced survival in patients with MM treated with denosumab versus ZOL in the phase III clinical trials program (HR = 2.26) [126], further investigations on the potential effects of RANKL inhibition on cancer immunosurveillance and response are warranted.

5. Conclusions

The skeletal and immune systems have a complex relationship under normal (physiologic) and pathologic conditions. The RANKL-RANK-OPG signal transduction pathway plays a key role in regulating osteoclastogenesis. However, the effects of RANKL signaling are not limited to the skeletal system; RANKL is also expressed in other regulatory systems including the immune, cardiovascular, endocrine, and nervous systems. Expression of RANKL in the immune system regulates antigen-specific T-cell and B-cell responses, as well as the ability of T cells to interact with dendritic cells. Furthermore, RANKL directly affects the survival of antigen-presenting dendritic cells, which help other cells in the immune system to recognize and destroy abnormal cells and foreign antigens. Because of the systemic nature of RANKL expression, RANKL inhibition to prevent bone destruction may result in unintended consequences outside of the bone, including immune suppression with resulting possible increases in risk of infection or new malignancies. The long-term safety profiles of agents targeting this pathway are not yet known.

Currently available therapies designed to reduce pathologic osteolysis may also result in modulation of the immune system. Nitrogen-containing bisphosphonates such as ZOL exert beneficial effects on the immune system, resulting in activation of anticancer responses, as demonstrated in several clinical studies in various malignancies. Careful consideration should be paid to the shared pathways in bone immunology to maximize beneficial and minimize potentially negative effects in the clinical setting.

6. References

[1] Lorenzo J, Horowitz M, Choi Y (2008) Osteoimmunology: interactions of the bone and immune system. Endocr Rev 29:403-440

[2] Takayanagi H (2007) Osteoimmunology: shared mechanisms and crosstalk between the immune and bone systems. Nat Rev Immunol 7:292-304

[3] Caetano-Lopes J, Canhao H, Fonseca JE (2009) Osteoimmunology — the hidden immune regulation of bone. Autoimmun Rev 8:250-255

[4] Gohda J, Akiyama T, Koga T, Takayanagi H, Tanaka S, Inoue J (2005) RANK-mediated amplification of TRAF6 signaling leads to NFATc1 induction during osteoclastogenesis. EMBO J 24:790-799

[5] Kadono Y, Okada F, Perchonock C, Jang HD, Lee SY, Kim N, Choi Y (2005) Strength of TRAF6 signalling determines osteoclastogenesis. EMBO Rep 6:171-176

[6] Kobayashi N, Kadono Y, Naito A, Matsumoto K, Yamamoto T, Tanaka S, Inoue J (2001) Segregation of TRAF6-mediated signaling pathways clarifies its role in osteoclastogenesis. EMBO J 20:1271-1280

[7] Koga T, Inui M, Inoue K, Kim S, Suematsu A, Kobayashi E, Iwata T, Ohnishi H, Matozaki T, Kodama T, Taniguchi T, Takayanagi H, Takai T (2004) Costimulatory signals mediated by the ITAM motif cooperate with RANKL for bone homeostasis. Nature 428:758-763

[8] Mao D, Epple H, Uthgenannt B, Novack DV, Faccio R (2006) PLCgamma2 regulates osteoclastogenesis via its interaction with ITAM proteins and GAB2. J Clin Invest 116:2869-2879

[9] Mocsai A, Humphrey MB, Van Ziffle JA, Hu Y, Burghardt A, Spusta SC, Majumdar S, Lanier LL, Lowell CA, Nakamura MC (2004) The immunomodulatory adapter proteins DAP12 and Fc receptor gamma-chain (FcRgamma) regulate development of functional osteoclasts through the Syk tyrosine kinase. Proc Natl Acad Sci U S A 101:6158-6163

[10] Ross FP, Teitelbaum SL (2005) alphavbeta3 and macrophage colony-stimulating factor: partners in osteoclast biology. Immunol Rev 208:88-105

[11] Sato K, Suematsu A, Nakashima T, Takemoto-Kimura S, Aoki K, Morishita Y, Asahara H, Ohya K, Yamaguchi A, Takai T, Kodama T, Chatila TA, Bito H, Takayanagi H (2006) Regulation of osteoclast differentiation and function by the CaMK-CREB pathway. Nat Med 12:1410-1416

[12] Simonet WS, Lacey DL, Dunstan CR, Kelley M, Chang MS, Luthy R, Nguyen HQ, Wooden S, Bennett L, Boone T, Shimamoto G, DeRose M, Elliott R, Colombero A, Tan HL, Trail G, Sullivan J, Davy E, Bucay N, Renshaw-Gegg L, Hughes TM, Hill D, Pattison W, Campbell P, Sander S, Van G, Tarpley J, Derby P, Lee R, Boyle WJ (1997) Osteoprotegerin: a novel secreted protein involved in the regulation of bone density. Cell 89:309-319

[13] Tsuda E, Goto M, Mochizuki S, Yano K, Kobayashi F, Morinaga T, Higashio K (1997) Isolation of a novel cytokine from human fibroblasts that specifically inhibits osteoclastogenesis. Biochem Biophys Res Commun 234:137-142

[14] Wagner EF, Eferl R (2005) Fos/AP-1 proteins in bone and the immune system. Immunol Rev 208:126-140

[15] Wong BR, Josien R, Lee SY, Vologodskaia M, Steinman RM, Choi Y (1998) The TRAF family of signal transducers mediates NF-kappaB activation by the TRANCE receptor. J Biol Chem 273:28355-28359

[16] Wong BR, Rho J, Arron J, Robinson E, Orlinick J, Chao M, Kalachikov S, Cayani E, Bartlett FS, 3rd, Frankel WN, Lee SY, Choi Y (1997) TRANCE is a novel ligand of

the tumor necrosis factor receptor family that activates c-Jun N-terminal kinase in T cells. J Biol Chem 272:25190-25194

[17] Gururajan P, Gurumurthy P, Nayar P, Babu S, Sarasabharati A, Victor D, Cherian KM (2009) Increased serum concentrations of soluble CD40 ligand as a prognostic marker in patients with acute coronary syndrome. Indian J Clin Biochem 24:229-233

[18] Montecucco F, Steffens S, Mach F (2007) The immune response is involved in atherosclerotic plaque calcification: could the RANKL/RANK/OPG system be a marker of plaque instability? Clin Dev Immunol 2007:75805

[19] Chakraborty S, Cheek J, Sakthivel B, Aronow BJ, Yutzey KE (2008) Shared gene expression profiles in developing heart valves and osteoblast progenitor cells. Physiol Genomics 35:75-85

[20] Takayanagi H, Kim S, Koga T, Nishina H, Isshiki M, Yoshida H, Saiura A, Isobe M, Yokochi T, Inoue J, Wagner EF, Mak TW, Kodama T, Taniguchi T (2002) Induction and activation of the transcription factor NFATc1 (NFAT2) integrate RANKL signaling in terminal differentiation of osteoclasts. Dev Cell 3:889-901

[21] Asagiri M, Sato K, Usami T, Ochi S, Nishina H, Yoshida H, Morita I, Wagner EF, Mak TW, Serfling E, Takayanagi H (2005) Autoamplification of NFATc1 expression determines its essential role in bone homeostasis. J Exp Med 202:1261-1269

[22] Crotti TN, Flannery M, Walsh NC, Fleming JD, Goldring SR, McHugh KP (2006) NFATc1 regulation of the human beta3 integrin promoter in osteoclast differentiation. Gene 372:92-102

[23] Kim Y, Sato K, Asagiri M, Morita I, Soma K, Takayanagi H (2005) Contribution of nuclear factor of activated T cells c1 to the transcriptional control of immunoreceptor osteoclast-associated receptor but not triggering receptor expressed by myeloid cells-2 during osteoclastogenesis. J Biol Chem 280:32905-32913

[24] Matsumoto M, Kogawa M, Wada S, Takayanagi H, Tsujimoto M, Katayama S, Hisatake K, Nogi Y (2004) Essential role of p38 mitogen-activated protein kinase in cathepsin K gene expression during osteoclastogenesis through association of NFATc1 and PU.1. J Biol Chem 279:45969-45979

[25] Herman S, Kronke G, Schett G (2008) Molecular mechanisms of inflammatory bone damage: emerging targets for therapy. Trends Mol Med 14:245-253

[26] Datta HK, Ng WF, Walker JA, Tuck SP, Varanasi SS (2008) The cell biology of bone metabolism. J Clin Pathol 61:577-587

[27] Takayanagi H, Ogasawara K, Hida S, Chiba T, Murata S, Sato K, Takaoka A, Yokochi T, Oda H, Tanaka K, Nakamura K, Taniguchi T (2000) T-cell-mediated regulation of osteoclastogenesis by signalling cross-talk between RANKL and IFN-gamma. Nature 408:600-605

[28] Takayanagi H, Kim S, Matsuo K, Suzuki H, Suzuki T, Sato K, Yokochi T, Oda H, Nakamura K, Ida N, Wagner EF, Taniguchi T (2002) RANKL maintains bone homeostasis through c-Fos-dependent induction of interferon-beta. Nature 416:744-749

[29] Lam J, Takeshita S, Barker JE, Kanagawa O, Ross FP, Teitelbaum SL (2000) TNF-alpha induces osteoclastogenesis by direct stimulation of macrophages exposed to permissive levels of RANK ligand. J Clin Invest 106:1481-1488

[30] Li P, Schwarz EM, O'Keefe RJ, Ma L, Boyce BF, Xing L (2004) RANK signaling is not required for TNFalpha-mediated increase in CD11(hi) osteoclast precursors but is essential for mature osteoclast formation in TNFalpha-mediated inflammatory arthritis. J Bone Miner Res 19:207-213

[31] Kim N, Kadono Y, Takami M, Lee J, Lee SH, Okada F, Kim JH, Kobayashi T, Odgren PR, Nakano H, Yeh WC, Lee SK, Lorenzo JA, Choi Y (2005) Osteoclast differentiation independent of the TRANCE-RANK-TRAF6 axis. J Exp Med 202:589-595

[32] Walsh MC, Kim N, Kadono Y, Rho J, Lee SY, Lorenzo J, Choi Y (2006) Osteoimmunology: interplay between the immune system and bone metabolism. Annu Rev Immunol 24:33-63

[33] Sato K, Suematsu A, Okamoto K, Yamaguchi A, Morishita Y, Kadono Y, Tanaka S, Kodama T, Akira S, Iwakura Y, Cua DJ, Takayanagi H (2006) Th17 functions as an osteoclastogenic helper T cell subset that links T cell activation and bone destruction. J Exp Med 203:2673-2682

[34] David JP (2007) Osteoimmunology: a view from the bone. Adv Immunol 95:149-165

[35] Askenasy N, Kaminitz A, Yarkoni S (2008) Mechanisms of T regulatory cell function. Autoimmun Rev 7:370-375

[36] Kim YG, Lee CK, Nah SS, Mun SH, Yoo B, Moon HB (2007) Human CD4+CD25+ regulatory T cells inhibit the differentiation of osteoclasts from peripheral blood mononuclear cells. Biochem Biophys Res Commun 357:1046-1052

[37] Kelchtermans H, Geboes L, Mitera T, Huskens D, Leclercq G, Matthys P (2009) Activated CD4+CD25+ regulatory T cells inhibit osteoclastogenesis and collagen-induced arthritis. Ann Rheum Dis 68:744-750

[38] Biswas SK, Lewis CE (2010) NF-κB as a central regulator of macrophage function in tumors. J Leukoc Biol 88:877-884

[39] Hagemann T, Biswas SK, Lawrence T, Sica A, Lewis CE (2009) Regulation of macrophage function in tumors: the multifaceted role of NF-kappaB. Blood 113:3139-3146

[40] Pantel K, Alix-Panabieres C, Riethdorf S (2009) Cancer micrometastases. Nat Rev Clin Oncol 6:339-351

[41] Raimondi C, Gradilone A, Gandini O, Petracca A, Nicolazzo C, Palazzo A, Naso G, Cortesi E, Gazzaniga P (2010) Circulating tumor cells in breast cancer: are currently available detection methods enough? (abstract 170PD). In: Presented at the 35th ESMO Congress; 8-12 October 2010, Milan, Italy

[42] De Giorgi U, Mego M, Scarpi E, Handy BC, Jackson SA, Reuben J, Valero V, Hortobagyi GN, Ueno N, Cristofanilli M (2010) Relationship between lymphopenia and circulating tumor cells as prognostic factors for overall survival in metastatic breast cancer (abstract 171PD). In: Presented at the 35th ESMO Congress; 8-12 October 2010, Milan, Italy

[43] Sastre J, Maestro ML, Gomez MA, Rivera Herrero F, Valladares M, Massuti B, Gallen M, Benavides M, Diaz Rubio E, Aranda E (2010) Enumeration circulating tumor cells (CTCs) is a prognostic and predictive factor for progression-free survival (PFS) and overall survival (OS) in colon cancer patients receiving first-line chemotherapy plus bevacizumab. A TTD Spanish Group Cooperative Study (abstract 173PD). In: Presented at the 35th ESMO Congress; 8-12 October 2010, Milan, Italy

[44] Seeliger H, Spatz H, Jauch KW (2003) Minimal residual disease in gastric cancer. Recent Results Cancer Res 162:79-87

[45] Passlick B (2001) Micrometastases in non-small cell lung cancer (NSCLC). Lung Cancer 34(suppl 3):S25-S29

[46] Morgan TM, Lange PH, Porter MP, Lin DW, Ellis WJ, Gallaher IS, Vessella RL (2009) Disseminated tumor cells in prostate cancer patients after radical prostatectomy and without evidence of disease predicts biochemical recurrence. Clin Cancer Res 15:677-683

[47] Roodman GD, Dougall WC (2008) RANK ligand as a therapeutic target for bone metastases and multiple myeloma. Cancer Treat Rev 34:92-101

[48] Kyle RA, Gertz MA, Witzig TE, Lust JA, Lacy MQ, Dispenzieri A, Fonseca R, Rajkumar SV, Offord JR, Larson DR, Plevak ME, Therneau TM, Greipp PR (2003) Review of 1027 patients with newly diagnosed multiple myeloma. Mayo Clin Proc 78:21-33

[49] Hjorth-Hansen H, Seifert MF, Borset M, Aarset H, Ostlie A, Sundan A, Waage A (1999) Marked osteoblastopenia and reduced bone formation in a model of multiple myeloma bone disease in severe combined immunodeficiency mice. J Bone Miner Res 14:256-263

[50] Orr W, Varani J, Gondex MK, Ward PA, Mundy GR (1979) Chemotactic responses of tumor cells to products of resorbing bone. Science 203:176-179

[51] Mori K, Le Goff B, Charrier C, Battaglia S, Heymann D, Redini F (2007) DU145 human prostate cancer cells express functional receptor activator of NFkappaB: new insights in the prostate cancer bone metastasis process. Bone 40:981-990

[52] Jones DH, Nakashima T, Sanchez OH, Kozieradzki I, Komarova SV, Sarosi I, Morony S, Rubin E, Sarao R, Hojilla CV, Komnenovic V, Kong YY, Schreiber M, Dixon SJ, Sims SM, Khokha R, Wada T, Penninger JM (2006) Regulation of cancer cell migration and bone metastasis by RANKL. Nature 440:692-696

[53] Manishen WJ, Sivananthan K, Orr FW (1986) Resorbing bone stimulates tumor cell growth. A role for the host microenvironment in bone metastasis. Am J Pathol 123:39-45

[54] Kostenuik PJ, Singh G, Suyama KL, Orr FW (1992) A quantitative model for spontaneous bone metastasis: evidence for a mitogenic effect of bone on Walker 256 cancer cells. Clin Exp Metastasis 10:403-410

[55] Kostenuik PJ, Singh G, Suyama KL, Orr FW (1992) Stimulation of bone resorption results in a selective increase in the growth rate of spontaneously metastatic Walker 256 cancer cells in bone. Clin Exp Metastasis 10:411-418

[56] Kearns AE, Khosla S, Kostenuik PJ (2008) Receptor activator of nuclear factor kappaB ligand and osteoprotegerin regulation of bone remodeling in health and disease. Endocr Rev 29:155-192

[57] Brown JM, Corey E, Lee ZD, True LD, Yun TJ, Tondravi M, Vessella RL (2001) Osteoprotegerin and rank ligand expression in prostate cancer. Urology 57:611-616

[58] Farrugia AN, Atkins GJ, To LB, Pan B, Horvath N, Kostakis P, Findlay DM, Bardy P, Zannettino AC (2003) Receptor activator of nuclear factor-kappaB ligand expression by human myeloma cells mediates osteoclast formation in vitro and correlates with bone destruction in vivo. Cancer Res 63:5438-5445

[59] Sezer O, Heider U, Zavrski I, Kuhne CA, Hofbauer LC (2003) RANK ligand and osteoprotegerin in myeloma bone disease. Blood 101:2094-2098

[60] Thomas RJ, Guise TA, Yin JJ, Elliott J, Horwood NJ, Martin TJ, Gillespie MT (1999) Breast cancer cells interact with osteoblasts to support osteoclast formation. Endocrinology 140:4451-4458

[61] Kitazawa S, Kitazawa R (2002) RANK ligand is a prerequisite for cancer-associated osteolytic lesions. J Pathol 198:228-236

[62] Mancino AT, Klimberg VS, Yamamoto M, Manolagas SC, Abe E (2001) Breast cancer increases osteoclastogenesis by secreting M-CSF and upregulating RANKL in stromal cells. J Surg Res 100:18-24

[63] Fizazi K, Yang J, Peleg S, Sikes CR, Kreimann EL, Daliani D, Olive M, Raymond KA, Janus TJ, Logothetis CJ, Karsenty G, Navone NM (2003) Prostate cancer cells-osteoblast interaction shifts expression of growth/survival-related genes in prostate cancer and reduces expression of osteoprotegerin in osteoblasts. Clin Cancer Res 9:2587-2597

[64] Giuliani N, Bataille R, Mancini C, Lazzaretti M, Barille S (2001) Myeloma cells induce imbalance in the osteoprotegerin/osteoprotegerin ligand system in the human bone marrow environment. Blood 98:3527-3533

[65] Okada T, Akikusa S, Okuno H, Kodaka M (2003) Bone marrow metastatic myeloma cells promote osteoclastogenesis through RANKL on endothelial cells. Clin Exp Metastasis 20:639-646

[66] Giuliani N, Colla S, Sala R, Moroni M, Lazzaretti M, La Monica S, Bonomini S, Hojden M, Sammarelli G, Barille S, Bataille R, Rizzoli V (2002) Human myeloma cells stimulate the receptor activator of nuclear factor-kappa B ligand (RANKL) in T lymphocytes: a potential role in multiple myeloma bone disease. Blood 100:4615-4621

[67] Standal T, Seidel C, Hjertner O, Plesner T, Sanderson RD, Waage A, Borset M, Sundan A (2002) Osteoprotegerin is bound, internalized, and degraded by multiple myeloma cells. Blood 100:3002-3007

[68] Grimaud E, Soubigou L, Couillaud S, Coipeau P, Moreau A, Passuti N, Gouin F, Redini F, Heymann D (2003) Receptor activator of nuclear factor kappaB ligand (RANKL)/osteoprotegerin (OPG) ratio is increased in severe osteolysis. Am J Pathol 163:2021-2031

[69] Schilbach K, Geiselhart A, Handgretinger R (2001) Induction of proliferation and augmented cytotoxicity of gammadelta T lymphocytes by bisphosphonate clodronate. Blood 97:2917-2918

[70] Lahtinen R, Laakso M, Palva I, Virkkunen P, Elomaa I (1992) Randomised, placebo-controlled multicentre trial of clodronate in multiple myeloma. Finnish Leukaemia Group. Lancet 340:1049-1052

[71] Laakso M, Lahtinen R, Virkkunen P, Elomaa I (1994) Subgroup and cost-benefit analysis of the Finnish multicentre trial of clodronate in multiple myeloma. Finnish Leukaemia Group. Br J Haematol 87:725-729

[72] McCloskey EV, MacLennan IC, Drayson MT, Chapman C, Dunn J, Kanis JA (1998) A randomized trial of the effect of clodronate on skeletal morbidity in multiple myeloma. MRC Working Party on Leukaemia in Adults. Br J Haematol 100:317-325

[73] McCloskey EV, Dunn JA, Kanis JA, MacLennan IC, Drayson MT (2001) Long-term follow-up of a prospective, double-blind, placebo-controlled randomized trial of clodronate in multiple myeloma. Br J Haematol 113:1035-1043

[74] Paterson AHG, Powles TJ, Kanis JA, McCloskey E, Hanson J, Ashley S (1993) Double-blind controlled trial of oral clodronate in patients with bone metastases from breast cancer. J Clin Oncol 11:59-65

[75] Dearnaley DP, Mason MD, Parmar MKB, Sanders K, Sydes MR (2009) Adjuvant therapy with oral sodium clodronate in locally advanced and metastatic prostate cancer: long-term overall survival results from the MRC PR04 and PR05 randomised controlled trials. Lancet Oncol 10:872-876

[76] Berenson JR, Lichtenstein A, Porter L, Dimopoulos MA, Bordoni R, George S, Lipton A, Keller A, Ballester O, Kovacs MJ, Blacklock HA, Bell R, Simeone J, Reitsma DJ, Heffernan M, Seaman J, Knight RD (1996) Efficacy of pamidronate in reducing skeletal events in patients with advanced multiple myeloma. Myeloma Aredia Study Group. N Engl J Med 334:488-493

[77] Menssen HD, Sakalova A, Fontana A, Herrmann Z, Boewer C, Facon T, Lichinitser MR, Singer CR, Euller-Ziegler L, Wetterwald M, Fiere D, Hrubisko M, Thiel E, Delmas PD (2002) Effects of long-term intravenous ibandronate therapy on skeletal-related events, survival, and bone resorption markers in patients with advanced multiple myeloma. J Clin Oncol 20:2353-2359

[78] Rosen LS, Gordon D, Kaminski M, Howell A, Belch A, Mackey J, Apffelstaedt J, Hussein M, Coleman RE, Reitsma DJ, Seaman JJ, Chen BL, Ambros Y (2001) Zoledronic acid versus pamidronate in the treatment of skeletal metastases in patients with breast cancer or osteolytic lesions of multiple myeloma: a phase III, double-blind, comparative trial. Cancer J 7:377-387

[79] Kohno N, Aogi K, Minami H, Nakamura S, Asaga T, Iino Y, Watanabe T, Goessl C, Ohashi Y, Takashima S (2005) Zoledronic acid significantly reduces skeletal complications compared with placebo in Japanese women with bone metastases from breast cancer: a randomized, placebo-controlled trial. J Clin Oncol 23:3314-3321

[80] Rosen LS, Gordon D, Tchekmedyian NS, Yanagihara R, Hirsh V, Krzakowski M, Pawlicki M, De Souza P, Zheng M, Urbanowitz G, Reitsma D, Seaman J (2004) Long-term efficacy and safety of zoledronic acid in the treatment of skeletal metastases in patients with nonsmall cell lung carcinoma and other solid tumors: a randomized, phase III, double-blind, placebo-controlled trial. Cancer 100:2613-2621

[81] Saad F, Gleason DM, Murray R, Tchekmedyian S, Venner P, Lacombe L, Chin JL, Vinholes JJ, Goas JA, Zheng M (2004) Long-term efficacy of zoledronic acid for the prevention of skeletal complications in patients with metastatic hormone-refractory prostate cancer. J Natl Cancer Inst 96:879-882

[82] Stopeck AT, Lipton A, Body JJ, Steger GG, Tonkin K, de Boer RH, Lichinitser M, Fujiwara Y, Yardley DA, Viniegra M, Fan M, Jiang Q, Dansey R, Jun S, Braun A (2010) Denosumab compared with zoledronic acid for the treatment of bone metastases in patients with advanced breast cancer: a randomized, double-blind study. J Clin Oncol Epub ahead of print

[83] Coxon FP, Thompson K, Rogers MJ (2006) Recent advances in understanding the mechanism of action of bisphosphonates. Curr Opin Pharmacol 6:307-312

[84] Thompson K, Roelofs AJ, Jauhiainen M, Monkkonen H, Monkkonen J, Rogers MJ (2010) Activation of gammadelta T cells by bisphosphonates. Adv Exp Med Biol 658:11-20

[85] Terpos E, Dimopoulos MA (2005) Myeloma bone disease: pathophysiology and management. Ann Oncol 16:1223-1231

[86] Berenson JR, Lichtenstein A, Porter L, Dimopoulos MA, Bordoni R, George S, Lipton A, Keller A, Ballester O, Kovacs M, Blacklock H, Bell R, Simeone JF, Reitsma DJ, Heffernan M, Seaman J, Knight RD (1998) Long-term pamidronate treatment of advanced multiple myeloma patients reduces skeletal events. Myeloma Aredia Study Group. J Clin Oncol 16:593-602

[87] Kunzmann V, Bauer E, Feurle J, Weissinger F, Tony HP, Wilhelm M (2000) Stimulation of gammadelta T cells by aminobisphosphonates and induction of antiplasma cell activity in multiple myeloma. Blood 96:384-392

[88] Terpos E, Viniou N, de la Fuente J, Meletis J, Voskaridou E, Karkantaris C, Vaiopoulos G, Palermos J, Yataganas X, Goldman JM, Rahemtulla A (2003) Pamidronate is superior to ibandronate in decreasing bone resorption, interleukin-6 and beta 2-microglobulin in multiple myeloma. Eur J Haematol 70:34-42

[89] Devitt B, McLachlan SA (2008) Use of ibandronate in the prevention of skeletal events in metastatic breast cancer. Ther Clin Risk Manag 4:453-458

[90] Berenson JR, Rosen LS, Howell A, Porter L, Coleman RE, Morley W, Dreicer R, Kuross SA, Lipton A, Seaman JJ (2001) Zoledronic acid reduces skeletal-related events in patients with osteolytic metastases. Cancer 91:1191-1200

[91] Rosen LS, Gordon D, Kaminski M, Howell A, Belch A, Mackey J, Apffelstaedt J, Hussein MA, Coleman RE, Reitsma DJ, Chen BL, Seaman JJ (2003) Long-term efficacy and safety of zoledronic acid compared with pamidronate disodium in the treatment of skeletal complications in patients with advanced multiple myeloma or breast carcinoma: a randomized, double-blind, multicenter, comparative trial. Cancer 98:1735-1744

[92] Rosen LS, Gordon D, Tchekmedyian S, Yanagihara R, Hirsh V, Krzakowski M, Pawlicki M, de Souza P, Zheng M, Urbanowitz G, Reitsma D, Seaman JJ (2003) Zoledronic acid versus placebo in the treatment of skeletal metastases in patients with lung cancer and other solid tumors: a phase III, double-blind, randomized trial — the Zoledronic Acid Lung Cancer and Other Solid Tumors Study Group. J Clin Oncol 21:3150-3157

[93] Naoe M, Ogawa Y, Takeshita K, Morita J, Shichijo T, Fuji K, Fukagai T, Iwamoto S, Terao S (2010) Zoledronate stimulates gamma delta T cells in prostate cancer patients. Oncol Res 18:493-501

[94] Lipton A (2008) Emerging role of bisphosphonates in the clinic — antitumor activity and prevention of metastasis to bone. Cancer Treat Rev 34(suppl 1):S25-S30

[95] Senaratne SG, Pirianov G, Mansi JL, Arnett TR, Colston KW (2000) Bisphosphonates induce apoptosis in human breast cancer cell lines. Br J Cancer 82:1459-1468

[96] Santini D, Martini F, Fratto ME, Galluzzo S, Vincenzi B, Agrati C, Turchi F, Piacentini P, Rocci L, Manavalan JS, Tonini G, Poccia F (2009) In vivo effects of zoledronic acid on peripheral gammadelta T lymphocytes in early breast cancer patients. Cancer Immunol Immunother 58:31-38

[97] Ferretti G, Fabi A, Carlini P, Papaldo P, Cordiali Fei P, Di Cosimo S, Salesi N, Giannarelli D, Alimonti A, Di Cocco B, D'Agosto G, Bordignon V, Trento E, Cognetti F (2005) Zoledronic-acid-induced circulating level modifications of

angiogenic factors, metalloproteinases and proinflammatory cytokines in metastatic breast cancer patients. Oncology 69:35-43

[98] Santini D, Vincenzi B, Galluzzo S, Battistoni F, Rocci L, Venditti O, Schiavon G, Angeletti S, Uzzalli F, Caraglia M, Dicuonzo G, Tonini G (2007) Repeated intermittent low-dose therapy with zoledronic acid induces an early, sustained, and long-lasting decrease of peripheral vascular endothelial growth factor levels in cancer patients. Clin Cancer Res 13:4482-4486

[99] Ottewell PD, Monkkonen H, Jones M, Lefley DV, Coleman RE, Holen I (2008) Antitumor effects of doxorubicin followed by zoledronic acid in a mouse model of breast cancer. J Natl Cancer Inst 100:1167-1178

[100] Neville-Webbe HL, Rostami-Hodjegan A, Evans CA, Coleman RE, Holen I (2005) Sequence- and schedule-dependent enhancement of zoledronic acid induced apoptosis by doxorubicin in breast and prostate cancer cells. Int J Cancer 113:364-371

[101] Rack B, Schindlbeck C, Strobl B, Sommer H, Friese K, Janni W (2008) [Efficacy of zoledronate in treating persisting isolated tumor cells in bone marrow in patients with breast cancer. A phase II pilot study]. Dtsch Med Wochenschr 133:285-289

[102] Solomayer E, Gebauer G, Hirnle P, Janni W, Lück H-J, Becker S, Huober J, Kraemer B, Fehm T (2009) Influence of zoledronic acid on disseminated tumor cells (DTC) in primary breast cancer patients (abstract 2048). Cancer Res 69(suppl):170s-171s

[103] Aft R, Naughton M, Ylagen L, Watson M, Chavez-MacGregor M, Trinkaus K, Zhai J, Weilbaecher K (2008) Effect of zoledronic acid on bone marrow micrometastases in women undergoing neoadjuvant chemotherapy for breast cancer (abstract 1021). In: Presented at the 44th Annual Meeting of the American Society of Clinical Oncology, 30 May-3 June 2008, Chicago, IL, USA

[104] Lin AY, Park JW, Scott J, Melisko M, Goga A, Moasser MM, Moore DH, Rugo HS (2008) Zoledronic acid as adjuvant therapy for women with early-stage breast cancer and disseminated tumor cells in bone marrow (abstract 559). In: Presented at the 44th Annual Meeting of the American Society of Clinical Oncology, 30 May-3 June 2008, Chicago, IL, USA

[105] Gnant M, Mlineritsch B, Schippinger W, Luschin-Ebengreuth G, Postlberger S, Menzel C, Jakesz R, Seifert M, Hubalek M, Bjelic-Radisic V, Samonigg H, Tausch C, Eidtmann H, Steger G, Kwasny W, Dubsky P, Fridrik M, Fitzal F, Stierer M, Rucklinger E, Greil R, Marth C (2009) Endocrine therapy plus zoledronic acid in premenopausal breast cancer. N Engl J Med 360:679-691

[106] Coleman RE, Winter MC, Cameron D, Bell R, Dodwell D, Keane MM, Gil M, Ritchie D, Passos-Coelho JL, Wheatley D, Burkinshaw R, Marshall SJ, Thorpe H (2010) The effects of adding zoledronic acid to neoadjuvant chemotherapy on tumour response: exploratory evidence for direct anti-tumour activity in breast cancer. Br J Cancer 102:1099-1105

[107] Coleman R, Bundred N, De Boer R, Llombarto A, Campbell I, Neven P, Barrios C, Dias R, Miller J, Brufsky A (2009) Impact of zoledronic acid in postmenopausal women with early breast cancer receiving adjuvant letrozole: Z-FAST, ZO-FAST, and E-ZO-FAST (abstract 4082). Cancer Res 69(suppl):733s

[108] Brufsky A, Graydon Harker W, Beck JT, Carroll R, Jin L, Warsi G, Argonza-Aviles E, Ericson S, Perez EA (2009) The effect of zoledronic acid on aromatase inhibitor-

associated bone loss in postmenopausal women with early breast cancer receiving adjuvant letrozole: the Z-FAST study 5-year final follow-up (abstract 4083). In: Presented at the 32nd Annual San Antonio Breast Cancer Symposium, 9-13 December 2009, San Antonio, TX, USA

[109] Costa L, Cook R, Body J-J, Brown J, Terpos E, Saad F, Lipton A, Coleman R (2009) Zoledronic acid treatment delays disease progression and improves survival in patients with bone metastases from solid tumors and elevated levels of bone resorption (abstract 50) In: Presented at the IX International Meeting on Cancer Induced Bone Disease, 28-31 October 2009, Arlington, VA, USA

[110] Body J-J, Cook R, Costa L, Brown J, Terpos E, Saad F, Lipton A, Coleman R (2009) Possible survival benefits from zoledronic acid treatment in patients with bone metastases from solid tumors and poor prognostic features (abstract 71). In: Presented at the IX International Meeting on Cancer Induced Bone Disease, 28-31 October 2009, Arlington, VA, USA

[111] Morgan GJ, Davies FE, Gregory WM, Cocks K, Bell SE, Szubert AJ, Navarro-Coy N, Drayson MT, Owen RG, Feyler S, Ashcroft AJ, Ross F, Byrne J, Roddie H, Rudin C, Cook G, Jackson GH, Child JA; National Cancer Research Institute Haematological Oncology Clinical Study Group (2010) First-line treatment with zoledronic acid as compared with clodronic acid in multiple myeloma (MRC Myeloma IX): a randomised controlled trial. Lancet 376:1989-1999

[112] Zaghloul MS, Boutrus R, El-Hosieny H, A-Kader Y, El-Attar I, Nazmy M (2008) A controlled prospective randomized placebo-controlled trial of zoledronic acid in bony metastatic bladder cancer patients (abstract 5033). J Clin Oncol 26(suppl):257s

[113] Zarogoulidis K, Boutsikou E, Zarogoulidis P, Eleftheriadou E, Kontakiotis T, Lithoxopoulou H, Tzanakakis G, Kanakis I, Karamanos NK (2009) The impact of zoledronic acid therapy in survival of lung cancer patients with bone metastasis. Int J Cancer 125:1705-1709

[114] Mystakidou K, Katsouda E, Parpa E, Kelekis A, Galanos A, Vlahos L (2005) Randomized, open label, prospective study on the effect of zoledronic acid on the prevention of bone metastases in patients with recurrent solid tumors that did not present with bone metastases at baseline. Med Oncol 22:195-201

[115] United States Food and Drug Administration. Background document for meeting of Advisory Committee for Reproductive Health Drugs (August 13, 2009). Available from: http://www.fda.gov/downloads/AdvisoryCommittees/CommitteesMeetingMate rials/Drugs/ReproductiveHealthDrugsAdvisoryCommittee/UCM176605.pdf [Accessed April 21, 2010].

[116] Anastasilakis AD, Toulis KA, Polyzos SA, Terpos E (2009) RANKL inhibition for the management of patients with benign metabolic bone disorders. Expert Opin Investig Drugs 18:1085-1102

[117] Cummings SR, San Martin J, McClung MR, Siris ES, Eastell R, Reid IR, Delmas P, Zoog HB, Austin M, Wang A, Kutilek S, Adami S, Zanchetta J, Libanati C, Siddhanti S, Christiansen C (2009) Denosumab for prevention of fractures in postmenopausal women with osteoporosis. N Engl J Med 361:756-765

[118] Stopeck A, Body JJ, Fujiwara Y, Lipton A, Steger GG, Viniegra M, Fan M, Braun A, Dansey R, Jun S (2009) Denosumab versus zoledronic acid for the treatment of

breast cancer patients with bone metastases: results of a randomized phase 3 study (abstract 2LBA). Eur J Cancer Suppl 7:2

[119] Fizazi K, Carducci M, Smith M, Damiao R, Brown J, Karsh L, Milecki P, Rader M, Shore N, Tadros S, Wang H, Jiang Q, Dansey R, Goessl C (2010) Denosumab compared with zoledronic acid for the treatment of bone metastases in patients with castration-resistant prostate cancer (abstract LBA4507). In: Presented at the 46th Annual Meeting of the Americal Society of Clinical Oncology, 4-8 June 2010, Chicago, IL, USA

[120] Thomas D, Henshaw R, Skubitz K, Chawla S, Staddon A, Blay JY, Roudier M, Smith J, Ye Z, Sohn W, Dansey R, Jun S (2010) Denosumab in patients with giant-cell tumour of bone: an open-label, phase 2 study. Lancet Oncol 11:275-280

[121] Gonzalez-Suarez E, Jacob AP, Jones J, Miller R, Roudier-Meyer MP, Erwert R, Pinkas J, Branstetter D, Dougall WC (2010) RANK ligand mediates progestin-induced mammary epithelial proliferation and carcinogenesis. Nature 468:103-107

[122] Anastasilakis AD, Toulis KA, Goulis DG, Polyzos SA, Delaroudis S, Giomisi A, Terpos E (2009) Efficacy and safety of denosumab in postmenopausal women with osteopenia or osteoporosis: a systematic review and a meta-analysis. Horm Metab Res 41:721-729

[123] Ellis GK, Bone HG, Chlebowski R, Paul D, Spadafora S, Smith J, Fan M, Jun S (2008) Randomized trial of denosumab in patients receiving adjuvant aromatase inhibitors for nonmetastatic breast cancer. J Clin Oncol 26:4875-4882

[124] Smith MR, Egerdie B, Hernandez Toriz N, Feldman R, Tammela TL, Saad F, Heracek J, Szwedowski M, Ke C, Kupic A, Leder BZ, Goessl C (2009) Denosumab in men receiving androgen-deprivation therapy for prostate cancer. N Engl J Med 361:745-755

[125] Fizazi K, Bosserman L, Gao G, Skacel T, Markus R (2009) Denosumab treatment of prostate cancer with bone metastases and increased urine N-telopeptide levels after therapy with intravenous bisphosphonates: results of a randomized phase II trial. J Urol 182:509-515; discussion follows

[126] Xgeva (denosumab) injection [prescribing information]. Amgen; Thousand Oaks, CA, USA; 2010.

Permissions

The contributors of this book come from diverse backgrounds, making this book a truly international effort. This book will bring forth new frontiers with its revolutionizing research information and detailed analysis of the nascent developments around the world.

We would like to thank Clio P. Mavragani, MD, for lending her expertise to make the book truly unique. She has played a crucial role in the development of this book. Without her invaluable contribution this book wouldn't have been possible. She has made vital efforts to compile up to date information on the varied aspects of this subject to make this book a valuable addition to the collection of many professionals and students.

This book was conceptualized with the vision of imparting up-to-date information and advanced data in this field. To ensure the same, a matchless editorial board was set up. Every individual on the board went through rigorous rounds of assessment to prove their worth. After which they invested a large part of their time researching and compiling the most relevant data for our readers. Conferences and sessions were held from time to time between the editorial board and the contributing authors to present the data in the most comprehensible form. The editorial team has worked tirelessly to provide valuable and valid information to help people across the globe.

Every chapter published in this book has been scrutinized by our experts. Their significance has been extensively debated. The topics covered herein carry significant findings which will fuel the growth of the discipline. They may even be implemented as practical applications or may be referred to as a beginning point for another development. Chapters in this book were first published by InTech; hereby published with permission under the Creative Commons Attribution License or equivalent.

The editorial board has been involved in producing this book since its inception. They have spent rigorous hours researching and exploring the diverse topics which have resulted in the successful publishing of this book. They have passed on their knowledge of decades through this book. To expedite this challenging task, the publisher supported the team at every step. A small team of assistant editors was also appointed to further simplify the editing procedure and attain best results for the readers.

Our editorial team has been hand-picked from every corner of the world. Their multi-ethnicity adds dynamic inputs to the discussions which result in innovative outcomes. These outcomes are then further discussed with the researchers and contributors who give their valuable feedback and opinion regarding the same. The feedback is then collaborated with the researches and they are edited in a comprehensive manner to aid the understanding of the subject.

Apart from the editorial board, the designing team has also invested a significant amount of their time in understanding the subject and creating the most relevant covers. They scrutinized every image to scout for the most suitable representation of the subject and create an appropriate cover for the book.

The publishing team has been involved in this book since its early stages. They were actively engaged in every process, be it collecting the data, connecting with the contributors or procuring relevant information. The team has been an ardent support to the editorial, designing and production team. Their endless efforts to recruit the best for this project, has resulted in the accomplishment of this book. They are a veteran in the field of academics and their pool of knowledge is as vast as their experience in printing. Their expertise and guidance has proved useful at every step. Their uncompromising quality standards have made this book an exceptional effort. Their encouragement from time to time has been an inspiration for everyone.

The publisher and the editorial board hope that this book will prove to be a valuable piece of knowledge for researchers, students, practitioners and scholars across the globe.

List of Contributors

Chang-Hee Suh
Rheumatology, Ajou University School of Medicine, Korea

Giannelou M., Gravani F., Papadaki I. and Ioakeimidis D.
Department of Rheumatology, Athens General Hospital "G.Gennimatas," Athens, Greece

Mavragani C.P.
Department of Experimental Physiology, School of Medicine, University of Athens, Athens, Greece

Sarah L. Brice, Andrew J. Sakko, Pravin Hissaria and Claudine S. Bonder
Human Immunology, Centre for Cancer Biology, SA Pathology, Co-operative Research Centre for Biomarker Translation, LaTrobe University, Australia

Erika Cristaldi, Giulia Malaguarnera, Alessandra Rando and Mariano Malaguarnera
University of Catania, Italy

Dolcetti R.
Cancer Bioimmunotherapy Unit, Dept. of Oncology, National Cancer Institute CRO-IRCCS, Italy

Ponzoni M.
Unit of Lymphoid Malignancies, Dept. of Onco-Hematology, Italy Pathology Unit, Italy

Mappa S.
Internal Medicine Unit, San Raffaele Scientific Institute, Italy Unit of Lymphoid Malignancies, Dept. of Onco-Hematology, Italy

Ferreri A.J.M.
Unit of Lymphoid Malignancies, Dept. of Onco-Hematology, Italy

Lotti Tajouri, Ekua W. Brenu and Sonya M. Marshall-Gradisnik
Population Health and Neuroimmunology Unit, Faculty of Health Science and Medicine, Bond University, Robina, Australia Faculty of Health Science and Medicine, Bond University, Robina, Australia

Donald R. Staines
Queensland Health, Gold Coast Population Health Unit, Southport, Australia

Gergely Toldi, András Treszl and Barna Vásárhelyi
Research Group of Pediatrics and Nephrology, Hungarian Academy of Sciences, Hungary

Evangelos Terpos, Maria Gkotzamanidou, Dimitrios Christoulas and Meletios A. Dimopoulos
Department of Clinical Therapeutics, University of Athens School of Medicine, Athens, Greece